Lecture Notes in Computer Science 10154

Commenced Publication in 1973
Founding and Former Series Editors:
Gerhard Goos, Juris Hartmanis, and Jan van Leeuwen

More information about this series at http://www.springer.com/series/7412

Alessandro Crimi · Bjoern Menze
Oskar Maier · Mauricio Reyes
Stefan Winzeck · Heinz Handels (Eds.)

Brainlesion: Glioma, Multiple Sclerosis, Stroke and Traumatic Brain Injuries

Second International Workshop, BrainLes 2016,
with the Challenges on BRATS, ISLES and mTOP 2016
Held in Conjunction with MICCAI 2016
Athens, Greece, October 17, 2016
Revised Selected Papers

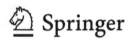 Springer

Editors

Alessandro Crimi
University of Zurich
Istituto Italiano di Tecnologia
Genoa
Italy

Bjoern Menze
TU München, Computer Science
Munich
Germany

Oskar Maier
Medical Informatics
University of Lübeck
Lübeck
Germany

Mauricio Reyes
Surgical Technology and Biomechanics
Universität Bern
Bern
Switzerland

Stefan Winzeck
Department of Medicine
University of Cambridge
Cambridge
UK

Heinz Handels
Institute of Medical Informatics
University of Lübeck
Lübeck
Germany

ISSN 0302-9743   ISSN 1611-3349   (electronic)
Lecture Notes in Computer Science
ISBN 978-3-319-55523-2   ISBN 978-3-319-55524-9   (eBook)
DOI 10.1007/978-3-319-55524-9

Library of Congress Control Number: 2017934457

LNCS Sublibrary: SL6 – Image Processing, Computer Vision, Pattern Recognition, and Graphics

Printed on acid-free paper

This Springer imprint is published by Springer Nature
The registered company is Springer International Publishing AG
The registered company address is: Gewerbestrasse 11, 6330 Cham, Switzerland

Preface

This volume contains articles from the BrainLesion Workshop as well as the Brain Tumor Segmentation (BRATS), the Ischemic Stroke Lesion Segmentation (ISLES), and Mild Traumatic Brain Injury Outcome Prediction (mTOP) challenges, which were held jointly at the Medical Image Computing for Computer-Assisted Intervention (MICCAI) Conference on October 17, 2016, in Athens, Greece.

The presented works are aimed at computer scientific and clinical researchers working on glioma, multiple sclerosis (MS), cerebral stroke and brain trauma injuries. This compilation does not claim to provide a comprehensive understanding from all points of view; however, the authors present their latest advances in segmentation, disease prognosis, and other applications to the clinical context.

The volume is divided into four parts: The first part comprises the submissions to the BrainLes Workshop, the second contains a selection of papers regarding methods presented at the BRATS challenge, followed by a selection of papers on methods presented at the ISLES challenge, and finally a selection of papers on methods presented at the mTOP challenge.

The aim of the first part is to provide an overview of new advances in medical image analysis in all of the aforementioned brain pathologies. This section brings together researchers from the medical image analysis domain, neurologists, and radiologists working on at least one of these diseases. The aim is to consider neuroimaging biomarkers used for one disease applied to the other diseases. This session did not have a specific dataset to be used.

The second part focuses on the papers from the BRATS challenge. In order to gauge the current state of the art in automated brain tumor segmentation and compare the different methods, a large dataset of magnetic resonance (MR) images of brain tumors was made available. The participants at the challenge compared the results obtained with their methods against manual segmentations.

The third part contains descriptions of the algorithms participating in ISLES, which aimed to provide a fair and direct comparison of methods for ischemic stroke lesion segmentation from multispectral MR images. A public dataset of diverse ischemic stroke cases and a suitable automatic evaluation procedure was made available for the following two tasks: sub-acute ischemic stroke lesion segmentation and acute stroke outcome/penumbra estimation.

The fourth part comprises approaches for semi-supervised outcome prediction after mild traumatic brain injury, submitted to the mTOP challenge. These aim to use early, multi-modal brain scans to classify subjects as healthy individuals or patients with different outcomes (assessed via the Glasgow outcome scale). The provided dataset included both structural and diffusional MR images.

We heartily hope that this volume will promote further exiting research on brain lesions.

February 2017   Alessandro Crimi
                                                                         Oskar Maier
                                                                       Bjoern Menze
                                                                     Mauricio Reyes
                                                                    Stefan Winzeck
                                                                     Heinz Handels

Organization

Organizing Committee

Spyridon Bakas	University of Pennsylvania, USA
Marta Correia	University of Cambridge, UK
Alessandro Crimi	Istituto Italiano di Tecnologia, Italy
	University of Zurich, Switzerland
Christos Davatzikos	University of Pennsylvania, USA
Keyvan Farahani	National Institute of Health, USA
Ben Glocker	Imperial College London, UK
Heinz Handels	Universität zu Lübeck, Germany
Jayashree Kalpathy-Cramer	Harvard Medical School, USA
Oskar Maier	Universität zu Lübeck, Germany
Richard McKinley	Universität Bern, Switzerland
Bjoern Menze	Technische Universität München, Germany
Mauricio Reyes	Universität Bern, Switzerland
Roland Wiest	Universität Bern, Switzerland
Stefan Winzeck	University of Cambridge, UK

Program Committee

Meritxell Bach Cuadra	University of Lausanne, Switzerland
Luca Dodero	Istituto Italiano di Tecnologia, Italy
Juan-Fruan Garamendi	Universitat Pompeu Fabra, Spain
Koen Van Leemput	Harvard Medical School, USA
Maria Preti	Ecole polythecnique federale de lausanne, Switzerland
Oula Puonti	Danmarks Tekniske Universitet, Denmark

Contents

Ischemic Stroke Lesion Image Segmentation

Mild Traumatic Brain Injury Outcome Prediction

Brain Lesion Image Analysis

Fully Automated Patch-Based Image Restoration: Application to Pathology Inpainting

Ferran Prados[1,2]([⊠]), M. Jorge Cardoso[1,4], Niamh Cawley[2],
Baris Kanber[1,2], Olga Ciccarelli[2], Claudia A.M. Gandini Wheeler-Kingshott[2,3],
and Sébastien Ourselin[1,4]

[1] Translational Imaging Group, Centre for Medical Image Computing (CMIC),
University College London, London WC1E 6BT, UK
f.carrasco@ucl.ac.uk
[2] NMR Research Unit, Queen Square MS Centre,
UCL Institute of Neurology, London WC1B 5EH, UK
[3] Brain MRI 3T Centre, C. Mondino National Neurological Institute, Pavia, Italy
[4] Dementia Research Centre, UCL Institute of Neurology, London WC1N 3BG, UK

Abstract. Pathology can have an important impact on MRI analysis. Specifically, white matter hyper-intensities, tumours, infarcts, etc., can influence the results of various image analysis techniques such as segmentation and registration. Several algorithms have been proposed for image inpainting and restoration, mainly in the context of Multiple Sclerosis lesions. These techniques commonly rely on a set of manually segmented pathological regions for inpainting. Rather than relying on prior segmentations for image restoration, we present a combined segmentation and inpainting algorithm for multimodal images. The proposed method is based on an iterative collaboration between two patch-based techniques, PatchMatch and Non-Local Means, where the former is used to estimate the most probable location of the pathological outliers and the latter to gradually fill the segmented areas with the most plausible multimodal texture. We demonstrate that the proposed method is able to automatically restore multimodal intensities in pathological regions within the context of Multiple Sclerosis.

1 Introduction

Abnormal image appearance due to pathological processes impacts the efficacy of image analysis. Several segmentation techniques have been developed recently for the detection of pathological outliers such as Multiple Sclerosis (MS) lesions [1], brain tumours [2], infarcts [3], *etc.* In all these scenarios, pathology significantly impacts image analysis procedures such as segmentation or registration. For example, from an image processing perspective, MS lesions influence tissue segmentation procedures, resulting in the misclassification of gray matter and white matter. The longitudinal differences in size and shape of pathology also hinders the registration between time points.

© Springer International Publishing AG 2016
A. Crimi et al. (Eds.): BrainLes 2016, LNCS 10154, pp. 3–15, 2016.
DOI: 10.1007/978-3-319-55524-9_1

To reduce the impact of these anatomical abnormalities, inpainting algorithms have been proposed, mainly in MS [4,5], to reduce the effect of lesions over the subsequent processing steps. While most inpainting methods rely on a single modality (commonly T1 images) [6–8] and fill the pathological region according to some regional statistic or intensity distribution, recent approaches have explored patch-based methodologies [9–12] for inpainting. This class of patch-based methodologies preserves the structural characteristics of the corrected image.

The original PatchMatch algorithm was designed to look for similarities between two 2D images [13]. Three different applications of the PatchMatch algorithm to MR images have been recently proposed. First, Shi et al. [14] used it for the estimation of high-resolution cardiac MR images from single short-axis cardiac MR image stacks. Secondly, Ta et al. [15,16] presented an optimised version of the PatchMatch algorithm, named Optimized PatchMatch Label fusion (OPAL), producing accurate and fast segmentation of the hippocampus. This method extended the concept to 3D data which, when combined with a library of associated segmented images, was able to speed up the process of multi-atlas label fusion. Finally, Prados et al. [17] proposed a generalization of OPAL for using with multimodal data and applied to MS lesion detection.

Traditionally, segmentation and inpainting techniques have been designed as two independent steps. First, the pathological region of interest (ROI) is segmented, and then this segmentation is used to inpaint the image without any feedback loop. This lack of feedback between the inpainting and segmentation processes is deleterious - we note that an imperfect segmentation results in poor inpainting, but automatically segmenting a poorly inpainted image is easier, from a model fit perspective, than segmenting the original pathological image. Recently, Xu et al. [18] proposed an iterative approach for simultaneous PET image denoising and segmentation, despite these two tasks are considered indepedent. The interaction between the two techniques significantly improved the performance and the results.

In this work, we propose to use the non-local means and PatchMatch algorithms for a fully automated iterative multi-modal image inpainting. We apply this algorithm within the context of MS lesion removal. The proposed algorithm does not require any prior input information to generate a pathology-free image and associated lesion localisation. More specifically, the method is based on a collaborative algorithm between the multimodal version of PatchMatch [17] for lesion segmentation and an improved version of a patch-based method [10] for image inpainting. The main contribution of this work is the first prior-free, regarding the target image, fully automated image restoration algorithm for medical data.

2   Method

The proposed method iterates over two main steps: (1) estimates the pathological ROI using PatchMatch, (2) restores the detected ROI with the most plausible multi-contrast values using the non-local means inpainting algorithm.

2.1   Optimized Multi-contrast PatchMatch

The original PatchMatch algorithm was designed to look for similarities between two 2D patches within the same image [13]. Later, OPAL extended patch correspondences between a target 3D image and reference library of different 3D training templates [15,16]. Finally, OPAL had a 4D version to match patches between multiple image modalities at the same time [17]. As in the reference [17], the multi-modal extension of the similarity term in OPAL is the l2-norm over the patches of the different modalities and the lesion probabilities are computed using an adaptive threshold value. Here, the PatchMatch algorithm is used to locate pathological regions through the use of a template library comprised of a series of multimodal images with manually segmented MS lesions. By matching patches between the target multimodal image and the multimodal images in the template library, PatchMatch can provide a rough estimate of the location of the lesions in the target image [17].

As the PatchMatch output is non-binary, we apply an adaptive threshold value to binarise the probabilistic mask obtained by the PatchMatch algorithm [17].

This section introduced an algorithm to localise pathological ROIs. These ROIs can then be used as the target for inpainting, presented in the next section.

2.2   Non-local Inpainting Extension

Most current lesion inpainting algorithms require accurate segmentations for ROI inpainting. Compared to other published methods, the non-local means inpainting algorithm presented by Prados et al. [10], and extended in Prados et al. [12], has the advantage of preserving the anatomical brain structures when lesions are neighbouring cortical grey matter and cerebrospinal fluid, making it robust to lesion over-segmentation. This method non-locally searches for the patches that can best inpaint the pathological ROI, only according to their intensity similarity. The robustness to over-segmentation makes this method ideal to use in combination with the rough segmentations obtained in Sect. 2.1 for pathology inpainting.

In practice, the inpainting method works replacing the voxel intensity with the intensity of the center voxel of the closest matching patch, and that a convolution operation is performed afterwards. However, a few problems with [10] still need to be addressed. Ventricular expansion can occur (see [10]) when limited anatomical structure and patch support exist in the pathological ROI neighbourhood. Also, when lesions are bigger than the patch size, the use of a fixed patch size introduces artefacts in the inpainting results.

To address these limitations, as in Prados et al. [12], we first propose to dynamically change the patch size. More specifically, for a voxel r inside the lesion $\mathcal{L}$, the Euclidean distance $\mathcal{E}$ to the closest voxel b in the boundary $\mathcal{B}$ of the pathological ROI is used to determine the patch size. Formally, the patch size w at location r, denoted $w(r)$, is defined as

$$w(r) = \arg\max_{\forall b \in B} (2 \times \mathcal{E}(r, b) + 1) \text{ with } \quad \mathcal{E}(r, b) = \arg\min_{b \in B \wedge b \in \mathcal{X} \wedge b \notin \mathcal{L}} ||r - b||_2 \quad (1)$$

where $\mathcal{X}$ is an inclusion region defined in Sect. 2.3.

Prados et al. [10] also proposes to solve the inpainting process layer by layer, from the outside to the inside of the patch, resulting in potential inpainting artefacts. To mitigate this problem, rather than using the full patch, we propose to use only non-lesion voxels (*i.e.* voxels $\notin \mathcal{L}$) to estimate the patch similarity. Note that we can guarantee that the patch similarity will always contain non-lesion voxels to estimate patch similarity due to the dynamic patch size.

Lastly, to increase the robustness in the inpainting patch search, we have also extended the non-local patch similarity to multimodal data as in Sect. 2.1, allowing the algorithm to jointly fill multiple image modalities at the same time. This improvement not only allows for better and more stable matches, but also makes the inpainting process consistent between multiple image modalities.

2.3   Iterative Algorithm

The proposed algorithm starts with a first PatchMatch. Using the pathological image, this step computes the probability for each voxel to be part of the pathological ROI. Any voxel with probability above λ is included in the current estimate of the pathological ROI. The current estimate of the pathological ROI is used as input for the inpainting method. The inpainted image is then used as the input for the PatchMatch pathology localisation algorithm. These two steps will be repeated until no voxels above λ are found after PatchMatch or until no changes are found between the pathological ROIs at two subsequent iterations.

Two minor improvements are also introduced at this stage: First, we constrain the inpainting method search through the use of a brain mask $\mathcal{X}$. This brain mask is estimated iteratively through the same process as the one used to localise the pathological ROI. In order to do so, brain segmentations are added to the template library containing the manual pathological ROIs. These brain segmentations are propagated jointly with the pathological ROIs during the first PatchMatch process. Here, the inclusion region $\mathcal{X}$ is defined as any voxel with probability above 0.01 to be part of the brain region. As a second improvement, the mask used for inpainting is morphologically dilated at every iteration to avoid inpainting problems due to pathological ROI undersegmentation.

3   Validation

Parameter tuning: All our experiments used the following parameters: Patch-Match was used with the parameters suggested by Ta et al. [15]; the patch size was $5 \times 5 \times 5$, the number of inner iterations 5, and, the number of threads and the number of best-matches, both to 10 [15,17]; the inpainting technique used as the minimum required percentage of the patch size $\alpha = 0.1$, for the cross-shape kernel $\mathcal{K} = 0.4$ [10,12], the patch size w was adaptively set up as described above, and the size of the search region Ω was calculated as $W = 4 \times w$ [10,12];

finally, the threshold value for the inpainting ROI was empirically set to $\lambda = 0.1$ as a pilot experiment.

Dataset: Data comprised of 25 patients with secondary progressive Multiple Sclerosis (SPMS) (mean age $= 52 \pm 9.75$ years), with a median expanded disability status scale (EDSS) of 6 (range of $4-6.5$) and 12 healthy controls (mean age $= 46 \pm 11.7$ years). Participants underwent axial PD/T2 image ($1 \times 1 \times 3\,\text{mm}^3$), and a sagittal 3D T1 ($1 \times 1 \times 1\,\text{mm}^3$), all on a 3 T scanner. One rater manually outlined T2-hyperintense lesions in all SPMS participants on the PD/T2 images using JIM v.6 (http://www.xinapse.com/).

Preprocessing: All the images were preprocessed through the following pipeline: correction of inhomogeneities using a robust version of the N3 algorithm [19], denoising using the non-local means filter [20], and linear registration to the MNI template ($1 \times 1 \times 1\,\text{mm}^3$).

Template library: Two template libraries were built. The first library was composed of 12 healthy individuals with no lesions and 25 patients with SPMS with associated manual segmentations of the visible MS lesions. Each subject had T1, PD and T2 images. The PD/T2 images and the associated segmentations were linearly registered to the T1 images using a pseudo-T1 contrast generated from the subtraction of the scanner-aligned PD and T2 images. In order to increase the size of the library, all the scans were left-right flipped, resulting in a template library with 74 datasets. For all of them, brain mask segmentations were obtained using GIF [21]. These template library masks were then used by the PatchMatch algorithm to define $\mathcal{X}$ described in Sect. 2.3. The second library was composed of 12 healthy individuals with synthetic lesions with their correspondent left-right flipped images, resulting in a template library with 24 datasets.

Generating synthetic lesions for validation: With the aim of comparing the performance of the algorithm with previous semi-automated approaches we generated synthetic MS lesions for the healthy control data. MS lesions were generated as follows: First, for each control subject, the white-matter (WM), grey-matter (GM) and cerebrospinal fluid (CSF) brain tissues were extracted using GIF [21]. Second, the T1 *BrainWeb* MS model (http://www.bic.mni.mcgill.ca/brainweb/) was registered to each of the healthy controls using a sequence of rigid, affine and then non-rigid registration steps. Using the same transformation, the binarised "severe" BrainWeb lesion mask was resampled to the respective healthy control data. The propagated lesion mask was intersected with the brain mask to ensure that all lesions were within the brain boundary. Gaussian noise was added to the lesion segmentation. This Gaussian noise corrupted image was then multiplied by 0.5, 2.5 and 2.0 to obtain T1, T2 and PD intensity profiles respectively. Finally, the T1, T2 and PD images of each subject were multiplied by their respective Gaussian corrupted and intensity scaled lesion mask only for voxels within the lesion region, thus resulting in MS lesion-like intensities for all modalities.

Methodological evaluation: The proposed fully automatic method, which jointly estimates the location of the pathological regions and performs the inpainting, was compared to the current state-of-the-art that consists in delinate the lesions manually by an expert and fill them automatically using an inpainting method [10]. With this comparison we would demonstrate that the proposed fully automated method can perform as well as the current state-of-the-art without the need for a manual lesion segmentation.

The healthy data with synthetic lesions was used for validation purposes. The lesion mask used to generate the synthetic lesions was used as input for the state-of-the-art [10] method used here for comparison. The original data without synthetic lesions was used as the ground-truth for the inpainting process.

To evaluate the performance of each method, we used the same estimation strategy as proposed in [7]. More specifically, the original healthy data and the inpainted data using both the proposed and state-of-the-art methods were segmented into WM/GM/CSF. The mean absolute volume error (MAE) was estimated per tissue and for the brain parenchyma fraction (BPF), demonstrating the bias and variance of the tissue volumes between the inpainted images and the original healthy data and their impact in a whole-brain atrophy measure. The MAE is defined as $MAE = 100 \times |V_T - V_0|/V_0$, where V_0 is the tissue volume for the original healthy data without synthetic lesions and V_T is the volume obtained from segmenting the inpainted data using the GIF algorithm [21]. To further assess the performance the dice score coefficient (DSC) between the mask of the corrected area and the original mask, and the mean squared error (MSE), between the inpainted and original intensities, was calculated to assess the error in the restoration process.

Finally, in order to remove possible bias, a leave one out strategy was used for the proposed method, i.e. when inpainting an image, this image and its left-right flipped version were removed from the template library that we were using.

4   Results

Table 1 shows the results of comparing the state of the art methodology (manual segmentation and inpaint) with our proposed fully automated method using the template library composed of datasets with synthetic lesions. The proposed method is able to find automatically the lesions and inpaint them in an accurate way without affecting tissue volumes, particularly BPF measures are not significantly different and have a high correlation using the proposed technique ($p < 0.05$ and correlation 0.99). Despite the performance of the method, it is affected by the gaussian noise of the synthetic lesions, which obscures similarities between patches. This effect is avoided when the SPMS template library is used with real data (see Figs. 1, 2, 3 and 4). Finally, Figs. 1, 2, 3 and 4 show the automated image inpainting results on different image modalities over an SPMS patient. After a set of iterations, the input images with MS lesions are successfully restored to resemble those of a healthy brain preserving the boundaries and restoring the original intensities of the anatomical structures.

Table 1. Evaluation results, with the mean (std) and paired t-test. First row, state-of-the-art technique based on manually delineate the lesions and then inpaint them. Second row, proposed fully automatic technique. Results obtained for the 12 controls with synthetic lesions using a template library composed of subjects with synthetic lesions applying a leave one out strategy.

	DSC	MSE $\times 10^{-5}$	MAE (GM)	MAE (WM)	MAE (CSF)	MAE (BPF)
Man. seg. + inpaint	-	3.0 (2.0)	0.1% (0.04)	0.1% (0.07)	0.1% (0.07)	0.0% (0.03)
Prop. aut. approach	0.91 (0.02)	3.7 (4.8) $p = 0.28$	0.1% (0.08) $p = 0.36$	0.1% (0.08) $p < 0.05$	0.2% (0.12) $p < 0.05$	0.1% (0.04) $p < 0.05$

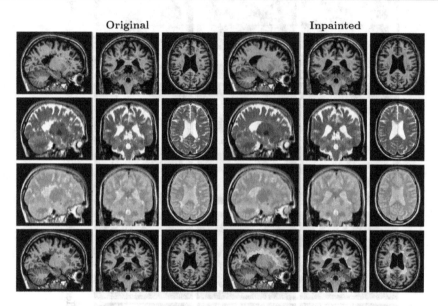

Fig. 1. Automated image inpainting results on different modalities of an SPMS patient. T1, T2 and PD images are shown on the first, second and third rows respectively, fourth row shows manual lesion segmentation (left/red) and automatic lesion detection (right/yellow). For more examples, see additional material. (Color figure online)

5   Discussion and Conclusion

In this paper, we have proposed a fully automated image inpainting method. We demonstrated that the proposed method is able to jointly restore the multimodal intensities in pathological regions in the context of Multiple Sclerosis.

The presented method does not require any prior information or manual segmentation of pathological regions for the target input image. It exploits the synergies between two patch-based methodologies to automatically inpaint the pathological regions of an image. The PatchMatch algorithm provides an accurate enough pathology localisation (see [17]), while the inpainting method, which

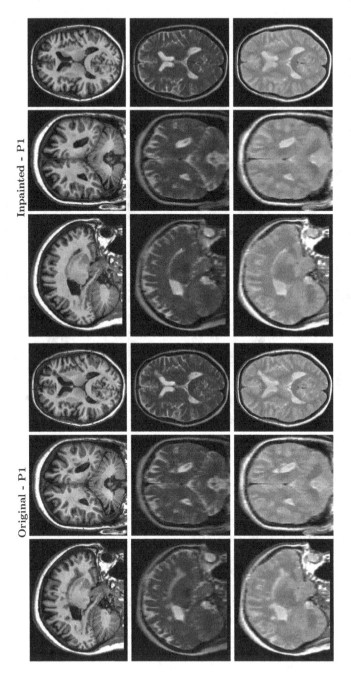

Fig. 2. Automated image inpainting results on different modalities. The input T1, T2 and PD images are shown on the first, second and third rows respectively.

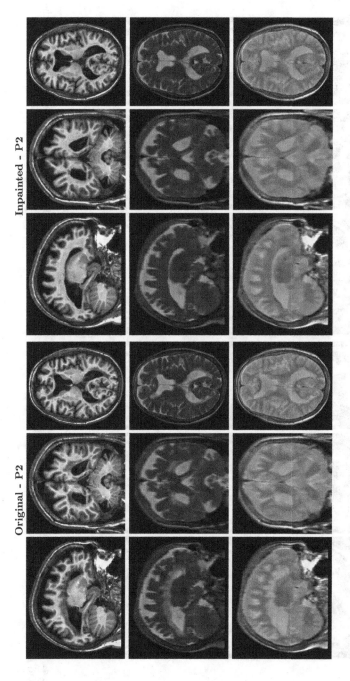

Fig. 3. Automated image inpainting results on different modalities of an SPMS patient. T1, T2 and PD images are shown on the first, second and third rows respectively.

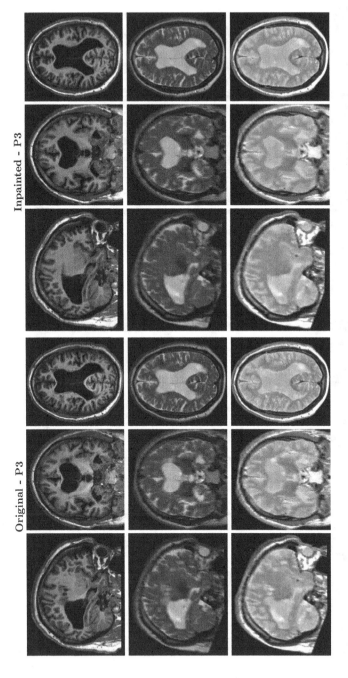

Fig. 4. Automated image inpainting results on different modalities of an SPMS patient. T1, T2 and PD images are shown on the first, second and third rows respectively.

is robust to lesion over-segmentation, inpaints the pathological ROI with the most plausible intensity pattern, without using a class-specific intensity model.

In the proposed algorithm, the lesions which are not inpainted after the first iteration are commonly detected in subsequent PatchMatch iterations. When two or more lesions are close, the PatchMatch random search tends to detect first the lesions most similar to the database library. Thus, this iterative update and feedback loop improves the robustness of the inpainting process by providing iteratively refined pathological regions. Moreover, in our 12 healthy individuals no lesions have been detected in the first iteration.

While the performance of the proposed methodology will depend on the size and quality of the template library, PatchMatch can find multiple matching patches even in relatively small template libraries. A limitation of this work is the need for similar acquisition parameters between the template library and target data due to the use of the l_2-norm in the patch matching process. Nonetheless, histogram matching techniques can be used to ameliorate this problem when the imaging data is significantly different. Future work will explore the application of the proposed method to different pathologies, extension to multi-centre data and model parameter and template library optimisation. Also, it could be used for lesion detection using a technique based on subtraction and using as baseline the inpainted image and as a follow-up the original image.

Acknowledgments. FP, BK and SO are funded by the National Institute for Health Research University College London Hospitals Biomedical Research Centre (NIHR BRC UCLH/UCL High Impact Initiative-BW.mn.BRC10269). SO receives funding from the EPSRC (EP/H046410/1, EP/J020990/1, EP/K005278), the MRC (MR/J01107X/1) and the NIHR Biomedical Research Unit (Dementia) at UCL. This work was also supported by the Medical Research Council, the UK Multiple Sclerosis Society (grant 892/08) and the Brain Research Trust.

References

1. Lladó, X., Oliver, A., Cabezas, M., Freixenet, J., Vilanova, J.C., Quiles, A., Valls, L., Ramió, L., Rovira, A.: Segmentation of multiple sclerosis lesions in brain MRI: a review of automated approaches. Inf. Sci. **186**(1), 164–185 (2012)
2. Gordillo, N., Montseny, E., Sobrevilla, P.: State of the art survey on MRI brain tumor segmentation. Magn. Reson. Imaging **31**(8), 1426–1438 (2013)
3. Rekik, I., Allassonnière, S., Carpenter, T.K., Wardlaw, J.M.: Medical image analysis methods in MR/CT-imaged acute-subacute ischemic stroke lesion: segmentation, prediction and insights into dynamic evolution simulation models. A critical appraisal. NeuroImage Clin. **1**(1), 164–178 (2012)
4. Ceccarelli, A., Jackson, J., Tauhid, S., Arora, A., Gorky, J., Dell'Oglio, E., Bakshi, A., Chitnis, T., Khoury, S., Weiner, H., Guttmann, C., Bakshi, R., Neema, M.: The impact of lesion in-painting and registration methods on voxel-based morphometry in detecting regional cerebral gray matter atrophy in multiple sclerosis. Am. J. Neuroradiol. **33**(8), 1579–1585 (2012)
5. Govindarajan, K.A., Datta, S., Hasan, K.M., Choi, S., Rahbar, M.H., Cofield, S.S., Cutter, G.R., Lublin, F.D., Wolinsky, J.S., Narayana, P.A., MRI Analysis Center

at Houston, T.C.I.G.: Effect of in-painting on cortical thickness measurements in multiple sclerosis: a large cohort study. Hum. Brain Mapp. **36**(10), 3749–3760 (2015)

6. Sdika, M., Pelletier, D.: Nonrigid registration of MS brain images using lesion inpainting for morphometry or lesion mapping. Hum. Brain Mapp. **30**(4), 1060–1067 (2009)

7. Chard, D.T., Jackson, J.S., Miller, D.H., Wheeler-Kingshott, C.: Reducing the impact of white matter lesions on automated measures of brain gray and white matter volumes. J. Magn. Reson. Imaging **32**(1), 223–228 (2010)

8. Battaglini, M., Jenkinson, M., De Stefano, N.: Evaluating and reducing the impact of white matter lesions on brain volume measurements. HBM **33**(9), 2062–71 (2012)

9. Guizard, N., Nakamura, K., Coupe, P., Arnold, D.L., Collins, D.L.: Non-local MS MRI lesion inpainting method for image processing. In: The endMS Conference (2013)

10. Prados, F., Cardoso, M.J., MacManus, D., Wheeler-Kingshott, C.A.M., Ourselin, S.: A modality-agnostic patch-based technique for lesion filling in multiple sclerosis. In: Golland, P., Hata, N., Barillot, C., Hornegger, J., Howe, R. (eds.) MICCAI 2014. LNCS, vol. 8674, pp. 781–788. Springer, Cham (2014). doi:10.1007/978-3-319-10470-6_97

11. Guizard, N., Nakamura, K., Coupé, P., Vladimir, S., Fonov, V., Arnold, D., Collins, D.: Non-local means inpainting of MS lesions in longitudinal image processing. Front. Neurosci. **9**, 456 (2015)

12. Prados, F., Cardoso, M.J., Kanber, B., Ciccarelli, O., Kapoor, R., Wheeler-Kingshott, C.A.G., Ourselin, S.: A multi-time-point modality-agnostic patch-based method for lesion filling in multiple sclerosis. NeuroImage **139**, 376–384 (2016)

13. Barnes, C., Shechtman, E., Goldman, D.B., Finkelstein, A.: The generalized patch-match correspondence algorithm. In: Daniilidis, K., Maragos, P., Paragios, N. (eds.) ECCV 2010. LNCS, vol. 6313, pp. 29–43. Springer, Heidelberg (2010). doi:10.1007/978-3-642-15558-1_3

14. Shi, W., Caballero, J., Ledig, C., Zhuang, X., Bai, W., Bhatia, K., Marvao, A.M.S.M., Dawes, T., O'Regan, D., Rueckert, D.: Cardiac image super-resolution with global correspondence using multi-atlas PatchMatch. In: Mori, K., Sakuma, I., Sato, Y., Barillot, C., Navab, N. (eds.) MICCAI 2013. LNCS, vol. 8151, pp. 9–16. Springer, Heidelberg (2013). doi:10.1007/978-3-642-40760-4_2

15. Ta, V.-T., Giraud, R., Collins, D.L., Coupé, P.: Optimized PatchMatch for near real time and accurate label fusion. In: Golland, P., Hata, N., Barillot, C., Hornegger, J., Howe, R. (eds.) MICCAI 2014. LNCS, vol. 8675, pp. 105–112. Springer, Cham (2014). doi:10.1007/978-3-319-10443-0_14

16. Giraud, R., Ta, V.T., Papadakis, N., Manjon, J.V., Collins, D.L., Coupe, P.: An optimized patchmatch for multi-scale and multi-feature label fusion. NeuroImage 124(Pt. A), 770–782 (2016)

17. Prados, F., Cardoso, M.J., Cawley, N., Ciccarelli, O., Wheeler-Kingshott, C.A., Ourselin, S.: Multi-contrast patchmatch algorithm for multiple sclerosis lesion detection. In: ISBI 2015 - Longitudinal MS Lesion Segmentation Challenge, pp. 1–2 (2015)

18. Xu, Z., Bagci, U., Seidel, J., Thomasson, D., Solomon, J., Mollura, D.J.: Segmentation based denoising of PET images: an iterative approach via regional means and affinity propagation. In: Golland, P., Hata, N., Barillot, C., Hornegger, J., Howe, R. (eds.) MICCAI 2014. LNCS, vol. 8673, pp. 698–705. Springer, Cham (2014). doi:10.1007/978-3-319-10404-1_87

19. Boyes, R.G., Gunter, J.L., Frost, C., Janke, A.L., Yeatman, T., Hill, D.L.G., Bernstein, M.A., Thompson, P.M., Weiner, M.W., Schuff, N., Alexander, G.E., Killiany, R.J., DeCarli, C., Jack, C.R., Fox, N.C.: Intensity non-uniformity correction using N3 on 3-T scanners. NeuroImage **39**(4), 1752–1762 (2008)
20. Buades, A., Coll, B., Morel, J.M.: A review of image denoising algorithms, with a new one. Multiscale Model. Simul. **4**(2), 490–530 (2005)
21. Cardoso, M.J., Wolz, R., Modat, M., Fox, N.C., Rueckert, D., Ourselin, S.: Geodesic information flows. In: Ayache, N., Delingette, H., Golland, P., Mori, K. (eds.) MICCAI 2012. LNCS, vol. 7511, pp. 262–270. Springer, Heidelberg (2012). doi:10. 1007/978-3-642-33418-4_33

Towards a Second Brain Images of Tumours for Evaluation (BITE2) Database

I.J. Gerard[1(✉)], C. Couturier[2], M. Kersten-Oertel[1], S. Drouin[1], D. De Nigris[3],
J.A. Hall[2], K. Mok[1], K. Petrecca[2], T. Arbel[1,3], and D.L. Collins[1,2,3]

[1] McConnell Brain Imaging Center, MNI, McGill University, Montreal, Canada
igerard1989@gmail.com
[2] Department of Neurology and Neurosurgery, McGill University, Montreal, Canada
[3] Centre for Intelligent Machines, McGill University, Montreal, Canada

Abstract. One of the main challenges facing members of the medical imaging community is the lack of real clinical cases and ground truth datasets with which to validate new registration, segmentation, and other image processing algorithms. In this work we present a collection of data from tumour patients acquired at the Montreal Neurological Institute and Hospital that will be released as a publicly available dataset to the image processing community. The database is comprised of 9 patient data sets, in its initial release, that consist of a preoperative and postoperative, gadolinium enhanced T1w MRI, pre- and post- resection tracked intra-operative ultrasound slices and volumes, expert tumour segmentations following the BRATS benchmark, and intra-operative ultrasound with/and MRI registration validation target points. This database extends the already widely used BITE database by improving the quality of registration validation and the variety of data being made available. By including addition features such as expert tumour segmentations, the database will appeal to a broader spectrum of image processing researchers and be useful for validating a wider range of techniques for image-guided neurosurgery.

Keywords: Database · Validation · Medical imaging · Intra-operative ultrasound

1 Introduction

Within the medical image processing community, one of the greatest challenges associated with the development of a new algorithm, be it for registration or segmentation, lies in the ability to validate the new method on real clinical data to demonstrate its superiority over existing methods and its applicability for clinical tasks. This challenge is amplified by the fact that technical laboratories are rarely located within a clinical environment making the access to appropriate validation data even more cumbersome. In addition, it is often difficult to find clinical experts who have the time to provide expertise in terms of creating a gold standard for validation purposes. A solution to some of these challenges lies in the creation of publicly available data sets that can be used by members of the medical image processing community for validation of new techniques that incorporate real clinical data. The data sets should be comprehensive in terms

© Springer International Publishing AG 2016
A. Crimi et al. (Eds.): BrainLes 2016, LNCS 10154, pp. 16–22, 2016.
DOI: 10.1007/978-3-319-55524-9_2

of modalities available, and offer data for validation of registration and segmentation. Over the last several years, imaging data for 25 patients undergoing neurosurgery for brain tumours has been collected at the Montreal Neurological Institute and Hospital. In this abstract we present 9 of these 25 cases that will be included in a publicly available database for use by the medical image processing community. Each patient underwent neurosurgery for a brain tumour and each patient included contains a pre- and post-operative T2 and T1 weighted, gadolinium enhanced MRIs, tracked intra-operative ultrasound (iUS) volumes and 2D slices, expert tumour segmentations following the BRATS [1] benchmark, and MRI-iUS registration validation target point sets. The work is an extension to the original Brain Images of Tumours for Evaluation (BITE) [2] database that has seen extensive use in the medical image processing literature and aims to improve on some of its critiques as described in other published work using the data for evaluation.

2   Methods

The patient information is summarized in Table 1. All patients consented to participate in the study and agreed to have their anonymized clinical data made publicly available. The complete study included 10 males and 15 females of which 3 and 6, respectively, are presented here. The mean age was 64. Both primary and metastatic brain tumours were included in the imaging study. All tumours included in the study were supraten-torial and varied amongst brain lobes.

Table 1. Patient information

Patient	Sex	Age	Tumour type	Lobe
1	F	72	Metastases	L–O/P
2	F	68	Glioblastoma	L–T
3	M	53	Glioblastoma	L–T/P
4	F	84	Glioma	R–P
5	F	41	Meningioma	L–F
6	M	63	Meningioma	R–F
7	F	77	Meningioma	R–F
8	F	62	Meningioma	L–O/P
9	M	55	Glioma	R–F

2.1   MR Images and Processing

Each patient in the series had a gadolinium enhanced 1.0 mm isotropic T1 weighted MRI, obtained on a 1.5 T MRI scanner (Ingenia Phillips Medical Systems). All images were processed in a custom image processing pipeline as follows [3]. First, the MRI is denoised, after estimating the standard deviation of the MRI Rician noise [4]. Next, intensity non-uniformity correction and normalization is done by estimating the non-uniformity field [5], followed by histogram matching with a reference image to normalize the intensities. The preoperative images were acquired on average 7 days prior to surgery. When available, T2w and FLAIR images were also included for the patient dataset, however the acquisition of these modalities was dependent on surgical need and not always included. Postoperative MR images were also T1w and were acquired within 48 h after surgery, however, slice thickness varied depending on the diagnostic request of the surgeon for the patient. All MR images were converted into the MINC format used at the McConnell Brain Imaging Centre, Montreal Neurological Institute and Hospital. All MINC tools can be found at packages.bic.mni.mcgill.ca and are publicly available.

2.2   Tracked Intraoperative Ultrasound

In each of the cases included in the database, tracked intraoperative ultrasound was acquired as part of a protocol for brain shift investigation [6]. Intraoperative ultrasound was acquired using our custom built prototype neuronavigation system, IBIS [7]. The workstation is equipped with an Intel Core i7-3820 @ 360 GHz x8 processor with 32 GB RAM, a GeForce GTX 670 graphics card and Conexant cx23800 video capture card. Tracking is performed using a Polaris N4 infrared optical system (Northern Digital, Waterloo, Canada). The Polaris infrared camera uses stereo triangulation to locate the passive reflective spheres on both the reference and pointing tools with an accuracy of 0.5 mm [8]. The ultrasound scanner, an HDI 5000 (ATL/Philips, Bothell, WA, USA) equipped with a 2D P7-4 MHz phased array transducer, enables intraoperative imaging during the surgical intervention. The ultrasound system transmits images using an S-video cable to the workstation at 30 frames/second and the ultrasound transducer probe is outfitted with a spatial tracking device with attached passive reflective spheres (Fig. 1) (Traxtal Technologies Inc., Toronto, Canada) and are tracked in the surgical environment.

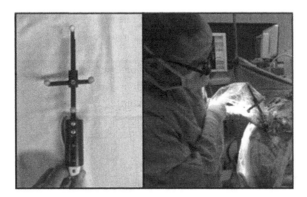

Fig. 1. Ultrasound probe with fitted tracking device (left) and use intraoperatively during neurosurgery (right).

For each case the surgeon acquired freehand ultrasound images in sweeps of 400 to 1000 2D images, moving the probe continuously in the plane of the craniotomy in a continuous forward motion in order to minimize any errors due to calibration. The sets of iUS series included in this database involved ultrasound images acquired at two time points during surgery: before and after resection. Pre-resection ultrasound images were acquired on the intact dura of the patient and post-resection ultrasound was acquired either in the resection cavity or on a dural graft attached to the patient after the resection was completed. During post-resection acquisition the cavity was filled with saline solution. For use in a volume-to-volume registration scheme the iUS series were reconstructed with a GPU implementation that looks for US pixels within a given search radius and that are no farther than 1.0 mm away from the point of interest. Each US voxel is weighted with a Gaussian function and normalized after all US pixels have been accumulated [9]. Both the original 2D series and the reconstructed volumes are available in the database. The tracking information for the individual slices is self-contained within the header of the ultrasound images which are also in the MINC format. An example of the included 2D and 3D iUS data can be seen in Fig. 2.

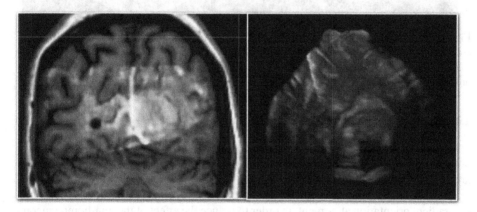

Fig. 2. Left: Example of a 2D US slice (orange) overlaid on the corresponding MR slice (grey) after registration. Right: 3D reconstructed volume of the iUS series. (Color figure online)

2.3 Tumour Segmentation

All tumour segmentations were performed by a senior neurosurgical resident (C. C.) using ITK Snap and followed the BRATS benchmark [1] in hopes of keeping consistent with a widely used system within the image processing community. For cases with gliomas, the labels included: (i) T2 tumour hyperintensities (edema), (ii) enhancing tumour core, and (iii) non-enhancing tumour core. For the other non-glioma tumour cases, all of these structures that were visible were segmented. An example of a segmentation for a glioblastoma and a meningioma can be seen in Fig. 3. The average solid tumour volume for the 9 cases was 28 cm^3. The intra-rater variability for the segmentations was measured by comparing two segmentations of the same tumour done on different days for both a glioblastoma and a meningioma. The intraclass correlations (ICC) for the solid tumour volume was 0.91 and 0.96 respectively for the Glioblastoma and meningioma cases, showing a consistent segmentation by the expert rater.

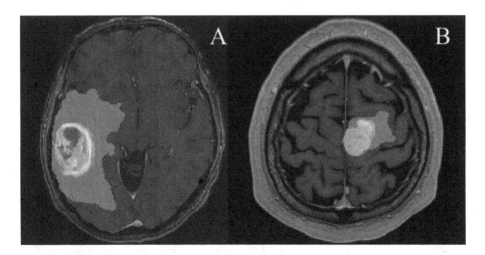

Fig. 3. Examples of expert segmentations that will be provided in the database of a GBM (A) and meningioma (B). In each segmentation, the same colour is used to differentiate between Edema (red), Enhancing tumour core (blue), and non-enhancing tumour core (green). (Color figure online)

2.4 Registration and Registration Validation

Since the intent of this database is to be useful to a broad image processing community both linear and non-linear registration transforms for the preoperative MRI and iUS data are included in the database.

Registration techniques to correct for brain shift have recently been developed, based on gradient orientation alignment, in order to reduce the effect of the non-homogeneous intensity response found in iUS images [9]. Once an iUS volume has been reconstructed the two volumes are registered using an algorithm based on gradient orientation alignment [9] which focuses on maximizing gradients with minimal uncertainty of the orientation estimates (i.e. locations with high gradient magnitude) within the set of images. This can be described mathematically as:

$$T^* = \arg \max_T \sum_{x \in \Omega} \cos(\Delta\theta)^2 \tag{1}$$

where T* is the transformation being determined, Ω is the overlap domain and $\Delta\theta$ is the inner angle between the fixed image gradient, ∇I_f, and the transformed moving image gradient $J^T \cdot \nabla I_m$:

$$\Delta\theta = < (\nabla I_f, J^T \cdot \nabla I_m) \tag{2}$$

The database includes the registration transforms obtained using this method.

Validation target sets for the MR-iUS registrations were obtained using the Validation Grid tool [10]. The tool is based on manually registering two images through manipulation of a series of target points that are placed as a regular shaped grid on both the target and fixed image. As the points are moved on the target image, the registration transform is updated based on the displacement of corresponding (target and fixed) grid points using a thin plate spline model. Due to the difficult nature of manually aligning images of different modalities the size of the validation grid can be changed from a coarse $2 \times 2 \times 2$ grid to a finer $7 \times 7 \times 7$ grid allowing the user to manually register the images in a hierarchical fashion from the largest deformations to small and local ones. Once complete, the set of points is exported and can be used as a large set to validate different registration procedures. A visual representation of this procedure can be seen in Fig. 4.

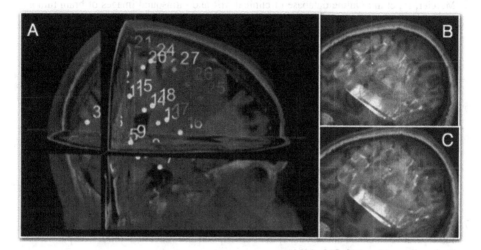

Fig. 4. Example of Validation Grid use for patient 9. A: 3D view of validation grid (yellow dots) on top of MRI volume (grey) and iUS volume (orange). B/C: 2D slice of unregistered iUS-MRI (B) and a target point (green) near a mis-registered sulcus being manipulated to facilitate registration (C). (Color figure online)

3   Discussion and Conclusion

We've presented here the structure and initial work towards a comprehensive tumour image database complete with multimodality imaging, intraoperative imaging, expert segmentation labels, linear and non-linear registration transformations, and registration validation target point sets with the goal of releasing 9 of the 25 patient sets publicly. The large range of data will enable comparison of a multitude of image processing techniques with a standard set of data for comparison with other techniques in the literature based on real clinical data.

The work here demonstrates an expansion on a previously popular brain tumour database [2] that has seen extensively used for validation in the literature. By adding a more reliable validation metric and through the introduction of expert segmentations following the BRATS benchmark it can be extended to both the registration and segmentation image processing communities. With further development and completion of the database we hope to inspire multiple future studies that will eventually benefit brain tumour patients through an easy and efficient resource to validate state-of-the-art image processing technologies. This will translate into tools and techniques that allow surgeons to better visualize tumours before, during, and after surgical interventions.

References

1. Menze, B.H., et al.: The multimodal brain tumor image segmentation benchmark (BRATS). IEEE Trans. Med. Imaging **34**(10), 1993–2024 (2015)
2. Mercier, L., et al.: Online database of clinical MR and ultrasound images of brain tumors. Med. Phys. **39**(6), 3253–3261 (2012)
3. Guizard, N., et al.: Robust individual template pipeline for longitudinal MR images. In: MICCAI 2012 Workshop on Novel Biomarkers for Alzheimer's Disease and Related Disorders (2012)
4. Coupe, P., et al.: An optimized blockwise nonlocal means denoising filter for 3-D magnetic resonance images. IEEE Trans. Med. Imaging **27**(4), 425–441 (2008)
5. Sled, J.G., Zijdenbos, A.P., Evans, A.C.: A nonparametric method for automatic correction of intensity nonuniformity in MRI data. IEEE Trans. Med. Imaging **17**(1), 87–97 (1998)
6. Gerard, I.J., Kersten-Oertel, M., Drouin, S., Hall, J.A., Petrecca, K., Nigris, D., Arbel, T., Louis Collins, D.: Improving patient specific neurosurgical models with intraoperative ultrasound and augmented reality visualizations in a neuronavigation environment. In: Oyarzun Laura, C., Shekhar, R., Wesarg, S., González Ballester, M.Á., Drechsler, K., Sato, Y., Erdt, M., Linguraru, M.G. (eds.) CLIP 2015. LNCS, vol. 9401, pp. 28–35. Springer, Heidelberg (2016). doi:10.1007/978-3-319-31808-0_4
7. Mercier, L., et al.: New prototype neuronavigation system based on preoperative imaging and intraoperative freehand ultrasound: system description and validation. Int. J. Comput. Assist. Radiol. Surg. **6**(4), 507–522 (2011)
8. Gerard, I.J., Collins, D.L.: An analysis of tracking error in image-guided neurosurgery. Int. J. Comput. Assist. Radiol. Surg. (2015)
9. De Nigris, D., Collins, D.L., Arbel, T.: Fast rigid registration of pre-operative magnetic resonance images to intra-operative ultrasound for neurosurgery based on high confidence gradient orientations. Int. J. Comput. Assist. Radiol. Surg. **8**(4), 649–661 (2013)
10. Gerard, I.J., et al.: The validation grid: a new tool to validate multimodal image registration. Int. J. CARS **11**(1), S1–S316 (2016)

Topological Measures of Connectomics
for Low Grades Glioma

Benjamin Amoah[1] and Alessandro Crimi[2(✉)]

[1] Lancaster University, Lancaster, UK
[2] Istituto Italiano di Tecnologia, Genoa, Italy
alecrimi@alice.it

Abstract. Recent advancements in neuroimaging have allowed the use of network analysis to study the brain in a system-based approach. In fact, several neurological disorders have been investigated from a network perspective. These include Alzheimer's disease, autism spectrum disorder, stroke, and traumatic brain injury. So far, few studies have been conducted on glioma by using connectome techniques. A connectome-based approach might be useful in quantifying the status of patients, in supporting surgical procedures, and ultimately shedding light on the underlying mechanisms and the recovery process.

In this manuscript, by using graph theoretical methods of segregation and integration, topological structural connectivity is studied comparing patients with low grade glioma to healthy control. These measures suggest that it is possible to quantify the status of patients pre- and post-surgical intervention to evaluate the condition.

1 Introduction

Glioma is the most common type of primary brain tumor which arises from glial cells. It is considered responsible for approximately 13000 deaths in the United States and more than 14000 in Europe each year [20]. It is considered one of the most aggressive types of cancer especially in its advanced stage termed glioblastoma multiforme (GBM). Tumor resection is the most effective therapy though generally complemented by chemo and radio therapies [19]. Nevertheless, resection of brain tumors involving relevant cortical areas is still a challenging task, as preservation of neuronal functions after surgery remains the goal [19]. Several studies have shown the potentiality of magnetic resonance imaging (MRI) in glioma patients for identifying pre-operatively their relationship with eloquent cortical areas, but individual significant variations in fiber structures and functional MRI (fMRI) activations have been reported [6,15,19]. Diffusion-tensor imaging (DTI) is used to track fibers combined with cortical stimulation as intra-operative support to preserve cognitive and motor functions, though this analysis might be subjective [1]. Moreover, analysis of functional activations highlights only the activations related to the task, but not the interaction among areas or the effect among the overall brain.

© Springer International Publishing AG 2016
A. Crimi et al. (Eds.): BrainLes 2016, LNCS 10154, pp. 23–31, 2016.
DOI: 10.1007/978-3-319-55524-9_3

A Connectome is the complete set of all neural connections of the human brain which can be structural or functional [22]. The human connectome has recently gained attention for its importance and possible implications for neuroscience as well as clinical neurology and psychology. It has already been used for studying stroke, autism spectrum disorders (ASD), Alzheimer's disease, schizophrenia, and other pathologies [9,24]. However, connectome analysis has not been extensively used for glioma patients. As for stroke, it is expected that specific cognitive and behavioral functions are not localized to anatomically restricted areas, but widespread across the neural networks of the injured brain, and specific symptoms are not necessarily localized in specific brain regions [11]. Hence, it can be hypothesized that connectomics can help to study cortical reorganization, functional recovery after resection, and help planning surgical interventions. Briganti et al. studied the functional connectivity of glioma affected patients by using a verb-generation task acquisition, and noticed that the patients had a statistically significant reduced degree of functional connectivity in the language related regions compared to healthy control [2]. Similarly, in another study functional connectivity exhibited chaotic changes in glioma patients compared to control correlating with language deficits [16]. It was also noticed that patients with gliomas have altered functional connectivity of the default mode network, and this was related to tumor grade, position and post-surgical status [12].

In this manuscript, topological measures are used to quantify the level of segregation and integration comparing low grade glioma patients and healthy control.

2   Method

An individual network measure may characterize one or several aspects of global and local brain connectivity. This study starts creating the tractography of the brain from DTI for patients and control, generating the related structural connectome, on which topological measures are computed to compare the two groups: low grade glioma patients and healthy control subjects.

Tractographies for all subjects have been generated processing DTI data with the Python library Dipy [7]. In particular, a deterministic algorithm called Euler Delta Crossings [7] has been used stemming from 2,000,000 seed-points and stopping when the fractional anisotropy (FA) was smaller than <0.1. Tracts shorter than 30 mm or in which a sharp angle occurred have been discarded. Linear registration has been applied between the automated anatomical labeling (AAL) atlas [23] and the first volume of the DTI acquisition by using linear registration with 12 degrees of freedom. Counting the fibers starting and ending in all $r = 90$ regions of the AAL atlas, a structural connectivity matrix of $r \times r$ elements is constructed for each subject. Connections with less than 4 fibers are neglected, and the matrix is afterwards binarized.

Once the connectome is constructed, the glioma patients and control subjects were characterized by the most common graph-topological measures. Topological measures are divided into measures of segregation and integration. Segregation measures are representations of densely connected network communities, while integration measures are related to network hubs that are rich in connections between the communities [4]. Simulations on artificial networks demonstrated that as the connectivity gradually changes from an ordered lattice to a pseudo-random network, perturbational integration decreases, and perturbational segregation increases [4]. However these decreases and increases are not easily quantifiable as different diseases might affect in different ways the brain or relevant nodes of it [3]. For this study, we chose the two most common measures of segregation (the Louvain modularity and clustering coefficient) and integration (characteristic path length and global efficiency) [17] computed for the n nodes of each graph.

The modularity of a network is the degree to which the network may be subdivided into non-overlapping groups. The Louvain algorithm is known for its efficiency in producing partitioned communities, and it is applicable to weighted and unweighted graphs. For weighted graphs, modularity is defined as

$$Q = \frac{1}{2m} \sum_{ij} \left[A_{ij} - \frac{k_i k_j}{2m} \right] \delta(c_i, c_j), \tag{1}$$

where A_{ij} is the weight between nodes i and j, k_i and k_j are the sum of weights of the edges connecting the nodes i and j respectively, m is the sum of all edge weights in the graph, c_i and c_j are the communities of the nodes, and δ is a simple delta function. For unweighted graphs, as in our case, the edge weights are just either 1 or 0. The algorithm starts with a true network and then performs random double edge swaps introducing an aleatory effect in the computation. Since modularity Q values might vary based on random differences in community assignments from run to run, Q values were averaged over 100 iterations of the algorithm. Clustering coefficient is the fraction of triangles around a node, and it can be defined as

$$C = \frac{1}{(n-1)(n-2)} \sum_{i \in N} \frac{2t}{k_i(k_i - 1)}, \tag{2}$$

where t_i and k_i is respectively the number of triangles around a node i, and the degree of the node i. It measures how much neighbors of a node are connected to each other. In the results, the mean value across the nodes are reported.

The characteristic path length d_{ij} is the average shortest path length in the network between each node i and j. The efficiency measure is given by the average inverse shortest path length. It can be computed globally or limited to the neighborhood of a node defining the local efficiency. Global efficiency is defined as

$$E = \frac{1}{n} \sum_{i \in N} \frac{\sum_{j \in N, j \neq i} d_{ij}^{-1}}{n - 1}. \tag{3}$$

Given the measures as features for representing the two populations of glioma patients and control, p-values were generated from a two-sample t-tests performed on each metric with the goal to assess difference between the two groups.

3   Data and Experimental Settings

The neuroimage data for the patients are from The Cancer Imaging Archive (TCIA)[1], which is a large and growing archive, comprising several hundreds volumes in different modalities. However, diffusion tensor and fMRI data available are very limited or acquired in different protocols. The brain volumes for the low grade glioma patients were acquired with a 1.5 T GE Signa Excite. In particular, the 20 available DTI volumes were acquired with an isotropic voxel-size of 2.6 mm, TR = 17 s, TE = 84.6 ms, and using 26 gradient directions. The mean age of the patients was 45.74 ± 13.35 years.

Being no control brain available in TCIA archive, those were matched with the 20 control volumes available from the NKI-Rockland Sample[2] randomly selected. Those DTI volumes were acquired with a Siemens 1.5 T scanner and isotropic voxel-size of 2 mm, TR = 10 s, TE = 91 ms, and using 35 gradient directions. The age of the healthy control was 38 ± 19.15 years.

All data had the skull stripped and eddy current correction performed before the tractography construction.

4   Results

The results of the network analysis for the two datasets and significance are reported in Table 1 as mean and variance value for the two groups. The last column reports the p-value of the discriminative test between the two groups. An example of resulting connectome for the healthy control subjects is shown in Fig. 1, while Figs. 2 and 3 depict axial slices for two cases subjects. In particular, those are T1 post gadolinium injection, FLAIR, tractography stopping the tracts if the FA was smaller than 0.25, and structural connectome using the tractography constructed stopping the tracts if the FA was smaller than 0.01.

Table 1. Topological network measures reported as mean and variance. The last column reports the p-value of the discriminative test between the two groups.

Features	Low grade glioma patients	Healthy controls	p-value
Modularity	0.491 ± 0.021	0.438 ± 0.026	1.15×10^{-7}
Clustering coefficient	0.605 ± 0.012	0.592 ± 0.017	0.0252
Char. path length	2.265 ± 0.058	2.139 ± 0.054	1.29×10^{-7}
Global efficiency	0.512 ± 0.010	0.540 ± 0.010	1.13×10^{-8}

---

[1] http://cancerimagingarchive.net.
[2] http://fcon_1000.projects.nitrc.org/indi/pro/nki.html.

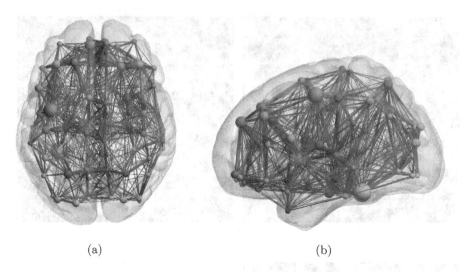

(a)   (b)

Fig. 1. Axial (a) and sagittal (b) view of a healthy control connectome (no slice). The size of the nodes represents the degree, while the number of tracts connecting the nodes is represented by the stroke of the edges. The tractography for these structural connections is constructed stopping the tracts if the FA was smaller than 0.01.

5 Discussions

The measures of segregation and integration used in this article have been already investigated for other diseases. In a study about ASD, all measures used in functional connectomes showed lower scores in ASD patients compared to healthy control [18]. In a study related to schizophrenia [5], connectomes of patients with psychotic episodes showed larger characteristic path length, but smaller global efficiency and clustering coefficients compared to schizophrenia subject without psychotic episodes. Another topological comparison between connectomes of schizophrenia patients and control subject showed smaller global efficiency and other integration metrics in the patients [10]. Conversely, other studies on schizophrenia showed elevated values of clustering coefficients and small values of characteristic shortest path, suggesting overall more segregated patterns in the network [13]. This lack of agreement can be related to different pre-processing steps, neglected local anatomical differences, or on the selecting criteria of the matching control group [13].

Our results for the case connectomes showed an increased modularity and clustering coefficient, and an increased characteristic path length and reduced related global efficiency compared to the control connectome scores. The increased path length and reduced global efficiency can be hypothetically explained as the destructive effect of low grade glioma being similar to the disconnecting impact of schizophrenia which share the same discrimination between case and control.

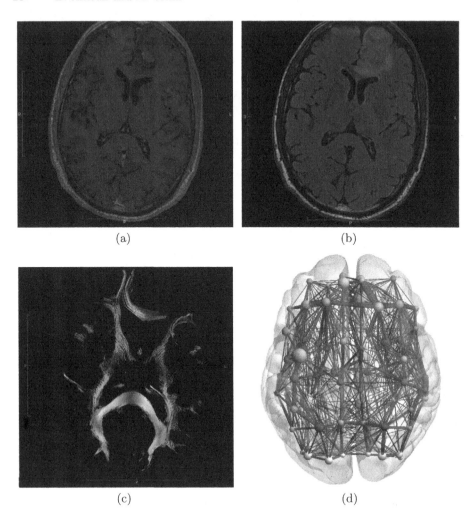

(a)

(b)

(c)

(d)

Fig. 2. Presurgical axial slices for one case subjects: (a) T1 post gadolinium injection, (b) FLAIR, (c) tractography stopping the tracts if the FA was smaller than 0.25, and (d) whole structural connectome using the tractography constructed stopping the tracts if the FA was smaller than 0.01 (no slice).

No clear difference was noticeable by visual inspection of the connectome, though an atlas with more detailed cortical subdivision might have allowed also this visual difference [8]. However, if the stopping threshold of the FA was moved from 0.01 to 0.25, the tracts crossing the tumor disappeared. This is a sign of damage in the area. It can hypothesized that due to the low grade of the tumors tracts are still presents and not completely damaged as with glioblastoma which is a brain tumor of higher grade. The main limitation of the study is the limited sample size and also the different type of acquisition for the case and control

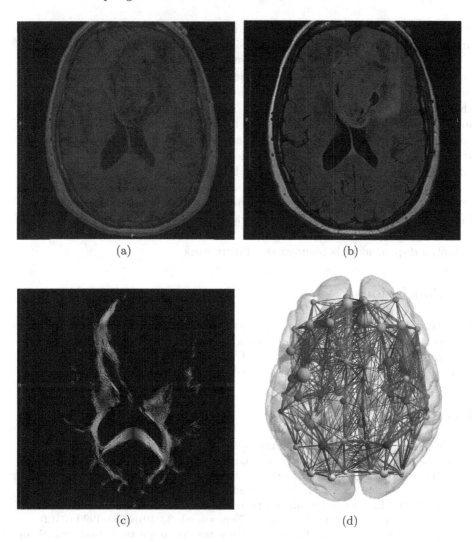

Fig. 3. Presurgical axial slices for one case subjects: (a) T1 post gadolinium injection, (b) FLAIR, (c) tractography stopping the tracts if the FA was smaller than 0.25, and (d) whole structural connectome using the tractography constructed stopping the tracts if the FA was smaller than 0.01 (no slice)

dataset which might have influenced the detected differences. Therefore, further studies with even more consistent datasets are required. Moreover, the measures give an indicative score of the status of the network to potentially correlate with health status, but they are not enough to help during surgical procedures, since population statistics to identify relevant areas or connections has only a relative meaning for pre-surgical planning [14]. However, the study of individual connectomes could be used jointly to existing procedure of cortical activation and stimulation to support surgical decisions.

Despite the registration of the volumes to the atlas was considered properly carried out as noticed by visual inspection, concerns remain about possible influence of the glioma in deforming the brain anatomy. In fact, it can be argued that due to the presence of the tumor some tracts might be pushed ending in a different location than expected by the atlas and therefore corrupting the subsequent analysis. The issue has been argued in tract based spatial statistics studies considering multiple sclerosis lesions, concluding that the misplacement effect is negligible [21]. Conversely, it has been argued that for high grade glioma located near the corticospinal tracts and eloquent areas, it is possible that such an effect has an impact [2]. Being this study mostly focused on the overall topological measures and using only low grade gliomas patients, this issue could be considered negligible, though an analysis with a model which take into account potential displacement is planned as a future work.

6   Conclusions

Understanding the brain connectome and dynamic network changes that occur due to tumor can give further information on the status of patients and evaluate rehabilitations. In fact, topological measures appear to differ in terms of segregation and integration in glioma patients compared to healthy control.

References

1. Berman, J.I., Berger, M.S., et al.: Diffusion-tensor imaging-guided tracking of fibers of the pyramidal tract combined with intraoperative cortical stimulation mapping in patients with gliomas. J. Neurosurg. **101**(1), 66–72 (2004)
2. Briganti, C., Sestieri, C., Mattei, P., Esposito, R., Galzio, R., Tartaro, A., Romani, G., Caulo, M.: Reorganization of functional connectivity of the language network in patients with brain gliomas. Am. J. Neuroradiol. **33**(10), 1983–1990 (2012)
3. Bullmore, E., Sporns, O.: Complex brain networks: graph theoretical analysis of structural and functional systems. Nat. Rev. Neurosci. **10**(3), 186–198 (2009)
4. Deco, G., Tononi, G., Boly, M., Kringelbach, M.L.: Rethinking segregation and integration: contributions of whole-brain modelling. Nat. Rev. Neurosci. **16**(7), 430–439 (2015)
5. Drakesmith, M., Caeyenberghs, K., Dutt, A., Zammit, S., Evans, C.J., Reichenberg, A., Lewis, G., David, A.S., Jones, D.K.: Schizophrenia-like topological changes in the structural connectome of individuals with subclinical psychotic experiences. Hum. Brain Mapp. **36**(7), 2629–2643 (2015)
6. Fandino, J., et al.: Intraoperative validation of functional magnetic resonance imaging and cortical reorganization patterns in patients with brain tumors involving the primary motor cortex. J. Neurosurg. **91**(2), 238–250 (1999)
7. Garyfallidis, E., Brett, M., Amirbekian, B., Rokem, A., Van Der Walt, S., Descoteaux, M., Nimmo-Smith, I.: Contributors, Dipy, a library for the analysis of diffusion MRI data. Frontiers Neuroinformatics **8** (2014)

8. Gordon, E.M., et al.: Generation and evaluation of a cortical area parcellation from resting-state correlations. Cerebral cortex, p. bhu239 (2014)
9. Griffa, A., Baumann, P.S., Thiran, J.P., Hagmann, P.: Structural connectomics in brain diseases. Neuroimage **80**, 515–526 (2013)
10. Griffa, A., Baumann, P.S., Ferrari, C., Do, K.Q., Conus, P., Thiran, J.P., Hagmann, P.: Characterizing the connectome in schizophrenia with diffusion spectrum imaging. Hum. Brain Mapp. **36**(1), 354–366 (2015)
11. Guggisberg, A.G., Honma, S.M., Findlay, A.M., Dalal, S.S., Kirsch, H.E., Berger, M.S., Nagarajan, S.S.: Mapping functional connectivity in patients with brain lesions. Ann. Neurol. **63**(2), 193–203 (2008)
12. Harris, R.J., Bookheimer, S.Y., Cloughesy, T.F., Kim, H.J., Pope, W.B., Lai, A., Nghiemphu, P.L., Liau, L.M., Ellingson, B.M.: Altered functional connectivity of the default mode network in diffuse gliomas measured with pseudo-resting state fmri. J. Neurooncol. **116**(2), 373–379 (2014)
13. van den Heuvel, M.P., Fornito, A.: Brain networks in Schizophrenia. Neuropsychol. Rev. **24**(1), 32–48 (2014)
14. Hou, B., et al.: Quantitative comparisons on hand motor functional areas determined by resting state and task bold fmri and anatomical mri for pre-surgical planning of patients with brain tumors. Neuroimage Clin. **11**, 378–387 (2016)
15. Kapsalakis, I.Z., et al.: Preoperative evaluation with FMRI of patients with intracranial gliomas. Radiology research and practice 2012 (2012)
16. Kinno, R., Ohta, S., Muragaki, Y., Maruyama, T., Sakai, K.L.: Differential reorganization of three syntax-related networks induced by a left frontal glioma. Brain **137**(4), 1193–1212 (2014)
17. Rubinov, M., Sporns, O.: Complex network measures of brain connectivity: uses and interpretations. Neuroimage **52**(3), 1059–1069 (2010)
18. Rudie, J.D., Brown, J., Beck-Pancer, D., Hernandez, L., Dennis, E., Thompson, P., Bookheimer, S., Dapretto, M.: Altered functional and structural brain network organization in autism. NeuroImage Clin. **2**, 79–94 (2013)
19. Sanai, N., Berger, M.S.: Glioma extent of resection and its impact on patient outcome. Neurosurgery **62**(4), 753–766 (2008)
20. Siegel, R.L., Miller, K.D., Jemal, A.: Cancer statistics, 2016. CA: A Cancer J. Clin. **66**(1), 7–30 (2016)
21. Smith, S.M., Jenkinson, M., Johansen-Berg, H., Rueckert, D., Nichols, T.E., Mackay, C.E., Watkins, K.E., Ciccarelli, O., Cader, M.Z., Matthews, P.M., et al.: Tract-based spatial statistics: voxelwise analysis of multi-subject diffusion data. Neuroimage **31**(4), 1487–1505 (2006)
22. Sporns, O., Tononi, G., Kötter, R.: The human connectome: a structural description of the human brain. PLoS Comput. Biol. **1**(4), e42 (2005)
23. Tzourio-Mazoyer, N., et al.: Automated anatomical labeling of activations in SPM using a macroscopic anatomical parcellation of the MNI MRI single-subject brain. Neuroimage **15**(1), 273–289 (2002)
24. Varoquaux, G., Craddock, R.C.: Learning and comparing functional connectomes across subjects. NeuroImage **80**, 405–415 (2013)

Multi-modal Registration Improves Group Discrimination in Pediatric Traumatic Brain Injury

Emily L. Dennis[1(✉)], Faisal Rashid[1], Julio Villalon-Reina[1], Gautam Prasad[1],
Joshua Faskowitz[1], Talin Babikian[2], Richard Mink[3], Christopher Babbitt[4],
Jeffrey Johnson[5], Christopher C. Giza[6], Robert F. Asarnow[2,7,8],
and Paul M. Thompson[1,2,9]

[1] Imaging Genetics Center, Keck USC School of Medicine, Marina del Rey, CA, USA
emily.dennis@ini.usc.edu
[2] Department of Psychiatry and Biobehavioral Sciences, Semel Institute for Neuroscience
and Human Behavior, UCLA, Los Angeles, CA, USA
[3] Department of Pediatrics, Harbor-UCLA Medical Center and Los Angeles BioMedical
Research Institute, Torrance, CA, USA
[4] Miller Children's Hospital, Long Beach, CA, USA
[5] Department of Pediatrics, LAC+USC Medical Center, Los Angeles, CA, USA
[6] Department of Neurosurgery and Division of Pediatric Neurology, UCLA Brain Injury Research
Center, Mattel Children's Hospital, Los Angeles, CA, USA
[7] Department of Psychology, UCLA, Los Angeles, CA, USA
[8] Brain Research Institute, UCLA, Los Angeles, CA, USA
[9] Departments of Neurology, Pediatrics, Psychiatry, Radiology, Engineering,
and Ophthalmology, USC, Los Angeles, USA

Abstract. Traumatic brain injury (TBI) can disrupt the white matter (WM) integrity in the brain, leading to functional and cognitive disruptions that may persist for years. There is considerable heterogeneity within the patient group, which complicates group analyses. Here we present improvements to a tract identification workflow, automated multi-atlas tract extraction (autoMATE), evaluating the effects of improved registration. Use of study-specific template improved group classification accuracy over the standard workflow. The addition of a multi-modal registration that includes information from diffusion weighted imaging (DWI), T_1-weighted, and Fluid-Attenuated Inversion Recovery (FLAIR) further improved classification accuracy. We also examined whether particular tracts contribute more to group classification than others. Parts of the corpus callosum contributed most, and there were unexpected asymmetries between bilateral tracts.

1 Introduction

Traumatic brain injury (TBI) is the leading cause of death and disability in children and adolescents. TBI can cause extensive white matter (WM) damage, which can still be detectable years post-injury. Diffusion weighted imaging (DWI) is useful in studying WM disruptions caused by brain injury, offering a non-invasive means to assess possible

© Springer International Publishing AG 2016
A. Crimi et al. (Eds.): BrainLes 2016, LNCS 10154, pp. 32–42, 2016.
DOI: 10.1007/978-3-319-55524-9_4

diffuse axonal injury (DAI). DAI is frequently associated with poor outcome, but can only be definitively diagnosed *post mortem* [1]. The structural damage and considerable heterogeneity within the TBI patient population can complicate brain imaging studies, especially inter-subject registration. Here we evaluated improvements in a DWI analytical workflow, automated multi-atlas tract extraction (autoMATE). We use study specific templates, and register images using information from three modalities (DWI, T1, and FLAIR) instead of one.

Fluid-Attenuated Inversion Recovery (FLAIR) is often collected in TBI research due to its sensitivity to lesions. The long inversion time (T_1) of FLAIR suppresses the signal from CSF leading to improved differentiation of lesions relative to some T_2-weighted sequences [2]. DWI has been applied in TBI research fairly recently, offering better anatomical resolution than conventional CT for detecting and localizing ischemia, DAI, and other TBI-associated neuropathologies [3, 4]. T_1-weighted imaging provides a high-resolution anatomical scan that offers a standard target for registration. By combining information from all three modalities, we hoped to leverage the benefits of each, resulting in a more accurate registration.

AutoMATE has been used to analyze WM integrity following TBI, and performs well even in injured tissue [5–8]. Here we sought to improve the workflow further. We tested the initial workflow and compared it with an intermediate workflow with one alteration, and the final process with two alterations on the same dataset of 31 moderate-to-severe TBI (msTBI) patients and well-matched healthy controls.

2   Methods

2.1   Subjects and Image Acquisition

TBI participants were recruited from 4 Pediatric Intensive Care Units (PICUs) at Level 1 Trauma Centers in Los Angeles County. Healthy controls, matched for age, sex, and educational level, were recruited from the community through flyers, magazines, and school postings. Participants were studied in the post-acute phase (2–6 months post-injury). We included 31 TBI participants (7 female, 14.3 average age) and 40 controls. *Inclusion criteria*: non-penetrating moderate-severe TBI (intake or post-resuscitation Glasgow Coma Scale (GCS) score between 3 and 12, or higher GCS with positive imaging findings), 8–18 years old at injury, right handed, normal vision, English proficiency. *Exclusion criteria*: history of neurological illness or injury, motor deficits or metal implant preventing safe MRI scanning, history of psychosis, ADHD, Tourette's, learning disability, mental retardation, or autism.

Participants were scanned with 3T MRI (Siemens Trio) with whole-brain anatomical and 66-gradient diffusion imaging. Diffusion-weighted images (DWI) were acquired with the following acquisition parameters: GRAPPA mode; acceleration factor PE = 2; TR/TE = 9500/87 ms; FOV = 256×256 mm; isotropic voxel size = 2 mm. 72 images were collected per subject: 8 b_0 and 64 diffusion-weighted images ($b = 1000$ s/mm^2).

2.2 Tractography

AutoMATE (automated multi-atlas tract extraction) is described fully in prior papers [9–11], and outlined in Fig. 1. Briefly, autoMATE labels tracts of interest from the whole brain tractography based on template atlases. While many tract labeling tools use only a single template, the strength of autoMATE is that it uses 5 templates, increasing the robustness and generalizability of results. Raw DWI images were visually checked for artifacts, resulting in 2 participants being excluded from all analyses due to extensive slice dropout (not included in above participant count). DWI images were corrected for eddy-current induced distortions using the FSL tool "eddy_correct" (http://fsl.fmrib.ox.ac.uk/fsl/). DWI scans were skull-stripped using FSL tool "BET" (default parameters). Eddy correct deformations were applied to the gradient vectors. Fractional anisotropy (FA) measures the degree to which water is diffusing preferentially in one direction (along axons). MD (mean diffusivity) is a measure of the average diffusivity across all 3 primary eigenvectors. RD (radial diffusivity) is the average of the eigenvalues corresponding to the 2 non-primary eigenvectors, and AD (axial diffusivity) is the eigenvalue corresponding to the primary eigenvector. FA, MD, RD, and AD maps were computed using FSL tool "dtifit". Whole-brain DWI tractography was performed with Camino (http://cmic.cs.ucl.ac.uk/camino/). The maximum fiber turning angle was set to 35°/voxel to limit biologically implausible results, and tracing stopped when FA dropped below 0.2, a threshold that is somewhat standard in the field.

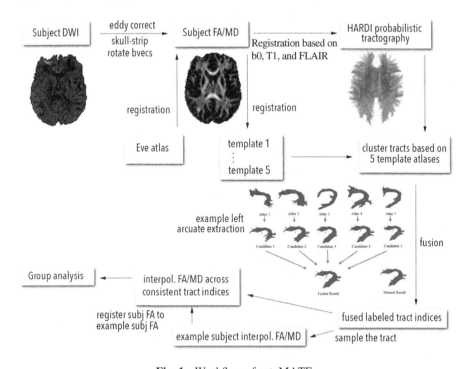

Fig. 1. Workflow of autoMATE.

2.3   Fiber Clustering and Label Fusion

The standard autoMATE templates are 5 WM tract atlases constructed from healthy 20–30 year olds, as detailed previously [9–11]. These templates will be referred to as the **standard template**. For this project, we also constructed 5 new WM atlases from 5 adolescents in the study (2F/3 M, 14–18 years old, all healthy controls). These templates will be referred to as the **study specific template**. The atlas used to identify tracts in the templates was based on the "Eve" brain atlas [12], and includes 19 major WM tracts: the bilateral corticospinal tract, bilateral cingulum, bilateral inferior fronto-occipital fasciculus, bilateral inferior longitudinal fasciculus, bilateral uncinate, bilateral parahippocampal cingulum, left arcuate fasciculus (the right arcuate is too asymmetric for population studies to be practical [13]), and corpus callosal tracts divided into 6 segments – frontal, precentral gyrus, postcentral gyrus, parietal, temporal, and occipital. The Eve atlas was registered, linearly and then non-linearly, to each subject's FA map using ANTs (Advanced Normalization Tools [14]) and its ROIs were correspondingly warped to extract 18 tracts of interest for each subject based on a look-up table [12]. ROI registration was visually checked for all subjects, and all passed quality control. While registration is difficult in injured brains, the registration tools in the ANTs library have been shown to work well [15].

Basic registration: Each subject's FA map was further registered non-linearly using ANTs SyN to each of the 5 *standard templates*. **Intermediate registration**: Each subject's FA map was further registered non-linearly to each of the 5 *study specific templates*. **Multi-modal registration**: Each subject's averaged b_0, FLAIR, and T_1-weighted image (T_1w) were registered linearly then non-linearly to each of the 5 *study specific template*'s b_0, FLAIR, and T_1w images respectively. Since each modality provides an improved resolution and is sensitive to different aspects of brain structure, they are expected to contribute different information during the registration process. First, each subject's FLAIR and T_1w images were linearly registered to their averaged b_0 image using the FSL tool "flirt" bringing all three modalities to a common space. ANTs SyN was then used to perform a multi-channel registration to simultaneously warp three images from each subject to the corresponding template images. The T_1w images were registered using a cross-correlation coefficient (CC) similarity metric and was also weighted the highest as it provided the best resolution, followed by FLAIR images registered using mutual information (MI) and weighted 2nd highest, and lastly the b_0 images were registered using MI and weighted the least. The transformations were then applied to each subject's FA map, resulting in finely registered FA images to each of the 5 *study specific templates*. This is shown in Fig. 2. All registrations were visually inspected for quality, and all passed quality control. At this point there are 3 separate processing streams. For each processing stream, the 18 tracts from each atlas were then warped to the subject space based on the deformation field from the above-referenced registration steps [16]. We refined fiber extractions of each tract based on the distance between the warped corresponding tract of each atlas and the subject's fiber candidates from ROI extraction. Individual results from the 5 atlases were fused. We visually inspected the resulting fiber bundles. For each of the 18 WM tracts, we selected one example subject to display group analysis results (this step was consistent across processing streams). We extracted FA, MD, RD, and AD along the tracts at this point, output as 8155×15 matrices, with each point in the matrix corresponding to tract coordinates.

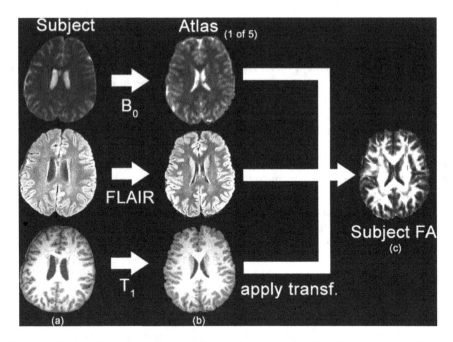

Fig. 2. (a) Each subject's b_0, FLAIR, and T_1-weighted image are first linearly then non-linearly registered to its respective atlas image. (b) This step is repeated for each of the five atlases. (c) The resulting transformations are then applied to each subject's FA image, resulting in an FA image finely registered to each of the five atlas FAs.

2.4 Support Vector Machine

Support vector machines (SVMs) [17] are one popular form of supervised learning model that we used to classify our connectivity features, to differentiate connectivity patterns in TBI and normal development. Clearly other machine learning models are possible, but here we chose SVMs as their properties are well understood. SVMs classify 2-class data by training a model, or classification function, to find the optimal hyperplane between the 2 classes in the data. Let $x_i \in \mathbb{R}^d$ represent the connectivity feature vectors, where d is the dimension of the feature set of interest and $Y_i = \pm 1$ be their label with -1 and 1 representing TBI and control. Our target hyperplane is:

$$\langle w, x \rangle + b = 0,$$

where $w \in \mathbb{R}^d$ should separate as many data points as possible. We find this hyperplane by solving the L2-norm problem:

$$\arg \min_{w,b,v} \left(\frac{1}{2} \langle w, w \rangle + D \sum_i v_i^2 \right),$$

such that

$$y_i(\langle w, x_i \rangle + b) \geq 1 - v_b \quad v_i \geq 0$$

where v_i are slack variables and D is a penalty parameter. In many instances, a hyperplane cannot be found that completely separates the 2 classes of data, and slack variables are added to create soft margins to separate most of the points.

Our classification design was to test the information provided by the point-wise WM integrity estimates with repeated stratified 10-fold cross-validation [18]. We repeated the cross-validation 10 times. Each repeat represents a different random grouping of dataset for 10-fold cross-validation. For cross-validation (CV), our performance metrics were balanced accuracy (average of sensitivity and specificity), accuracy (number of correctly identified subjects divided by the total number of subjects), sensitivity (true positives [TP] divided by total positives), specificity (true negatives [TN] divided by total negatives), and F1 (2 * ((precision * sensitivity)/(precision + sensitivity)), where precision is TP divided by total positive calls). We used the linear SVM implementation in scikit-learn 0.16.1 (http://scikit-learn.org/) with the default parameters. The input for the SVM was the point-wise estimates of FA, MD, RD, and AD across all tract indices, input as 8155 × 15 matrices for each subject.

Table 1. Differences in proportional volume of subcortical structures between workflows. For example, in the native space, the thalamus represented 0.479% of the brain volume, averaged across subjects, whereas in the basic workflow, this value was 0.523%, giving a difference of 0.044% (or an increase of 9.2%).

	Basic	Intermediate	Multi-modal
Thalamus	0.044% (9.2%)	−0.026% (−5.0%)	−0.048% (−10.6%)
Caudate	0.022% (9.0%)	−0.014% (−5.4%)	−0.016% (−6.9%)
Putamen	0.035% (9.3%)	−0.022% (−5.3%)	−0.035% (−10.0%)
GP	0.011% (10.1%)	−0.008% (−6.7%)	−0.006% (−6.0%)
Hippocampus	0.019% (8.1%)	−0.014% (−5.4%)	−0.028% (−12.6%)
Amygdala	0.008% (8.8%)	−0.005% (−5.6%)	−0.008% (−10.1%)
Accumbens	0.004% (10.2%)	−0.002% (−5.5%)	−0.003% (−9.2%)
Ventral DC	0.024% (9.2%)	−0.016% (−5.6%)	−0.016% (−6.8%)

3   Results

We calculated the average displacement across all subjects, across all 5 template atlases, across the whole brain, for each of the 3 registrations tested. For the single channel registration with the standard templates, the average displacement magnitude across all subjects was 3.0%. For the single-channel registration with the study specific templates, the average displacement magnitude across all subjects was 3.1%. For the multi-channel registration with the study specific templates, the average displacement magnitude across all subjects was 3.7%. As another check of registration, we extracted the volume of 8 subcortical structures in native space and compared it to the volumes extracted after each transformation. This was done across 9 healthy controls. The differences in volumes, expressed as a percent of the total brain volume are shown in Table 1.

3.1 Study Specific Template – Intermediate Registration

The creation of a study specific template was the first improvement to the workflow. The standard autoMATE templates are taken from 20–30 year old healthy controls, while the study specific templates include 5 14–18 year olds (2F/3 M, all healthy controls). Use of a more age-appropriate template, taken from the sample, improved nearly all measures of group discrimination across FA, MD, and RD. SVM based on AD gave mixed results. The classification outputs can be seen in Table 2. T-tests of the 10 CV repeats showed these improvements were largely significant.

Table 2. Comparison of SVM outputs from the basic, intermediate, and multi-modal registration protocols. **Bolded** entries are significantly improved over the previous step, *italicized* entries for the multi-modal step are significantly improved over the initial step, as shown in *t*-tests of the 10 CV repeats.

	Single channel registration/Standard template				
	BAC	*Accuracy*	*Sensitivity*	*Specificity*	*F1*
FA	0.7995	0.8039	0.8640	0.7350	0.8222
MD	0.7621	0.7692	0.8525	0.6717	0.7992
RD	0.7823	0.7892	0.8670	0.6975	0.8143
AD	0.7475	0.7580	0.8525	0.6425	0.7920
	Single channel registration/Study specific template				
	BAC	*Accuracy*	*Sensitivity*	*Specificity*	*F1*
FA	0.8012	0.8118	0.8850	0.7175	0.8414
MD	**0.8004**	**0.8043**	**0.8350**	**0.7658**	**0.8228**
RD	**0.8042**	**0.8132**	0.8775	**0.7308**	**0.8405**
AD	0.7325	0.7520	**0.8775**	**0.5875**	0.7978
	Multi-modal registration/Study specific template				
	BAC	*Accuracy*	*Sensitivity*	*Specificity*	*F1*
FA	0.8038	0.8146	*0.8900*	0.7175	*0.8437*
MD	*0.8104*	*0.8143*	0.8450	0.7758	*0.8328*
RD	*0.8029*	*0.8134*	*0.8875*	*0.7183*	*0.8432*
AD	0.7379	0.7751	*0.8850*	*0.5908*	*0.8031*

3.2 Multi-modal Registration

The second improvement to the workflow involved the inclusion of multiple image modalities for the template registration, as well as the same study specific templates used in the intermediate registration. This step brought further improvement to the classification outputs for all measures. These results can be seen in Table 2. T-tests of the 10 CV repeats showed the improvements over single channel were only significant for one measure (indicated in **bold** in the table), but over the original registration they were highly significant (indicated in *italics* in the table).

3.3 Most Robust Tracts

The analysis to this point was completed using all tract data, but we were interested to see whether specific tracts aided in classification more than others. We ran a separate classification examining each tract alone. For this, we ran SVM as above, but with data from each tract separately input into the SVM. The balanced accuracy across all 19 tracts is depicted in Fig. 3, averaged across the tract. We computed this on FA, MD, RD, and AD, but we display results here only for RD. The CC frontal, CC postcentral, and right inferior longitudinal fasciculus (ILF) had the highest BAC. There appeared to be an asymmetry as well, with right hemisphere tracts having higher average BAC than left hemisphere tracts (0.664 vs. 0.615).

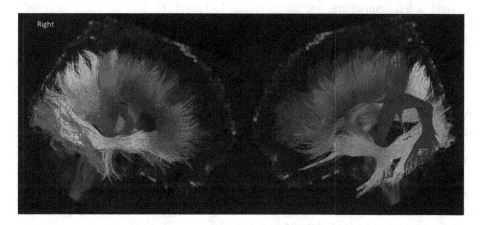

Fig. 3. Balanced accuracy (BAC) across the 19 tracts computed from MD along tract. Colors correspond to BAC, according to the legend.

4 Discussion

TBI can cause widespread damage to the brain, but the pattern of injury can differ based on severity, location, type, and any number of unknown premorbid patient characteristics. This heterogeneity can complicate inter-subject registration, which is critical for accurate and generalizable results. Here we aimed to improve this step, by including templates generated from subjects in the study, and by using a multi-modal registration.

Using study-specific templates improved the classification accuracy from resulting tract-wise WM integrity measures. This is an expected outcome, as templates matched for age and scan protocol should be more similar to the patient images to be registered. The images we selected for the multi-modal registration were chosen for their particular sensitivity to detecting pathology caused by brain injury. Conventional MRI (T_1w) identifies lesions more accurately than computed tomography (CT) does. DWI can indicate possible DAI, ischemia, and demyelination post-injury. FLAIR, one of the sequences most commonly used by neuroradiologists for clinical purposes, can detect contusions, edema, and subarachnoid and intraventricular hemorrhage [19]. Other researchers have used multi-modal approaches for segmentation and registration [20–22]. Creating study-specific templates and choosing disease-specific sequences tailors this workflow to the study of TBI and improves our ability to study its effects on the brain.

We also examined how tracts differed in their individual contributions to the classification, finding considerable variation in classification accuracy across the tracts. The tracts with the highest balanced accuracy were the CC frontal segment, CC postcentral gyrus, and right ILF. The corpus callosum is one of the most well-documented areas of disruption following a brain injury, so it is not surprising that callosal segments had high BAC [23]. Of our 31 TBI patients, 3 had large space occupying lesions on the left hemisphere 1 had a large lesion on the right hemisphere, 10 had small lesions on either the right or left hemisphere, and the remainder had no visible lesions. These large left hemisphere lesions likely increased the within-group variance, affecting the accuracy classification based on information from left hemisphere tracts.

5   Conclusion

We present step-wise changes to the DWI processing workflow, including use of study-specific templates and incorporating information from multiple modalities when registering images. Each step improved on the previous method in our ability to accurately classify subjects, ending with accuracy around 0.81 for FA, MD, and RD. Additionally, we show that certain tracts aid more in this classification than others, with the CC frontal segment, CC postcentral gyrus segment, and right ILF emerging as providing the most discriminative information. This improved workflow will aid us in further multi-modal investigations of recovery following pediatric TBI.

Acknowledgements.   This study was supported by the NICHDS (R01 HD061504). ELD is supported by a grant from the NINDS (K99 NS096116). ELD, FR, JV, GP, JF and PT are also supported by NIH grants to PT: U54 EB020403, R01 EB008432, R01 AG040060, and R01 NS080655. CCG is supported by the UCLA BIRC, NS027544, NS05489, Child Neurology Foundation, and the Jonathan Drown Foundation. Scanning was supported by the Staglin IMHRO Center for Cognitive Neuroscience. We gratefully acknowledge the contributions of Alma Martinez and Alma Ramirez in assisting with recruitment and study coordination. Finally, the authors thank the participants and their families for contributing their time.

References

1. Parizel, P., Özsarlak, Ö., Van Goethem, J., Van Den Hauwe, L., Dillen, C., Verlooy, J., Cosyns, P., De Schepper, A.: Imaging findings in diffuse axonal injury after closed head trauma. Eur. Radiol. **8**, 960–965 (1998)
2. Ashikaga, R., Araki, Y., Ishida, O.: MRI of head injury using FLAIR. Neuroradiology **39**, 239–242 (1997)
3. Ashwal, S., Holshouser, B.A., Tong, K.A.: Use of advanced neuroimaging techniques in the evaluation of pediatric traumatic brain injury. Dev. Neurosci. **28**, 309–326 (2006)

4. Xu, J., Rasmussen, I.-A., Lagopoulos, J., Håberg, A.: Diffuse axonal injury in severe traumatic brain injury visualized using high-resolution diffusion tensor imaging. J. Neuroatraum **24**, 753–765 (2007)
5. Dennis, E.L., Jin, Y., Villalon-Reina, J., Zhan, L., Kernan, C., Babikian, T., Mink, R., Babbitt, C., Johnson, J., Giza, C.C.: White matter disruption in moderate/severe pediatric traumatic brain injury: advanced tract-based analyses. NeuroImage Clin. **7**, 493–505 (2015)
6. Dennis, E.L., Ellis, M.U., Marion, S.D., Jin, Y., Moran, L., Olsen, A., Kernan, C., Babikian, T., Mink, R., Babbitt, C., Johnson, J., Giza, C.C., Thompson, P.M., Asarnow, R.F.: Callosal function in pediatric traumatic brain injury linked to disrupted white matter integrity. J. Neurosci. **35**, 10202–10211 (2015)
7. Dennis, E.L., Rashid, F., Ellis, M.U., Babikian, T., Villalon-Reina, J.E., Jin, Y., Olsen, A., Mink, R., Babbitt, C., Johnson, J., Giza, C.C., Thompson, P.M., Asarnow, R.F.: Diverging White Matter Trajectories in Children after Traumatic Brain Injury: The RAPBI Study Neurology. In Press, New York (2016)
8. Dennis, E., Jin, Y., Villalon-Reina, J., Kernan, C., Babikian, T., Mink, R., Babbitt, C., Johnson, J., Giza, C., Asarnow, R.F., Thompson, P.: Tract-based analysis of white matter integrity in pediatric TBI: mapping individual abnormalities. In: Organization for Human Brain Mapping. Honolulu, HI (2015)
9. Jin, Y., Shi, Y., Zhan, L., de Zubicaray, G.I., McMahon, K.L., Martin, N.G., Wright, M.J., Thompson, P.M.: Labeling white matter tracts in hardi by fusing multiple tract atlases with applications to genetics. In: Proceedings of 10th IEEE ISBI, pp. 512–515, San Francisco, CA (2013)
10. Jin, Y., Shi, Y., Zhan, L., Gutman, B., de Zubicaray, G.I., McMahon, K.L., Wright, M.J., Toga, A.W., Thompson, P.M.: Automatic clustering of white matter fibers in brain diffusion MRI with an application to genetics. NeuroImage **100**, 75–90 (2014)
11. Jin, Y., Shi, Y., Zhan, L., Li, J., Zubicaray, Greig, I., McMahon, Katie, L., Martin, Nicholas, G., Wright, Margaret, J., Thompson, Paul, M.: Automatic population hardi white matter tract clustering by label fusion of multiple tract atlases. In: Yap, P.-T., Liu, T., Shen, D., Westin, C.-F., Shen, L. (eds.) MBIA 2012. LNCS, vol. 7509, pp. 147–156. Springer, Heidelberg (2012). doi: 10.1007/978-3-642-33530-3_12
12. Zhang, Y., Zhang, J., Oishi, K., Faria, A.V., Jiang, H., Li, X., Akhter, K., Rosa-Neto, P., Pike, G.B., Evans, A., Toga, A.W., Woods, R., Mazziotta, J.C., Miller, M.I., van Zijl, P.C.M., Mori, S.: Atlas-guided tract reconstruction for automated and comprehensive examination of the white matter anatomy. NeuroImage **52**, 1289–1301 (2010)
13. Catani, M., Allin, M.P., Husain, M., Pugliese, L., Mesulam, M.M., Murray, R.M., Jones, D.K.: Symmetries in human brain language pathways correlate with verbal recall. Proc. Natl. Acad. Sci. **104**, 17163–17168 (2007)
14. Avants, B.B., Tustison, N.J., Song, G., Cook, P.A., Klein, A., Gee, J.C.: A reproducible evaluation of ANTs similarity metric performance in brain image registration. NeuroImage **54**, 2033–2044 (2011)
15. Kim, J., Avants, B., Patel, S., Whyte, J., Coslett, B.H., Pluta, J., Detre, J.A., Gee, J.C.: Structural consequences of diffuse traumatic brain injury: a large deformation tensor-based morphometry study. NeuroImage **39**, 1014–1026 (2008)
16. Jin, Y., Shi, Y., Jahanshad, N., Aganj, I., Sapiro, G., Toga, A.W., Thompson, P.M.: 3D elastic registration improves HARDI-derived fiber alignment and automated tract clustering. In: 8th Proceedings of IEEE International Symposium on Biomed Imaging, Chicago, IL, pp. 822–826. IEEE (2011)
17. Cortes, C., Vapnik, V.: Support-vector networks. Mach. Learn. **20**, 273–297 (1995)

18. Kohavi, R.: A study of cross-validation and bootstrap for accuracy estimation and model selection. In: IJCAI, pp. 1137–1145 (1995)
19. Weiss, N., Galanaud, D., Carpentier, A., Naccache, L., Puybasset, L.: Clinical review: prognostic value of magnetic resonance imaging in acute brain injury and coma. Crit. Care **11**, 230 (2007)
20. Irimia, A., Wang, B., Aylward, S.R., Prastawa, M.W., Pace, D.F., Gerig, G., Hovda, D.A., Kikinis, R., Vespa, P.M., Van Horn, J.D.: Neuroimaging of structural pathology and connectomics in traumatic brain injury: toward personalized outcome prediction. Neuroimage Clin. **1**, 1–17 (2012)
21. Wang, B., Prastawa, M., Irimia, A., Chambers, M.C., Sadeghi, N., Vespa, P.M., Van Horn, J.D., Gerig, G.: Analyzing imaging biomarkers for traumatic brain injury using 4D modeling of longitudinal MRI. In: 2013 IEEE 10th International Symposium on Biomedical Imaging, pp. 1392–1395 (2013)
22. Wang, B., Liu, W., Prastawa, M., Irimia, A., Vespa, P.M., van Horn, J.D., Fletcher, P.T. and Gerig, G.: 4D active cut: an interactive tool for pathological anatomy modeling. In: Proceedings/IEEE International Symposium on Biomedical Imaging: From Nano to Macro, pp. 529–532 (2014)
23. Hulkower, M.B., Poliak, D.B., Rosenbaum, S.B., Zimmerman, M.E., Lipton, M.L.: A decade of DTI in traumatic brain injury: 10 years and 100 articles later. AJNR. Am. J. Neuroradiol. **34**(11), 2064–2074 (2013)

An Online Platform for the Automatic Reporting of Multi-parametric Tissue Signatures: A Case Study in Glioblastoma

Javier Juan-Albarracín[✉], Elies Fuster-Garcia, and Juan M. García-Gómez

Instituto de Aplicaciones de las Tecnologías de la Información y de las Comunicaciones Avanzadas (ITACA), Universitat Politècnica de València, Camino de Vera s/n, 46022 Valencia, Spain
jajuaal1@ibime.upv.es
http://mtsimaging.com/

Abstract. Glioblastomas are infiltrative and deeply invasive neoplasms characterized by high vascular proliferation and diffuse margins. As a consequence, this lesion presents a high degree of heterogeneity that requires being studied through a multiparametric combination of several imaging sequences. Nowadays few systems are available to perform a relevant multiparametric analysis of this tumour. In this work, we present the study of GBM by means of http://mtsimaging.com, an online platform for the automatic reporting of multiparametric tissue signatures. The platform implements two full automated GBM pipelines: (1) the anatomical pipeline, which involves MRI preprocessing and tumour segmentation; and (2) the hemodynamic MTS pipeline, which adds the quantification of perfusion parameters and a nosologic segmentation map of the vascular habitats of the GBM. A radiologic report summarizes the findings of both analysis and provides volumetric and perfusion statistics of each tissue and habitat of the tumour.

Keywords: Glioblastoma · Segmentation · Perfusion quantification · Vascular habitats · On-line service

1 Introduction

Cancer heterogeneity has become the focus of research interest in the past few years, as it has been claimed to be the key to understand the response of the tumour against treatment [1]. Specifically, heterogeneity is one of the most important hallmarks that characterizes Glioblastoma (GBM) [2]. GBMs are heterogeneous malignant masses, characterized by hypercellularity, pleomorphism, vascular proliferation and high necrosis mitotic activity, in which different areas of malignancy grade can co-exist. Therefore, the analysis of such complex behaviour requires the combined analysis of multiparametric sequences such as anatomical and quantitative Magnetic Resonance Imaging (MRI) [3]. Due to the

© Springer International Publishing AG 2016
A. Crimi et al. (Eds.): BrainLes 2016, LNCS 10154, pp. 43–51, 2016.
DOI: 10.1007/978-3-319-55524-9_5

high vascular proliferation and angiogenic nature of the GBM, most of radiological protocols have included Perfusion Weighted Imaging (PWI) [4,5] besides the anatomical modalities. PWI parameters such as Cerebral Blood Volume (CBV), Cerebral Blood Flow (CBF), volume transfer coefficient (K^{trans}) and extravascular extracellular space volume fraction (v_e) have demonstrated their potential to characterize the behaviour of these malignant masses.

In the last years, a great effort has been done in the academic context to generate automatic segmentation systems for GBM based on anatomical information [6]. However, to improve the characterization of the tumour it is required studies combining anatomical and quantitative or functional MRI. To contribute to this, we have recently developed a methodology for the anatomical and hemodynamic characterization of the GBM called Hemodynamic Tissue Signature (HTS). Such technology is based on the patent ES-P201431289 [7] for nosologic imaging generation, and aims to provide a method to describe the heterogeneity of the GBM in terms of the anatomical properties and angiogenic process located at each tissue.

To facilitate the clinical use of Multi-parametric Tissue Signatures (MTSs), easy-to-use and practice-adjusted software is required. Currently there are large enterprises offering basic image processing and biomarker quantification products together with their scanning technologies, and small-medium enterprises focused on more sophisticated biomarker quantification services. However, to date, there are very few available applications able to perform a complete analysis of GBM employing both anatomical and quantitative imaging information of the tumour.

In these sense, we present an on-line platform for the automatic reporting of MTS called MTSimaging (http://mtsimaging.com). MTSimaging implements two image analysis pipelines to study the GBM: the conventional anatomical analysis, where MRI images are pre-processed and segmented to obtain a GBM tissue segmentation; and the hemodynamic MTS pipeline, which extends the anatomical pipeline by combining such information with perfusion quantification to provide a new nosologic map where GBM tissues are grouped in different vascular habitats with different angiogenic and hemodynamic behaviour.

2   GBM Analysis Pipelines

Figure 1 summarizes the two services that MTSimaging offers for GBM: the anatomical pipeline and the hemodynamic MTS pipeline. The different modules included in each service and the output generated by each one are detailed in the following sections.

2.1   Anatomical Pipeline

The anatomical pipeline provides the conventional GBM analysis that includes: the MRI pre-processing module and the GBM segmentation module. This pipeline performs a morphological study of the tumour by identifying and

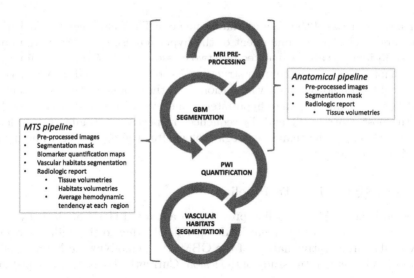

Fig. 1. Services included in http://mtsimaging.com

segmenting the different tissues of the GBM and generating a radiologic report with a summary of the analysis and a volumetric study of each tissue.

The pre-processing module consist of the following steps: (1) Resampling at $1 \times 1 \times 1 \, \text{mm}^3$, (2) Denoising, (3) Bias field correction, (4) Registration and (5) Skull-stripping. Image resampling is performed at $1 \, \text{mm}^3$ through a cubic b-spline interpolation method. Denoising is carried out using the adaptive Non Local Means (NLM) filter [8] with a search window of $7 \times 7 \times 7$ voxels and a patch window of $3 \times 3 \times 3$ voxels. Magnetic field inhomogeneities are removed with the N4 software [9]. Affine registration is conducted with the Advanced Normalization Tools (ANTS) software [10], taking the contrast enhancement T1-weighted sequence as patient's reference. Finally, brain extraction is performed with an in-house pipeline based on a on-linear registration of the T_{1c} sequence to a template with a known intra-cranial mask.

MTSimaging GBM segmentation considers three tissues to be segmented: Enhancing tumour, oedema and necrosis. Segmentation is performed through an automated unsupervised segmentation system based on the methods proposed in [11,12]. The system employs the Directional Class Adaptive Spatially Varying Finite Mixture Model (DCA-SVFMM) algorithm [13], which remains the state of the art of classification algorithms from the unsupervised learning family. Moreover, this algorithm is also enclosed in the family of structured learning methods, as it introduces statistical dependencies between the random variables of the model through a continuous Markov Random Field (MRF) in the form of a prior distribution over the parameters of the model. The system builds over this algorithm and follows a hierarchical strategy for the segmentation that identifies the pathological structures from most general to most specific. First the whole lesion area is detected through a 2-class segmentation (hypo-intense and hyper-intense areas) of the T_2 and Flair sequences. The lesion region $\mathcal{L}$ is defined as the largest connected component of the hyper-intense class. Next, the post-contrast T_1 image is also segmented into two classes and the $\mathcal{L}$ region is employed to search for the enhancing tumour structure. Necrosis is detected through a combination of morphological binary operations over the enhancing tumour structure and through a segmentation of hypo-intense and hyper-intense structures within $\mathcal{L}$ in the post-contrast T_1 and T_2 sequences respectively. Finally, the oedema tissue is defined as the remaining region of $\mathcal{L}$ after the enhancing tumour and necrosis delineations.

2.2   Hemodynamic MTS Pipeline

The hemodynamic MTS pipeline provides an advanced GBM analysis by combining anatomical and functional MRI. Specifically, due to the high angiogenic and vascular proliferative nature of the GBM, the hemodynamic MTS pipeline employs PWI to enrich the study of the lesion. Currently, Dynamic Susceptibility Contrast (DSC) perfusion is supported by MTSimaging. Automated quantification of DSC parameters is conducted and employed to generate a nosologic map of the GBM where tissues are divided in vascular habitats sharing a common hemodynamic behaviour. A more complete automated radiological report is also generated to inform about the findings of the process. Volumetry analysis and quantitative perfusion statistics at each tissue and habitat are reported.

The hemodynamic MTS pipeline includes all the modules of the anatomical pipeline plus the modules referred to perfusion quantification and vascular habitats segmentation. Several pre-processing modules are adapted to handle the DSC sequence: a temporal denoising based on Principal Component Analysis (PCA) is performed to remove the noise of the concentration curves, while bias field correction is computed with a common bias intensity map for all the sequence to not alter the morphology of the curves.

DSC quantification involves the computation of the hemodynamic parameters obtained from the kinetic analysis of the concentration-time curves retrieved from the first pass of a intravenously injected paramagnetic contrast agent [14]. MTSimaging implements the two main models usually employed to quantify the hemodynamic parameters: the mono-compartmental model and the pharmacokinetic (bi-compartmental) model [15]. Our system quantifies both the mono-compartmental maps: Cerebral Blood Volume (CBV), Cerebral Blood Flow (CBF) and Mean Transit Time (MTT); and the pharmacokinetic maps: K^{trans}, v_e and K_{ep} from DSC sequence following the recommendations proposed in [16]. The Arterial Input Function (AIF) is also automatically computed by selecting those curves with highest area under the curve, earliest Time To Peak (TTP), highest peak height and quickly wash-out.

GBM tumour present a high degree of heterogeneity which is manifested into different patterns of hemodynamic behaviour related to the neovascularity of each area. The hemodynamic MTS pipeline intends to capture this heterogeneity by searching for different vascular habitats inside the GBM that present common hemodynamic properties.

Four patterns of hemodynamic activity are considered by MTSimaging to generate the vascular habitats segmentation. Such patterns are mainly focused to describe the following regions inside the GBM: (1) the more angiogenic enhancing tumour region, (2) the less angiogenic enhancing tumour region, (3) the tumour infiltrated oedema area and (4) the vasogenic oedema.

The vascular habitats segmentation allows to visualize the vascular heterogeneity of the GBM and distinguish regions within a tissue with different imaging properties that would otherwise be obscured. Hence, it could be considered as an objective methodology to define ROIs within the GBM based on a multiparametric combination of morphological and functional imaging criteria. We called this analysis *Hemodynamic Tissue Signature*. In addition to the segmentation, a signature graph is generated in the form of a radar chart, where the hemodynamic properties of each habitat are summarized and compared with each other.

3   MTS On-Line Service

MTSimaging evaluation version is hosted at http://mtsimaging.com and is free for non-commercial research purposes. MTSimaging is not available for clinical purpose yet. A simple registration is required to start using the platform. The registration requests a user name, a valid email and the user institution of origin. The email is required to inform the user about the status of their jobs and to provide the links to access to the results. For practical reasons, result files will only be accessible in the system for a week from the end of the job. MTSimaging currently supports NIfTI, compressed NIfTI and DICOM medical imaging formats.

3.1   Platform Architecture

The on-line service architecture is divided in two blocks: the orchestrator and the slaves. The orchestrator controls the user requests and manages the work flows to assign the jobs to the slaves. The slaves group comprises a cluster of 7 Intel Xeon servers, each one with two physical processors and 12 threads per processor, 64 GB of RAM and 1 TB of hard disk drive. In total, 168 threads and up to 448 GB of RAM are available to supply the requirements of the service.

MTSimaging software implementation can be organized into 3 main levels: the web service level, the orchestrator level and the algorithms and computational methods level. The web service layer and user GUI is implemented in Wordpress, PHP and Java. The orchestrator layer, which is the responsible of the data work flows, is implemented in MATLAB and python. Finally, the algorithms for pre-processing, segmentation and image analysis are mainly developed in C++ with ITK and Eigen libraries, and MATLAB scripting. Radiological reports are written in LaTeX.

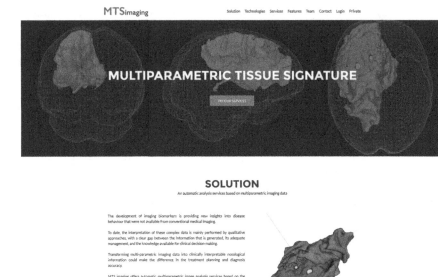

Fig. 2. MTS imaging landing webpage.

3.2 System Output and Results

Anatomical and hemodynamic MTS results can be accessed trough a link provided to the user via email. Such link points to a compressed file with the resulting images and masks. All images are returned in compressed NIfTI format. Additionally, an independent link is also provided to download the radiological report of the corresponding pipeline.

Anatomical pipeline. MTSimaging anatomical pipeline has been tested with 100 cases from the training set of BRATS 2015 dataset, and 20 cases from the BRATS 2013 test set. Consider that MTSimaging segmentation system employs an unsupervised classification approach, thus no training set is employed. Hence, results obtained with the BRATS 2015 training set are as fair as the results obtained with the BRATS 2013 test set.

The median Dice segmentation results for the BRATS 2015 training set were: 0.73 for the enhancing tumour + oedema + necrosis segmentation, 0.82 for the enhancing tumour + necrosis segmentation and 0.83 for the enhancing tumour segmentation. The results obtained for the BRATS 2013 test set were: 0.76 for the enhancing tumour + oedema + necrosis segmentation, 0.85 for the enhancing tumour + necrosis segmentation and 0.81 for the enhancing tumour segmentation.

The anatomical pipeline output includes the pre-processed original images, the brain extraction intra-cranial mask and the GBM tissue segmentation mask. The anatomical report summarizes the information of the segmentation process and extends the study by including a volumetry analysis of the GBM tissues. Volumetry results are provided in absolute units (mL of tissue) and in relative percentage with respect to the complete intra-cranial cavity. The analysis takes approximately 50 mins.

Hemodynamic MTS pipeline. The hemodynamic MTS pipeline includes all the results of the anatomical pipeline and extends it with the quantified biomarker maps, the vascular habitats segmentation and the HTS information. The pipeline has been evaluated on a retrospective dataset comprising cases within 2012 to 2013 from Hospital La Fe from Spain. Cox proportional hazard modelling and linear regressions were conducted to examine the relationship between the perfusion parameters located at each vascular habitat and the patient's overall survival. Strong relationships were found with hazard ratios $\gg 1$ and R^2 between 0.45 and 0.75 with p-values < 0.05 corrected for multiple hypothesis testing with False Discovery Rate at level < 0.05. In contrast, perfusion parameters located at the conventional GBM tissue segmentation did not yield statistically significant results for the study of patient's overall survival. The pipeline outputs the CBV, CBF, MTT, K^{trans}, v_e, K_{ep} and $K2$ maps in addition to the pre-processed original images, the brain extraction intra-cranial mask and the segmentation masks. The analysis takes approximately 1 h.

The report is also upgraded including perfusion statistics at each tissue and habitat of the GBM, and the HTS diagrams that quickly summarizes the vascular properties of each habitat. An example of hemodynamic MTS report is shown in Fig. 3.

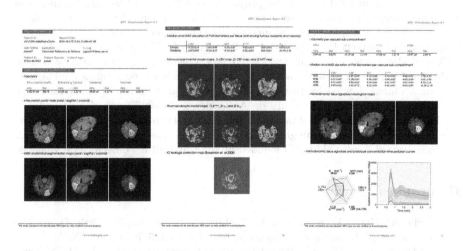

Fig. 3. Example of several pages of the hemodynamic MTS report.

4   Conclusions

The high complexity of the GBM requires the combined analysis of different imaging techniques that allows the complete characterization of the lesion and the improvement in the clinical decision making. To facilitate the use of multiparametric analyses into the clinical routine, it is important to develop easily accessible and completely automated services that can generate clinical knowledge integrable into the daily routine. In this work, we present the evaluation version of a GBM analysis service called MTSimaging (http://mtsimaging.com), that implements an anatomical analysis and an advanced hemodynamic MTS analysis which combines anatomical and perfusion biomarker information. The system generates a radiologic report that summarizes the relevant findings detected in the analysis, and returns the conventional segmentation of the GBM tissues, the vascular habitats map and the pre-processed images without MR artefacts. Currently, we are conducting a multi-center evaluation of the MTSimaging service to consolidate the platform.

Acknowledgments. This work was partially supported by project TIN2013-43457-R: Caracterización de firmas biológicas de glioblastomas mediante modelos no-supervisados de predicción estructurada basados en biomarcadores de imagen, co-funded by the Ministerio de Economía y Competitividad of Spain; by project DPI2016-80054-R: Biomarcadores dinamicos basados en firmas tisulares multiparametricas para el seguimiento y evaluacion de la respuesta a tratamiento de pacientes con glioblastoma y cancer de prostata; by project Spanish EIT Proof of Concept grant (PoC-2016-SPAIN-07) entitled MULTIBIOIM: Multiparametric nosological images for supporting clinical decisions in solid tumors; by project CON2016-C05 UPV-IISLaFe: Inclusión de las tecnologías de firma tisular y modelos mutiescala para el soporte a la planificación de la radioterapia en el tratamiento del glioblastoma, funded by Instituto de Investigación Sanitaria H. Universitario y Politécnico La Fe; by project CON2014002 UPV-IISLaFe: Empleo de segmentación no supervisada multiparamétrica basada en perfusión RM para la caracterización del edema peritumoral de gliomas y metástasis cerebrales únicas, funded by Instituto de Investigación Sanitaria H. Universitario y Politécnico La Fe; and by Instituto de Aplicaciónes de las Tecnologías de la Información y las Comunicaciones Avanzadas (ITACA). E. Fuster-Garcia acknowledges the financial support from the program PAID- 10-14: Ayudas para la Contratación de Doctores para el Acceso al SECTI founded by the Universitat Politécnica de Valéncia.

References

1. Soeda, A., Hara, A., Kunisada, T., Yoshimura, S., Iwama, T., Park, D.M.: The evidence of glioblastoma heterogeneity. Nat. Sci. Rep. **5**(7979), 1–7 (2015)
2. von Deimling, A.: Gliomas. Recent Results in Cancer Research, vol. 171. Springer, Heidelberg (2009)
3. Fuster-Garcia, E., García-Gómez, J.M., De Angelis, E., Sraum, A., Molnar, A., Van Huffel, S., Stamatakos, G.: Use case II: imaging biomarkers and new trends for integrated glioblastoma management. In: Martí-Bonmatí, L., Alberich-Bayarri, A. (eds.) Imaging Biomarkers, pp. 181–194. Springer, Heidelberg (2017)

4. Knopp, E.A., Cha, S., Johnson, G., Mazumdar, A., Golfinos, J.G., Zagzag, D., Miller, D.C., Kelly, P.J., Kricheff, I.I.: Glial neoplasms: dynamic contrast-enhanced T2*-weighted MR imaging. Radiology **211**(3), 791–798 (1999)
5. Shah, M.K., Shin, W., Parikh, V.S., Ragin, A., Mouannes, J., Bernstein, R.A., Walker, M.T., Bhatt, H., Carroll, T.J.: Quantitative cerebral MR perfusion imaging: preliminary results in stroke. J. Magn. Reson. Imaging **32**(4), 796–802 (2010)
6. Menze, B.H., Jakab, A., Bauer, S., Kalpathy-Cramer, J., Farahani, K., Kirby, J., Burren, Y., Porz, N., Slotboom, J., Wiest, R., Lanczi, L.: The multimodal brain tumor image segmentation benchmark (BRATS). IEEE Trans. Med. Imaging **34**(10), 1993–2024 (2015)
7. Juan-Albarracín, J., Fuster-Garcia, E., Robles, M., Manjón-Herrera, J.V., Sáez-Silvestre, C., Esparza-Manzano, M., García-Gómez, J.M.: Patent ESP201431289: Método y sistema de generación de imágenesnosológicas multiparamétricas, 19 October 2015
8. Manjón, J.V., Coupé, P., Martí-Bonmatí, L., Collins, D.L., Robles, M.: Adaptive non-local means denoising of MR images with spatially varying noise levels. J. Magn. Reson. Imaging **31**(1), 192–203 (2010)
9. Tustison, N.J., Avants, B.B., Cook, P.A., Zheng, Y., Egan, A., Yushkevich, P.A., Gee, J.C.: N4ITK: improved N3 bias correction. IEEE Trans. Med. Imaging **29**(6), 1310–1320 (2010)
10. Avants, B.B., Epstein, C.L., Grossman, M., Gee, J.C.: Symmetric diffeomorphic image registration with cross-correlation: evaluating automated labeling of elderly and neurodegenerative brain. Med. Image Anal. **12**(1), 26–41 (2008)
11. Juan-Albarracín, J., Fuster-Garcia, E., Manjón, J.V., Robles, M., Aparici, F., Martí-Bonmatí, L., García-Gómez, J.M.: Automated glioblastoma segmentation based on a multiparametric structured unsupervised classification. PLOS One **10**(5), 1–20 (2015)
12. Juan-Albarracín, J., Fuster-Garcia, E., García-Gómez, J.M.: Glioblastoma tissue-guided segmentation through unsupervisedstructured classification. In: Proceedings of II International Symposium onClinical and Basic Investigation in Glioblastoma, vol. 1, no. 3, p. 101 (2015)
13. Nikou, C., Galatsanos, N.P., Likas, C.L.: A class-adaptive spatially variant mixture model for image segmentation. IEEE Trans. Image Process. **16**(4), 1121–1130 (2007)
14. Boxerman, J.L., Schmainda, K.M., Weisskoff, R.M.: Relative cerebral blood volume maps corrected for contrast agent extravasation significantly correlate with glioma tumor grade, whereas uncorrected maps do not. Am. J. Neuroradiol. **27**(4), 859–867 (2006)
15. Tofts, P.S.: Quantitative MRI of the Brain: Measuring Changes Caused by Disease, vol. 1. Wiley, England (2005). West Sussex PO19 8SQ
16. Quarles, C.C., Gore, J.C., Xu, L., Yankeelov, T.E.: Comparison of dual-echo DSC-MRI- and DCE-MRI-derived contrast agent kinetic parameters. Magn. Reson. Imaging **30**(7), 944–953 (2012)

A Fast Approach to Automatic Detection
of Brain Lesions

Subhranil Koley[1,2], Chandan Chakraborty[2], Caterina Mainero[1,3],
Bruce Fischl[1,3,4], and Iman Aganj[1,3(✉)]

[1] Athinoula A. Martinos Center for Biomedical Imaging, Radiology Department,
Massachusetts General Hospital, Charlestown, MA, USA
subhranil.bmi.smst@gmail.com
[2] School of Medical Science and Technology,
Indian Institute of Technology Kharagpur, Kharagpur 721302, WB, India
drchandanc@gmail.com
[3] Radiology Department, Harvard Medical School, Boston, MA, USA
{caterina,fischl,iman}@nmr.mgh.harvard.edu
[4] Computer Science and Artificial Intelligence Laboratory,
Massachusetts Institute of Technology, Cambridge, MA, USA

Abstract. Template matching is a popular approach to computer-aided detection of brain lesions from magnetic resonance (MR) images. The outcomes are often sufficient for localizing lesions and assisting clinicians in diagnosis. However, processing large MR volumes with three-dimensional (3D) templates is demanding in terms of computational resources, hence the importance of the reduction of computational complexity of template matching, particularly in situations in which time is crucial (e.g. emergent stroke). In view of this, we make use of 3D Gaussian templates with varying radii and propose a new method to compute the normalized cross-correlation coefficient as a similarity metric between the MR volume and the template to detect brain lesions. Contrary to the conventional fast Fourier transform (FFT) based approach, whose runtime grows as $O(N \log N)$ with the number of voxels, the proposed method computes the cross-correlation in $O(N)$. We show through our experiments that the proposed method outperforms the FFT approach in terms of computational time, and retains comparable accuracy.

1 Introduction

A brain lesion is typically a region with abnormal tissue due to brain infection, malformation, injury, or disease. Lesions appear in various types of diseases including brain abscesses, tumors, stroke, and multiple sclerosis (MS). Brain imaging plays a pivotal role in early diagnosis and treatment of such diseases. The identification of the exact location of a lesion helps to determine the lesion characteristics and clinical implications, on the basis of which clinicians make diagnosis and plan treatment. Magnetic resonance imaging (MRI) is widely regarded as one of the most Preferred imaging modalities for visualizing brain lesions, because it is free of ionizing radiation and yields high soft-tissue contrast. In conventional clinical diagnosis, two-dimensional

© Springer International Publishing AG 2016
A. Crimi et al. (Eds.): BrainLes 2016, LNCS 10154, pp. 52–61, 2016.
DOI: 10.1007/978-3-319-55524-9_6

(2D) slices from the MR volume are visually screened, which is a time-consuming task and prone to inter-observer variations. A fully automatic lesion detection tool can make the screening task considerably faster, easier, and potentially more accurate.

Researchers have shown interest in template matching for computer-aided detection of abnormal regions from medical images. In template matching, the image is searched and locally compared with a template image, until the locations in the image that best match the template are found. This process can then be repeated for a set of templates with various lesion sizes, eventually revealing the optimum location and size of the lesion. This technique has been explored in detecting masses from mammogram images [1, 2]. Nodules [3, 4] and metastatic lesions [5] in the lungs have also been detected by template matching algorithms from computed tomography images. In other work, an anatomical template was used to develop an 'adaptive, template moderated, spatially varying statistical classification' framework for segmentation of MS lesions and brain tumors [6]. The normalized cross-correlation coefficient (NCCC), which can be computed in the frequency domain, is a suitable choice for the similarity measure between three-dimensional (3D) templates and the MR volumes [7]. The cross-correlation coefficient has also been employed as a similarity metric in contrast-enhanced MRI to detect small metastatic lesions [8], where the tumor growth pattern was simulated by a 3D spherical-shell template. The different characteristics of lesions, e.g. shape, size, and brightness, were explored to set up rule-based criteria, and a nodule enhancement strategy was introduced to improve the overall performance of the proposed technique. In a different study, NCCC was used to measure the similarity between a black-blood MR pulse sequence and 3D spherical templates, and finally artificial neural network driven pattern classifier was adapted to characterize the metastatic lesions and non-tumor regions [9]. In another study, NCCC was adopted as a similarity measure between MRI images and templates, where various steps such as noise reduction, brain extraction and ROI selection, 3D template building, and matching with the tumor region were followed for detection of brain tumors [10]. A challenging issue in existing template matching techniques is the determination of the optimal template size, especially since the runtime of the algorithm increases proportionally to the number of tried sizes. Designing an efficient mathematical framework for faster computation of NCCC is therefore a critical task in the field of computer-aided lesion detection.

In this work, we focus on reducing the time complexity of the computation of NCCC with a 3D Gaussian template. Inspired by a fast method of computation of the continuous wavelet transform [11], we consider the convolution with the 3D Gaussian template as multiple convolutions with a box kernel per the principle of central limit theorem, which takes linear time, $O(N)$, with respect to the number of voxels (Sect. 2). This is in contrast to the conventional fast Fourier transform (FFT) based method for NCCC computation, with the computational complexity of $O(N \log N)$. We show through our experiments that the proposed method speeds up the computation of NCCC noticeably, while practically keeping the same accuracy as the FFT-based approach (Sect. 3).

2 Proposed Methodology

Let $f\left(\vec{X}\right)$ be the D-dimensional input image, the lesions of which are to be detected. In this work, the D-dimensional Gaussian is proposed as the template, which is approximated, following the central limit theorem, by convolving a D-dimensional symmetric and normalized box kernel, $h_D(\cdot)$, with itself $n-1$ times, denoted as $h_D^{(n)}(\cdot)$ (aka B-splines). In our experiments, a small value of $n=2$ or $n=3$ turned out to be sufficient. The sizes of the box kernel and the engulfing template are $2a$ and $2b$ in all dimensions, respectively; i.e. $h_D\left(\vec{X}\right)$ is $1/(2a)^D$ if $\vec{X} \in \Omega_a$, and 0 otherwise, where $\Omega_l := \left\{\vec{X} \mid |X_1|, \ldots, |X_D| \leq l\right\}$. To ensure that the box kernel fits in the engulfing template after the convolutions, we restrict its size as: $0 < a \leq a_{\max} < b/n$. The similarity between the given image and the symmetric template with a varying a can be computed from the following formula for the NCCC:

$$\mathrm{NCCC}\left(\vec{X}\right) := \frac{\int_{\Omega_b} \left(f\left(\vec{X}+\vec{X'}\right) - \bar{f}\left(\vec{X}\right)\right)\left(h_D^{(n)}\left(\vec{X'}\right) - \overline{h_D^{(n)}}\right)\mathrm{d}\vec{X'}}{\sqrt{\int_{\Omega_b}\left(f\left(\vec{X}+\vec{X'}\right) - \bar{f}\left(\vec{X}\right)\right)^2 \mathrm{d}\vec{X'}}\sqrt{\int_{\Omega_b}\left(h_D^{(n)}\left(\vec{X'}\right) - \overline{h_D^{(n)}}\right)^2 \mathrm{d}\vec{X'}}},$$

(1)

where $\bar{f}\left(\vec{X}\right)$ and $\overline{h_D^{(n)}}$ represent the mean of the image inside the template centered at $\vec{X}$, and the mean of the template, respectively. Our goal is to maximize NCCC with respect to both a and $\vec{X}$, to accurately localize the lesions. Since by definition $\int_{\Omega_b}\left(h_D^{(n)}(\vec{X'}) - \overline{h_D^{(n)}}\right)\mathrm{d}\vec{X'} = 0$, we can omit $\bar{f}\left(\vec{X}\right)$ from the numerator of Eq. (1). We compute $\int_{\Omega_b} f\left(\vec{X}+\vec{X'}\right)h_D^{(n)}\left(\vec{X'}\right)\mathrm{d}\vec{X'} = \int_{\mathbb{R}^D} f\left(\vec{X}+\vec{X'}\right)h_D^{(n)}\left(\vec{X'}\right)\mathrm{d}\vec{X'} = \left(f * h_D^{(n)}\right)\left(\vec{X}\right)$. Thanks to the separability property of the template, i.e. $h_D^{(n)}\left(\vec{X}\right) = \prod_{j=1}^{D} h_1^{(n)}(X_j)$, we can first find the solution to this convolution for $D=1$ and then apply it sequentially for each dimension. For $D=1$, we note that:

$$f * h_1^{(n+1)} = \left(f * h_1^{(n)}\right) * h_1.$$

(2)

We assume (and then verify) the following solution for the convolution:

$$\left(f * h_1^{(n)}\right)(X) = \frac{1}{(2a)^n}\sum_{k=-n}^{n} \gamma_{n,k} F_n(X+ka),$$

(3)

where $F_n(X) = \int_{-\infty}^{X} F_{n-1}(X')dX'$, with $F_0 = f$. Let $\gamma_{n,k} = 0$ for $|k| > n$, and also $\gamma_{0,0} = 1$ for the case with no convolution. Now we substitute Eq. (3) in Eq. (2):

$$
\begin{aligned}
\left(f * h_1^{(n+1)}\right)(X) &= \left(\frac{1}{(2a)^n} \sum_{k=-n}^{n} \gamma_{n,k} F_n(X + ka)\right) * h_1(X) \\
&= \frac{1}{(2a)^n} \sum_{k=-n}^{n} \gamma_{n,k} \int_{-\infty}^{\infty} F_n(X + ka + X') h_1(X') dX' \\
&= \frac{1}{(2a)^{n+1}} \sum_{k=-n}^{n} \gamma_{n,k} \{F_{n+1}(X + a(k+1)) - F_{n+1}(X + a(k-1))\} \\
&= \frac{1}{(2a)^{n+1}} \sum_{k=-n+1}^{n+1} \gamma_{n,k-1} F_{n+1}(X + ak) - \frac{1}{(2a)^{n+1}} \sum_{k=-n-1}^{n-1} \gamma_{n,k+1} F_{n+1}(X + ak) \\
&= \frac{1}{(2a)^{n+1}} \sum_{k=-(n+1)}^{n+1} (\gamma_{n,k-1} - \gamma_{n,k+1}) F_{n+1}(X + ak).
\end{aligned}
\tag{4}
$$

According to Eq. (3):

$$
\left(f * h_1^{(n+1)}\right)(X) = \frac{1}{(2a)^{n+1}} \sum_{k=-(n+1)}^{n+1} \gamma_{n+1,k} F_{n+1}(X + ak).
\tag{5}
$$

This validates our assumption in Eq. (3) by induction, as it is true for the base case $n = 0$, and provided that it is true for n, it holds for $n+1$ with the following recursive relationship for γ, which is obtained by coefficient matching between Eqs. (4) and (5):

$$
\gamma_{n+1,k} = \gamma_{n,k-1} - \gamma_{n,k+1}.
\tag{6}
$$

For example, $\gamma_{1,\{-1,0,1\}} = \{-1, 0, 1\}$ and $\gamma_{2,\{-2,\dots,2\}} = \{1, 0, -2, 0, 1\}$. Being closely related to Pascal's triangle, Eq. (6) is solved as follows:

$$
\gamma_{n,k} =
\begin{cases}
(-1)^{(n+s)} \dbinom{n}{s} & n + k = 2s \\
0 & n + k = 2s + 1
\end{cases}
, \quad s \in \mathbb{Z}.
\tag{7}
$$

We now extend this to D dimensions and solve the first numerator term of Eq. (1):

$$
\int_{\Omega_b} f\left(\vec{X} + \vec{X}'\right) h_D^{(n)}\left(\vec{X}'\right) d\vec{X}' = \frac{1}{(2a)^{nD}} \sum_{k_1,\dots,k_D=-n}^{n} \left(\prod_{j=1}^{D} \gamma_{n,k_j}\right) F_{n,D}\left(\vec{X} + a\vec{k}\right),
\tag{8}
$$

where $F_{n,j}\left(\vec{X}\right) := \int_{-\infty}^{X_j} F_{n-1,j}\left(X_1, \dots, X_j', \dots, X_D\right) dX_j'$, with $F_{0,j} := F_{n,j-1}$ for $j > 1$, and $F_{0,1} := f$. The remainder of the numerator of Eq. (1) can be computed similarly to Eq. (8) (with $n = 1$):

$$-\overline{h_D^{(n)}} \int_{\Omega_b} f\left(\vec{X}+\vec{X'}\right)d\vec{X'} = -\frac{1}{(2b)^D} \sum_{k_1,\ldots,k_D=-1}^{1} \left(\prod_{j=1}^{D}\gamma_{1,k_j}\right) F_{1,D}\left(\vec{X}+b\vec{k}\right). \quad (9)$$

Next, we rewrite the first factor of the denominator of Eq. (1) using the popular expansion of the variance as $\int_{\Omega_b}\left(f(\vec{X}+\vec{X'})-\bar{f}(\vec{X})\right)^2 d\vec{X'} = (2b)^D\left(\overline{f^2}(\vec{X})-\bar{f}(\vec{X})^2\right)$, where both $\overline{f^2}\left(\vec{X}\right)$ and $\bar{f}\left(\vec{X}\right)$ are calculated similarly to Eq. (8) as follows:

$$\bar{f}\left(\vec{X}\right) = \frac{1}{(2b)^D} \sum_{k_1,\ldots,k_D=-1}^{1} \left(\prod_{j=1}^{D}\gamma_{1,k_j}\right) F_{1,D}\left(\vec{X}+b\vec{k}\right),$$

$$\overline{f^2}\left(\vec{X}\right) = \frac{1}{(2b)^D} \sum_{k_1,\ldots,k_D=-1}^{1} \left(\prod_{j=1}^{D}\gamma_{1,k_j}\right) G_{1,D}\left(\vec{X}+b\vec{k}\right), \quad (10)$$

where $G_{n,j}$ is defined similarly to $F_{n,j}$, except that $G_{0,1}=f^2$. Lastly, we calculate the second factor in the denominator of Eq. (1):

$$\int_{\Omega_b}\left(h_D^{(n)}(\vec{X'})-\overline{h_D^{(n)}}\right)^2 d\vec{X'} = (2b)^D\left(\overline{h_D^{(n)^2}}-\overline{h_D^{(n)}}^2\right). \quad (11)$$

The Fourier transform of the box function is $\mathcal{F}\{h_D\} = \prod_{j=1}^{D}\text{sinc}\left(a\omega_j\right)$, which leads to the Fourier transform of the kernel $\mathcal{F}\left\{h_D^{(n)}\right\} = \mathcal{F}\{h_D\}^n = \prod_{j=1}^{D}\text{sinc}^n\left(a\omega_j\right)$ via the convolution theorem. The integral of the template is $\int_{\Omega_b} h_D^{(n)}\left(\vec{X'}\right)d\vec{X'} = \int_{\mathbb{R}^D} h_D^{(n)}\left(\vec{X'}\right)d\vec{X'} = \mathcal{F}\left\{h_D^{(n)}\right\}\Big|_{\vec{\omega}=0} = 1$, from which the template mean is computed as $\overline{h_D^{(n)}} = 1/(2b)^D$. As for the mean of the square of the template, we use Parseval's theorem as follows:

$$\int_{\Omega_b} h_D^{(n)^2}\left(\vec{X'}\right)d\vec{X'} = \int_{\mathbb{R}^D} h_D^{(n)^2}\left(\vec{X'}\right)d\vec{X'} = \frac{1}{(2\pi)^D}\int_{\mathbb{R}^D} \mathcal{F}\left\{h_D^{(n)}\right\}^2\left(\vec{\omega}\right)d\vec{\omega}$$

$$= \prod_{j=1}^{D}\frac{1}{2\pi}\int_{-\infty}^{\infty}\text{sinc}^{2n}\left(a\omega_j\right)d\omega_j = \left(\frac{1}{2\pi a}\int_{-\infty}^{\infty}\text{sinc}^{2n}\omega\,d\omega\right)^D. \quad (12)$$

We now define and compute [12]:

$$\beta_n := \frac{1}{2\pi}\int_{-\infty}^{\infty}\text{sinc}^{2n}\omega\,d\omega = n\sum_{i=0}^{n-1}\frac{(-1)^i(n-i)^{2n-1}}{i!(2n-i)!}. \quad (13)$$

Therefore, $\overline{h_D^{(n)^2}} = \left(\frac{\beta_n}{2ab}\right)^D$, and substituting in Eq. (11) leads to:

$$\int_{\Omega_b} \left(h_D^{(n)}(\vec{X}') - \overline{h_D^{(n)}} \right)^2 d\vec{X}' = \left(\frac{\beta_n}{a} \right)^D - \frac{1}{(2b)^D}. \tag{14}$$

Substituting all of the above in Eq. (1) and simplifying results in the following formula for the proposed fast approach of computing NCCC:

$$\mathrm{NCCC}(\vec{X}) = \frac{\left(\frac{2b}{(2a)^n} \right)^D \sum_{\vec{k}=-n}^{n} \left(\prod_{j=1}^{D} \gamma_{n,k_j} \right) F_{n,D}(\vec{X}+a\vec{k}) - \sum_{\vec{k}=-1}^{1} \left(\prod_{j=1}^{D} \gamma_{1,k_j} \right) F_{1,D}(\vec{X}+b\vec{k})}{\sqrt{(2b)^D \sum_{\vec{k}=-1}^{1} \left(\prod_{j=1}^{D} \gamma_{1,k_j} \right) G_{1,D}(\vec{X}+b\vec{k}) - \left(\sum_{\vec{k}=-1}^{1} \left(\prod_{j=1}^{D} \gamma_{1,k_j} \right) F_{1,D}(\vec{X}+b\vec{k}) \right)^2} \sqrt{\left(\frac{2\beta_n b}{a} \right)^D - 1}}, \tag{15}$$

where $\sum_{\vec{k}=-n}^{n} (\cdot)$ is short for $\sum_{k_1,\dots,k_D=-n}^{n} (\cdot)$. NCCC values range from -1 to 1.

Note that $F_{n,D}$, $F_{1,D}$, and $G_{1,D}$ are independent of a and can be pre-computed, along with the second term in the numerator and the first factor in the denominator of Eq. (15). Furthermore, the second factor in the denominator is a scalar that is computed fast in $O(1)$ for each a. Thus, in the proposed approach to estimate NCCC with the Gaussian template, the bulk of the computational cost is only due to the first term in the numerator of Eq. (15), which can be computed in $O(N)$ for each a, with N the number of voxels in the image. On the contrary, the computational complexity of FFT is $O(N \log N)$ [13], making the overall computational cost of lesion detection noticeably higher for the FFT-based algorithm (template has to be zero-padded to the size of the image) than the proposed approach. This difference in computational cost is particularly amplified given that the NCCC needs to be repeatedly computed for many values of a.

3 Experimental Results

We evaluated the proposed template matching approach by comparing its performance with that of the conventional FFT-based approach. We used both artificial volumes, and real brain T2-weighted Fluid Attenuation Inversion Recovery (FLAIR) MRI volumes containing MS lesions. To avoid boundary artifacts, the images were zero-padded with b elements on the positive side of each dimension. In each experiment, the NCCC was computed for $a = 1,\dots,a_{max}$. Both algorithms were implemented in MATLAB.

3.1 Experiments on Synthetic Data

We first evaluated the performance of the proposed approach on synthetic data. Twenty artificial volumes of the size $513 \times 513 \times 513$ voxels were created, each of which contained an enhancing sphere with random radius (from 8 to 21 pixels) and random location in the volume. We used both our algorithm ($n = 2$, $b = 50$, $a_{max} = 24$) and the FFT-based approach (similar parameters, using the exact Gaussian kernel) to detect the sphere from the volume. We computed the NCCC for 24 values for the radius and found its maximum with respect to the location and the radius. Both methods accurately

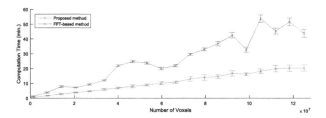

Fig. 1. Runtime analysis of proposed (red) and FFT-based (blue) approaches. (Color figure online)

recovered the locations of all of the spheres i.e. the centers of the detected spheres are identical to the original ones for all 20 volumes. Since the standard deviation of the Gaussian is proportional, but not necessarily equal to the size of the sphere that it detects, we conducted a regression analysis on the liner relationship between the original radius and the detected radius. Their ratio was 1.61 ± 0.05 and 1.74 ± 0.06 for the proposed and the FFT methods, respectively, both values significant (p = 9×10^{-18}).

We performed a different experiment on volumes with varying dimensions to compare the computational costs of the proposed and the FFT-based algorithms for NCCC computation.[1] We made 20 volumes with linearly increasing number of voxels, from 10^6 ($100 \times 100 \times 100$) to 1.25×10^8 ($500 \times 500 \times 500$), with each volume containing a bright sphere of radius 17 pixels at the center. For each volume, each algorithm was run 10 times on a Xeon 5472 3.0 GHz processor ($n = 2$, $b = 50$, $a_{max} = 24$). The mean and the standard deviation of the runtimes are shown in Fig. 1. Our method (red curve) was 2.4 ± 0.4 times faster than the conventional FFT-based method (blue curve), while using $38\% \pm 4\%$ less resident memory. The irregularity in the FFT runtime is partly because it is fastest when each dimension is a power of two (e.g., the valley at 9.9×10^7).

3.2   Lesion Detection Experiments on Real MR Volumes

Next, we tested the two algorithms on a T2-FLAIR 1 mm^3 isotropic-voxel human brain MR volume that contained MS lesions. We used $n = 2$, $b = 7$, and $a_{max} = 3$ due to the small size of the lesions (according to Sect. 3.1, $a = 3$ corresponds to a radius of 5). For each voxel, we computed the maximum value of NCCC across all a. Then, to locate the top 10 most probable lesion areas on this a-maximized volume, we found the voxel with the maximum value, masked a sphere around it (with a radius twice the optimal a), then repeated this process to find the next maxima. The true positive (red circle) and false positive (blue circle) lesions from top 10 detected areas are shown in their respective slices in Fig. 2 for the proposed (two top rows) and the FFT-based (two

---

[1] We ran the experiments on a Linux computing cluster. Although we used MATLAB with the singleCompThread option, it still multithreaded the codes on multiple cores. Therefore, here for each experiment we report the total time spent by the cores (CPU time), as opposed to the real-world time elapsed between the start and end times of the code (wall time).

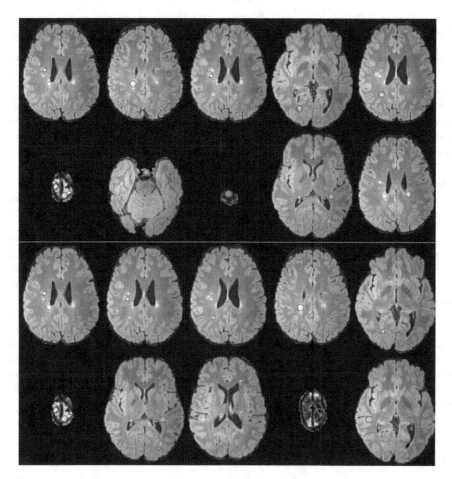

Fig. 2. The top 10 (from left to right) detected lesions by the proposed method (top two rows) and the FFT-based approach (bottom two rows) are each represented in their corresponding slices by a red (true positive) or a blue (false positive) circle. Green circles are intersections with other detected spheres in nearby slices. (Color figure online)

bottom rows) approaches. The green circles are the intersection of the slice with the spheres that represent detected lesions centered in other slices. Essentially, these results show the ability of proposed algorithm in efficient detection of non-rounded lesions, which is utterly useful for the clinicians. Both methods equally identified six true lesions and four false lesions. Among the true positives, five were commonly identified by both algorithms. The results suggest that the accuracies of the two methods are similar for brain lesion detection from MRI. In this experiment, we detected the lesions from the entire brain; however, if desired, one can restrict the detection to the white matter (or any other region of interest) using a mask.

4   Conclusions

In this work, we have presented a fast NCCC-based template-matching framework, with an approximated multi-dimensional Gaussian kernel. The proposed algorithm significantly reduces the computational complexity of automatic detection of brain lesions compared to the FFT-based approach, virtually without compromising the accuracy. As part of the future work, we will extend the proposed framework to use more flexible templates, especially those suitable for the detection of ring enhancing lesions containing non-enhancing region in the center from MRI with contrast agents.

Acknowledgments. Support for this research was provided in part by the National Institute of Diabetes and Digestive and Kidney Diseases (K01DK101631, R21DK108277), the National Institute for Biomedical Imaging and Bioengineering (P41EB015896, R01EB006758, R21EB018907, R01EB019956), the National Institute on Aging (5R01AG008122, R01AG016495), the National Institute for Neurological Disorders and Stroke (R01NS0525851, R21NS072652, R01NS070963, R01NS083534, 5U01NS086625), the National Institutes of Health (NIH) Blueprint for Neuroscience Research (5U01-MH093765; part of the multi-institutional Human Connectome Project), and was made possible by the resources provided by the NIH Shared Instrumentation Grants (S10RR023401, S10RR019307, and S10RR023043). Additionally, SK was supported by a Fulbright-Nehru Doctoral Research Fellowship (Award no: 2098/DR/2015-2016), and CC was supported by the DAE-Young Scientist Research Award Scheme (2013/36/38-BRNS/2350, dt.25-11-2013) by Board of Research in Nuclear Sciences (BRNS), Dept. of Atomic Energy, Govt. of India. BF has a financial interest in CorticoMetrics, a company whose medical pursuits focus on brain imaging and measurement technologies. BF's interests were reviewed and are managed by Massachusetts General Hospital and Partners HealthCare in accordance with their conflict of interest policies.

References

1. Tourassi, G.D., Vargas-Voracek, R., Catarious, D.M., Floyd, C.E.: Computer-assisted detection of mammographic masses: a template matching scheme based on mutual information. Med. Phys. **30**, 2123–2130 (2003)
2. Lochanambal, K.P., Karnan, M., Sivakumar, R.: Identifying masses in mammograms using template matching. In: Proceedings of the Second International Conference on Communication Software and Networks (ICCSN 2010), pp. 339–342 (2010)
3. Osman, O., Ozekes, S., Ucan, O.N.: Lung nodule diagnosis using 3D template matching. Comput. Biol. Med. **37**, 1167–1172 (2007)
4. Moltz, J.H., Schwier, M., Peitgen, H.-O.: A general framework for automatic detection of matching lesions in follow-up CT. In: Proceedings of the IEEE International Symposium on Biomedical Imaging: From Nano to Macro (ISBI 2009), pp. 843–846 (2009)
5. Wang, P., DeNunzio, A., Okunieff, P., O'Dell, W.G.: Lung metastases detection in CT images using 3D template matching. Med. Phys. **34**, 915–922 (2007)
6. Warfield, S.K., Kaus, M., Jolesz, F.A., Kikinis, R.: Adaptive, template moderated, spatially varying statistical classification. Med. Image Anal. **4**, 43–55 (2000)
7. Ambrosini, R.D., Wang, P., O'Dell, W.G.: Computer-aided detection of metastatic brain tumors using automated three-dimensional template matching. J. Magn. Reson. Imaging **31**, 85–93 (2010)

8. Farjam, R., Parmar, H.A., Noll, D.C., Tsien, C.I., Cao, Y.: An approach for computer-aided detection of brain metastases in post-Gd T1-W MRI. Magn. Reson. Imaging **30**, 824–836 (2012)

9. Yang, S., Nam, Y., Kim, M.-O., Kim, E.Y., Park, J., Kim, D.-H.: Computer-aided detection of metastatic brain tumors using magnetic resonance black-blood imaging. Invest. Radiol. **48**, 113–119 (2013)

10. Wang, X.-F., Gong, J., Bu, R.-R., Nie, S.-D.: A 3D adaptive template matching algorithm for brain tumor detection. In: Ma, S., Jia, L., Li, X., Wang, L., Zhou, H., Sun, X. (eds.) LSMS/ICSEE 2014. CCIS, vol. 461, pp. 50–61. Springer, Heidelberg (2014). doi:10.1007/978-3-662-45283-7_6

11. Muñoz, A., Ertlé, R., Unser, M.: Continuous wavelet transform with arbitrary scales and O(N) complexity. Sig. Process. **82**, 749–757 (2002)

12. Kogan, S.: A note on definite integrals involving trigonometric functions (1999). http://mathworld.wolfram.com/SincFunction.html

13. Cooley, J.W., Tukey, J.W.: An algorithm for the machine calculation of complex fourier series. Math. Comput. **19**, 297–301 (1965)

Brain Tumor Image Segmentation

Improving Boundary Classification for Brain Tumor Segmentation and Longitudinal Disease Progression

Ramandeep S. Randhawa[1(✉)], Ankit Modi[2],
Parag Jain[3], and Prashant Warier[2]

[1] University of Southern California, Los Angeles, USA
ramandeep.randhawa@marshall.usc.edu
[2] Fractal Analytics, Mumbai, India
[3] Dhristi Inc., Palo Alto, USA

Abstract. Tracking the progression of brain tumors is a challenging task, due to the slow growth rate and the combination of different tumor components, such as cysts, enhancing patterns, edema and necrosis. In this paper, we propose a Deep Neural Network based architecture that does automatic segmentation of brain tumor, and focuses on improving accuracy at the edges of these different classes. We show that enhancing the loss function to give more weight to the edge pixels significantly improves the neural network's accuracy at classifying the boundaries. In the BRATS 2016 challenge, our submission placed third on the task of predicting progression for the complete tumor region.

Keywords: Deep neural networks · Segmentation · Loss functions · Glioblastoma

1 Introduction

Accurate quantification of gross tumor volumes of brain tumor is an important factor in the assessment of therapy response in patients — it is also important to quantify the volume of the different tumor components, e.g., cysts, enhancing patterns, edema and necrotic regions. In particular, identifying the edges of these tumor components and observing their evolution over time is critical to an accurate assessment of disease progression. Multi-modal MRI is often used to detect, monitor and quantify this progression [1].

Most automatic segmentation models use traditional machine learning approaches — features are manually defined and fed to a classifier, and the algorithms focus on learning the best weights for the classifier. Over the past couple of years, deep learning models have enabled automatic learning of features in addition to the weights used for classification. Several methods using deep neural networks (DNNs) for brain tumor segmentation have already been proposed [2–6]. Our work builds upon the work by Pereira et al. [4] which uses a

© Springer International Publishing AG 2016
A. Crimi et al. (Eds.): BrainLes 2016, LNCS 10154, pp. 65–74, 2016.
DOI: 10.1007/978-3-319-55524-9_7

DNN that comprises a combination of convolutional and fully connected layers, where the convolutional layers have small 3×3 kernels and max-pooling layers.

In addition to standard accuracy measures such as dice scores that determine classification accuracy across the entire segment, we focus our efforts to improve performance at the boundaries between segments. To this end, we propose a pixel-wise weighted cross-entropy loss function, where pixels that are at the boundary of different classes are given more weight and hence the DNN learns to classify them better. We find that incorporating such a weighted function improves the performance of the DNN by 1.4–4.5% measured as an average of out-of-sample dice scores for each of the three regions of interest. It also lowers the standard deviation of the out-of-sample dice scores by 4–18% for each of the three regions. Further, visual inspections of the DNN's predictions also show that our approach leads to much better classification of the tumor at the boundaries between different regions.

2 Dataset

The training dataset of BRATS 2015 [1] comprises brain MRIs for 274 patients — each MRI scan has four modalities: *T1*, *T1c*, *T2*, and *FLAIR*. All images are of dimension $240 \times 240 \times 155$ voxels. All images are already aligned with the *T1c* modality and are skull stripped. Ground truth is provided for each voxel in terms of one of 5 labels: non-tumor, necrosis, edema, non-enhancing tumor and enhancing tumor. Three tumor regions of interest are defined in this problem:

- Complete tumor region that includes all tumor voxels.
- Core tumor region that includes all tumor voxels except *edema*.
- Enhancing tumor region that consists of only the enhancing tumor voxels.

We measure accuracy using the Dice score, which measures the overlap between the ground truth and predictions over each region of interest, and is formally defined as:

$$Dice\ Score = \frac{|P_1 \cap T_1|}{\frac{1}{2}(|P_1| + |T_1|)},$$

where P_1 and T_1 denote the predicted and ground-truth positives, respectively. We compute three dice scores, one for each tumor region: complete, core, and enhancing.

3 DNN Architecture for MRI Segmentation

DNN Architecture. For our submission to the challenge, we used the same DNN proposed by Pereira et al. [4], whose network architecture is illustrated in Fig. 2. This DNN takes a 2-dimensional patch-based approach. That is, each patient's MRI is converted to 155 axial slices, and within each slice, every pixel's class is predicted by taking as input a 33×33 patch around the pixel, and combining this across all four modalities. Thus, the input to the DNN has dimensionality

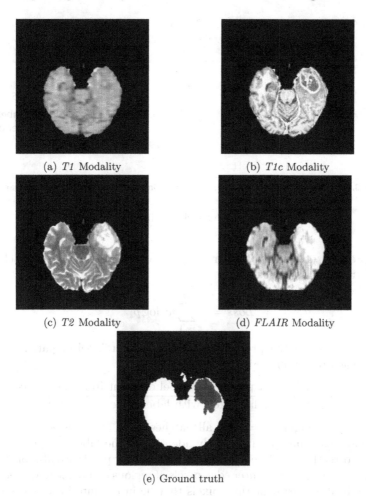

(a) *T1* Modality

(b) *T1c* Modality

(c) *T2* Modality

(d) *FLAIR* Modality

(e) Ground truth

Fig. 1. (a–d) Different modalities of a sample MRI (axial slice) and (e) ground-truth: the tumor region is most clearly identified on the *T1c* modality. The label-color mapping for the ground-truth is: necrosis (blue), edema (green), non-enhancing tumor (red), enhancing tumor (pink). (Color figure online)

$4 \times 33 \times 33$, and the output is the class of the pixel: non-tumor, necrosis, edema, non-enhancing or enhancing tumor. The network uses 8 layers, and has about 28 million parameters.

We also considered two other DNN architectures (U-net [7] and Tri-planar version of the above DNN). However, as we discuss in Sect. 5, the above described DNN (Fig. 2) dominated both these architectures, and so we focused our study on it.

Pixel-Wise Weighted Loss Function. In order to improve accuracy of prediction around the edges, we modify the cross-entropy loss function to weigh pixels based

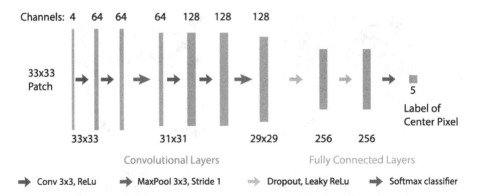

Fig. 2. Network architecture

on their proximity to pixels of other classes. For a mini-batch of M patches, our proposed training loss function is:

$$Loss = -\sum_{i=1}^{M} w_i \log p_i, \qquad (1)$$

where p_i is the predicted probability for the correct label of patch i and the weight for each patch w_i is given by:

$$w_i = \frac{N + \#\ \text{patch-}i\ \text{pixels with label different from center pixel}}{N + \#\ \text{patch-}i\ \text{pixels with label same as center pixel}} \qquad (2)$$

If we set the weight $w_i = 1$ for all patches, then (1) reduces to the regular cross-entropy loss function. Intuitively, identifying the label of the center pixel of a patch correctly would be easier if its neighboring pixels are also of the same label. This implies that the outer edge pixels of regions of a particular label would be more difficult to segment than pixels that lie in the interior of such regions. The weights w_i measure this difficulty by computing a ratio of the number of pixels in the patch with labels different from the center pixel to the number of pixels in the patch with the same label as the center pixel. The weights w_i weight the "more difficult" patches that have more pixels in the patch that are different from the center pixel, higher than patches that are "easier." The constant N is a "smoothing" hyper-parameter that is added to ensure the weights remain bounded in a reasonable range so that the DNN learns consistently from all patches, and is only slightly leaned toward the difficult patches.

We also add L_1- and L_2-regularization to the loss function to prevent over-fitting.

Pre-processing. We perform very limited pre-processing. In particular, we perform $N4$ bias correction on the *T1* and *T1c* modalities. We transform each input channel on a per image basis by first thresholding intensities lower than 1-percentile and greater than 99-percentile and then normalizing all values to have zero mean and unit standard deviation.

Training and Testing. We train the network using a combination of High-Grade Glioblastoma (HGG) and Low-Grade Glioblastoma (LGG) images. We train using 243 MRIs, and reserve the remaining 27 MRIs for out-of-sample testing (approximately 90/10 split). We maintain the same training and testing datasets throughout the experiments.

Our dataset is highly skewed: with most voxels healthy (approximately 92.4%), and only few with tumors. In particular, we had approximately 0.4% necrosis, 5.1% edema, 0.7% non-enhancing tumor and 1.3% enhancing tumor on average. When dealing with such skewed data, a common practice is to perform two-stage training [2]. In this, the first-stage is an equiprobable stage in which the patches are sampled from the training dataset in a manner so that each label (non-tumor, necrosis, edema, enhancing tumor and non-enhancing tumor) is equally-likely to be chosen. The second-stage is a fine-tuning stage, in which the patches are sampled according to the actual distribution with which they occur in the dataset, but the training is used to train only the fully-connected layers of the DNN. That is, the higher convolutional layers are fixed, or frozen, during the fine-tuning stage. Intuitively, the convolutional layers build a latent representation of the patch, and the fully-connected layers use this latent representation to classify the patch. The equiprobable training phase exposes the convolutional layers to patches of all labels to help build better latent representations, and the fine-tuning phase then helps in refining the classification ability of the fully connected layers.

We train the equiprobable phase for 500 epochs, and the fine-tuning phase for 250 epochs. The overall training takes about 9 h, and segmenting an MRI image takes about 6 min. For our submission to the BRATS 2016 challenge, we used an ensemble of three such trained nets.

When comparing the baseline DNN (with regular cross-entropy loss function) with the (pixel-wise) weighted DNN, we use all the same hyper-parameters except N. We also used data-augmentation by flipping the input patches both horizontally and vertically.

Post-processing. As in [4], we remove small regions of voxels with predicted tumor (of any label) below a cumulative voxel size of certain threshold. We found that a threshold of 3,000 voxels worked best.

4   Results

Table 1 compares the dice scores for the three regions as described in Sect. 2 for the test data for the proposed DNN trained with (pixel-wise) weighted loss function ($N = 10,000$) and the baseline DNN, in which the usual cross-entropy loss function is used. We observe that when using the DNN trained with the weighted loss function, the average dice score improves for all three regions: complete, core and enhancing (tumor). The improvement is the highest for the core region. Further, the standard deviation of the dice scores across all images is lower when using the weighted loss function. For the complete and core regions,

Table 1. Test-set dice scores reported as mean (standard deviation). DNN with weighted loss function ($N = 10,000$) has a higher mean dice score, and lower standard deviation compared with the non-weighted baseline DNN.

DNN	Complete	Core	Enhancing
Baseline	0.85 (0.11)	0.72 (0.22)	0.70 (0.26)
Weighted	**0.87** (0.09)	**0.75** (0.19)	**0.71** (0.25)

the performance improvement was statistically significant with $p = .038$ and $p = .030$, respectively; for the enhancing region, we obtained $p = .080$, which suggests that with a larger test set, the performance improvement could potentially be statistically established.

Table 2 displays the same results separated by the glioblastoma grade (HGG and LGG). We observe that using the weighted loss function leads to consistent improvement in the dice score in all cases. The improvement is in fact higher for the LGG images. We also notice that the dice scores are quite low for both methods for the enhanced tumor in LGG images (some LGG images have no enhanced tumor, which leads to a low dice score for the prediction).

Table 2. Dice scores for test images separated by tumor grade (HGG and LGG).

DNN	Complete	Core	Enhancing
HGG			
Baseline	0.86	0.73	0.78
Weighted	**0.87**	**0.76**	**0.79**
LGG			
Baseline	0.83	0.65	0.36
Weighted	**0.86**	**0.68**	**0.37**

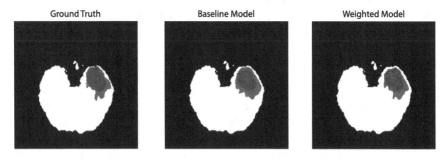

Fig. 3. Groundtruth, prediction without weights and with weights ($N = 10,000$). The images depict 5 classes; the label-color mapping is: necrosis (blue), edema (green), non-enhancing tumor (red), enhancing tumor (pink). (Color figure online)

Figure 3 displays the ground truth, predictions of the baseline and weighted models for the image slice of Fig. 1. Looking at the predictions of the baseline model, we see that there are a large number of misclassifications at the edges of the various regions. The pixel-wise weighted loss function is quite successful at correctly classifying the edge pixels. We do see some misclassifications between the blue (necrosis) and pink (enhancing tumor) regions, which may explain the fact that for the enhancing region, the dice score is only marginally better for the weighted model.

We also compare the specificity and sensitivity of both methods. Tables 3 and 4 displays these results across all images, and separated by grade. We observe that the specificity is marginally higher for the DNN with pixel-wise weighted loss function with the most significant improvement for LGG complete tumor region. For sensitivity, the results are mixed. Across all images, the sensitivity is slightly higher for the DNN with pixel-wise weighted loss function for core and enhancing regions, but slightly lower for complete tumor. When segregating the

Table 3. Specificity scores for test images separated by tumor grade (HGG and LGG).

DNN	Complete	Core	Enhancing
All			
Baseline	0.987 (0.010)	0.997 (0.002)	0.997 (0.002)
Weighted	**0.992** (0.006)	0.997 (0.003)	0.997 (0.002)
HGG			
Baseline	0.988	0.997	0.997
Weighted	**0.991**	0.997	0.997
LGG			
Baseline	0.984	0.996	0.999
Weighted	**0.993**	0.996	0.999

Table 4. Sensitivity scores for test images separated by tumor grade (HGG and LGG).

DNN	Complete	Core	Enhancing
All			
Baseline	**0.86** (0.13)	0.70 (0.24)	0.78 (0.23)
Weighted	0.84 (0.13)	**0.71** (0.22)	**0.80** (0.21)
HGG			
Baseline	0.75	0.71	0.80
Weighted	**0.83**	**0.73**	**0.82**
LGG			
Baseline	**0.89**	**0.71**	**0.73**
Weighted	0.84	0.66	0.69

images by glioblastoma grade, we see that DNN with pixel-wise weighted loss function performs better for all regions for HGG images, but worse for all regions for LGG images. These results suggest that there may be benefits to training separate networks for HGG and LGG images.

5   Discussion

Selecting N. For our results in the previous section, we used $N = 10,000$, which is approximately ten times the number of pixels per patch. With this choice of N, the weights per pixel range from 0.9 to 1.1. It is interesting that such a small change in weights leads to the improved performance in the DNN. We tried various other values for the hyper-parameter N (as reported in Table 5). We also tried $N = 100$, however this performed quite poorly. The table also provides, as a reference, the baseline case which can be considered as setting $N = \infty$.

Table 5. Dice scores for different values of hyper-parameter N.

N	Complete	Core	Enhancing
1,000	0.85 (0.13)	**0.75** (0.19)	**0.72** (0.25)
10,000	**0.87** (0.09)	**0.75** (0.19)	0.71 (0.25)
20,000	0.86 (0.10)	**0.75** (0.18)	0.71 (0.25)
100,000	0.85 (0.11)	0.73 (0.19)	0.70 (0.25)
Baseline	0.85 (0.11)	0.72 (0.22)	0.70 (0.26)

Value of Two-Stage Training. As mentioned earlier, we perform training of the DNN in two stages. To understand the value of the fine-tuning phase, we computed the dice scores for the DNN (weighted) after only completing the equiprobable training phase. In this case, we obtained dice scores of: 0.77 (complete), 0.65 (core) and 0.60 (enhanced). Comparing this with the dice scores in Table 1, we see that there is significant benefit to the fine-tuning phase of training: about 10% for complete region, 15% for core region, and 20% for the enhanced region.

Comparison with Other Architectures. Before embarking on our study we compared three different DNN architectures (with the regular cross-entropy loss function), to pick the best candidate for studying the effect of introducing the pixel-wise weighted loss function. In particular, we considered a tri-planar version of the DNN displayed in Fig. 2, in which for each patch, the sagittal and coronal slices containing the center pixel of interest were also used as input (so the input was 12 channels instead of 4); such an architecture has been referred to as 2.5D [8,9]. We also considered the popular U-net architecture [7]. For this we did not obtain good results for direct segmentation, but instead we trained three different networks, one for each region of interest, in a one-versus-rest fashion. Table 6 displays the results. Our baseline DNN clearly dominates the tri-planar

Table 6. Comparison of different unweighted architectures.

DNN	Complete	Core	Enhancing
Baseline	0.85 (0.11)	**0.72** (0.22)	**0.71** (0.26)
U-net	**0.87** (0.08)	0.63 (0.19)	0.60 (0.28)
Tri-planar	0.77 (0.22)	0.65 (0.27)	0.60 (0.29)

architecture. Turning to the U-net, it performs slightly better than our baseline architecture for the complete tumor region, but performed worse for the core and enhancing regions. Thus, put together with the fact that the U-net was trained in a one-versus-rest fashion for each region, we chose to proceed our study with the baseline architecture. The lower performance of the U-net was surprising, and would make for an interesting future study.

6 Conclusions

In this paper, we propose a pixel-wise weighted loss function that focuses on improving classification accuracy at edges of regions of different labels. This loss function is a modification of the traditional cross-entropy loss function that gives more weight to pixels that are surrounded by a large number of pixels of different labels. Our out-of-sample results show that a small such modification (with weights ranging from 0.9–1.1) improves the performance of the DNN by 1.5–4.5% on average. In the BRATS 2016 challenge, our submission placed third on the task of predicting progression for the complete tumor region.

References

1. Menze, B.H., Jakab, A., Bauer, S., Kalpathy-Cramer, J., Farahani, K., Kirby, J., Burren, Y., Porz, N., Slotboom, J., Wiest, R., et al.: The multimodal brain tumor image segmentation benchmark (BRATS). IEEE Trans. Med. Imaging **34**(10), 1993–2024 (2015)
2. Havaei, M., Davy, A., Warde-Farley, D., Biard, A., Courville, A., Bengio, Y., Pal, C., Jodoin, P.-M., Larochelle, H.: Brain tumor segmentation with deep neural networks. Med. Image Anal. **35**, 18–31 (2016)
3. Havaei, M., Dutil, F., Pal, C., Larochelle, H., Jodoin, P.-M.: A convolutional neural network approach to brain tumor segmentation. In: Crimi, A., Menze, B., Maier, O., Reyes, M., Handels, H. (eds.) BrainLes 2015. LNCS, vol. 9556, pp. 195–208. Springer, Cham (2016). doi:10.1007/978-3-319-30858-6_17
4. Pereira, S., Pinto, A., Alves, V., Silva, C.A.: Deep convolutional neural networks for the segmentation of gliomas in multi-sequence MRI. In: Crimi, A., Menze, B., Maier, O., Reyes, M., Handels, H. (eds.) BrainLes 2015. LNCS, vol. 9556, pp. 131–143. Springer, Cham (2016). doi:10.1007/978-3-319-30858-6_12
5. Urban, G., Bendszus, M., Hamprecht, F., Kleesiek, J.: Multi-modal brain tumor segmentation using deep convolutional neural networks. In: proceedings of the BRATS-MICCAI (2014)

6. Zikic, D., Ioannou, Y., Brown, M., Criminisi, A.: Segmentation of brain tumor tissues with convolutional neural networks. In: Proceedings of the MICCAI-BRATS, pp. 36–39 (2014)
7. Ronneberger, O., Fischer, P., Brox, T.: U-net: convolutional networks for biomedical image segmentation. In: Navab, N., Hornegger, J., Wells, W.M., Frangi, A.F. (eds.) MICCAI 2015. LNCS, vol. 9351, pp. 234–241. Springer, Cham (2015). doi:10.1007/978-3-319-24574-4_28
8. Rao, V., Sarabi, M.S., Jaiswal, A.: Brain tumor segmentation with deep learning. In: MICCAI BraTS (Brain Tumor Segmentation) Challenge, pp. 31–35 (2014)
9. Shin, H.-C., Roth, H.R., Gao, M., Lu, L., Xu, Z., Nogues, I., Yao, J., Mollura, D.J., Summers, R.M.: Deep convolutional neural networks for computer-aided detection: CNN architectures, dataset characteristics and transfer learning. CoRR abs/1602.03409 (2016). http://dblp.uni-trier.de/rec/bib/journals/corr/ShinRGLXNYMS16

Brain Tumor Segmentation
Using a Fully Convolutional Neural Network
with Conditional Random Fields

Xiaomei Zhao[1](✉), Yihong Wu[1](✉), Guidong Song[2], Zhenye Li[3],
Yong Fan[4], and Yazhuo Zhang[2,3,5,6]

[1] National Laboratory of Pattern Recognition, Institute of Automation,
Chinese Academy of Sciences, Beijing, China
zhaoxiaomei14@mails.ucas.ac.cn, yhwu@nlpr.ia.ac.cn
[2] Beijing Neurosurgical Institute, Capital Medical University, Beijing, China
[3] Department of Neurosurgery, Beijing Tiantan Hospital,
Capital Medical University, Beijing, China
[4] Department of Radiology, Perelman School of Medicine,
University of Pennsylvania, Philadelphia, USA
[5] Beijing Institute for Brain Disorders Brain Tumor Center, Beijing, China
[6] China National Clinical Research Center for Neurological Diseases, Beijing, China

Abstract. Deep learning techniques have been widely adopted for learning task-adaptive features in image segmentation applications, such as
brain tumor segmentation. However, most of existing brain tumor segmentation methods based on deep learning are not able to ensure appearance and spatial consistency of segmentation results. In this study we
propose a novel brain tumor segmentation method by integrating a
Fully Convolutional Neural Network (FCNN) and Conditional Random
Fields (CRF), rather than adopting CRF as a post-processing step of
the FCNN. We trained our network in three stages based on image
patches and slices respectively. We evaluated our method on BRATS
2013 dataset, obtaining the second position on its Challenge dataset and
first position on its Leaderboard dataset. Compared with other top ranking methods, our method could achieve competitive performance with
only three imaging modalities (Flair, T1c, T2), rather than four (Flair,
T1, T1c, T2), which could reduce the cost of data acquisition and storage. Besides, our method could segment brain images slice-by-slice, much
faster than the methods patch-by-patch. We also took part in BRATS
2016 and got satisfactory results. As the testing cases in BRATS 2016
are more challenging, we added a manual intervention post-processing
system during our participation.

Keywords: Brain tumor segmentation · Magnetic resonance image ·
Fully Convolutional Neural Network · Conditional Random Fields ·
Recurrent Neural Network

© Springer International Publishing AG 2016
A. Crimi et al. (Eds.): BrainLes 2016, LNCS 10154, pp. 75–87, 2016.
DOI: 10.1007/978-3-319-55524-9_8

1   Introduction

Accurate automatic or semi-automatic brain tumor segmentation is very helpful in clinical, however, it remains a challenging task up to now [1]. Gliomas are the most frequency primary brain tumors in adults [2]. Therefore, the majority of brain tumor segmentation methods focus on gliomas. So do we in this paper. Accurate segmentation of gliomas is very difficult for the following reasons: (1) in MR images, gliomas may have the same appearance with gliosis, stroke and so on [3]; (2) gliomas have a variety of shape, appearance, and size, and may appear in any position in the brain; (3) gliomas invade the surrounding tissue rather than displacing it, causing fuzzy boundaries [3]; (4) there exists intensity inhomogeneity in MR images.

The existing brain tumor segmentation methods can be roughly divided into two groups: generative models and discriminative models. Generative models usually acquire prior information through probabilistic atlas image registration [4,5]. However, the image registration is unreliable when the brain is deformed due to large tumors. Discriminative models typically segment brain tumors by classifying voxels based on image features [6,7]. Their segmentation performance is hinged on the image features and classification models. Since deep learning techniques are capable of learning high level and task-adaptive features from training data, they have been adopted in brain tumor segmentation studies [8–14]. However, most of the existing brain tumor segmentation methods based on deep learning do not yield segmentation results with appearance and spatial consistency [15]. To overcome such a limitation, we propose a novel deep network by integrating a fully convolutional neural network (FCNN) and a CRF to segment brain tumors. Our model is trained in three steps and is able to segment brain images slice-by-slice, which is much faster than the segmentation method patch-by-patch [14]. Moreover, our method requires only three MR imaging modalities (Flair, T1c, T2), rather than four modalities (Flair, T1, T1c, T2) [1,6–14], which could help reduce the cost of data acquisition and storage.

2   The Proposed Method

The proposed brain tumor segmentation method consists of three main steps: pre-processing, segmentation using the proposed deep network model, and post-processing. In the following, we will introduce each step in detail respectively.

2.1   Pre-processing

As magnetic resonance imaging devices are not perfect and each imaging object is specific, the intensity ranges and bias fields of different MR images are different. Therefore, the absolute intensity values in different MR images or even in the same MR image do not have fixed tissue meanings. It is necessary to pre-process MR images in an appropriate way.

In this paper, we firstly use N4ITK [16] to correct the bias field of each MR image. Then, we normalize the intensity by subtracting the gray-value of the highest frequency and dividing the revised deviation. We denote the revised deviation by $\tilde{\sigma}$ and the MR image ready to be normalized by V, which is composed by a set of voxels $\{v_1, v_2, v_3, \ldots, v_N\}$. The intensity value of each voxel v_k is denoted as I_k. Then, the revised deviation $\tilde{\sigma}$ can be calculated by $\tilde{\sigma} = \sqrt{\sum_{k=1}^{N}(I_k - \hat{I})^2/N}$, where $\hat{I}$ denotes the gray-value of the highest frequency. Besides, in order to process the MR images as common images, we also change their intensity range to 0–255 linearly.

We take T2 for an example to show the effect of our normalization method. Figure 1 shows 30 T2 MR images' intensity histograms before and after normalization. The 30 T2 MR images come from BRATS 2013 training dataset. It can be seen from Fig. 1 that our normalization method can try to make different MR images have similar intensity distributions, while guarantee their histogram shapes unchanged. In most cases, the gray value of the highest frequency is close to the intensity of white matter. Therefore, transforming the gray value of the highest frequency to the same level is equivalent to transforming the intensity of white matter to the same level. Then, after normalizing the revised deviation, the similar intensities in different MR images can roughly have the similar tissue meaning.

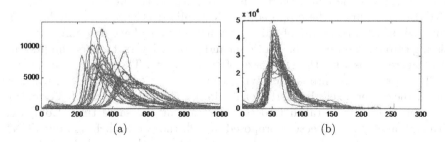

Fig. 1. Comparison of 30 T2 intensity histograms before and after intensity normalization. (a). Before normalization (after N4ITK); (b). After normalization

2.2   Brain Tumor Segmentation Model

Our brain tumor segmentation model consists of two parts, a Fully Convolutional Neural Network (FCNN) and Conditional Random Field (CRF), as shown in Fig. 2. The proposed model was trained by three steps, using image patches and slices respectively. In the testing phase, it can segment brain images slice by slice. Next, we will introduce each part of the proposed segmentation model in detail.

FCNN. FCNN contains the majority of parameters in our whole segmentation model. It was trained based on image patches, which were extracted from slices

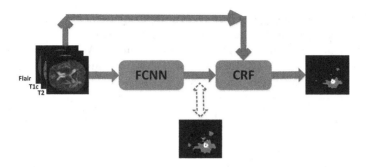

Fig. 2. The structure of our brain tumor segmentation model

of the axial view. Training FCNN by patches can avoid the problem of lacking training samples, as thousands of patches can be extracted from one image. It can also help to avoid the training sample imbalance problem, because the number and position of training samples for each class can be easily controlled by using different patch sampling schemes. In our experiment, we sampled training patches randomly from each training subject and kept the number of training samples for each class equal (5 classes in total, including normal tissue, necrosis, edema, non-enhancing core, and enhancing core). As we didn't reject patches sampled in the same place, there existed duplicated training samples. Figure 3 shows the structure of the proposed FCNN. Similar to the cascaded architecture proposed in [12], the inputs of our FCNN network also have two different sizes. Passing through a series of convolutional and pooling layers, the large inputs turn into feature maps with the same size of small inputs. These feature maps and small inputs are sent into the following network together. In this way, when we predict the center pixel's label, the local information and the context information in larger scale can be taken into consideration at the same time. Compared with the cascaded architecture proposed in [12], the two branches in our FCNN was trained simultaneously, while the two branches in the cascaded architecture in [12] was trained in different steps. Besides, our FCNN network has more convolutional layers.

FCNN is a fully convolutional neural network and the stride of each layer is set to 1. Therefore, even though it was trained by patches, it can segment brain images slice by slice.

CRF. Let's briefly review conditional random field first. Consider an image I composed by a set of pixels $\{I_1, I_2, \ldots, I_M\}$, where M denotes the number of pixels in this image. Each pixel I_i has a label x_i, $x_i \in L = \{l_1, l_2, \ldots, l_k\}$. L is a set of labels, showing the range of value for x_i. The energy function of CRF is written as:

$$E(x) = \sum_i \Phi(x_i) + \sum_{i,j \in N_i} \Psi(x_i, x_j), i \in \{1, 2, 3, \ldots, M\}, j \in N_i \qquad (1)$$

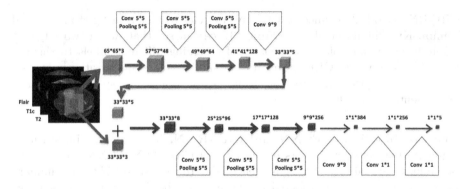

Fig. 3. The structure of our FCNN network

$\Phi(x_i)$ is the unary term, representing the cost of assigning label x_i to the pixel I_i. $\Psi(x_i, x_j)$ is the pairwise term, representing the cost of assigning label x_i and x_j to I_i and I_j respectively. N_i represents the neighborhood of pixel I_i. Using CRF to segment an image is to find a set of x_i to make the energy function have minimum value. In order to improve segmentation accuracy and get a global optimized result, fully connected CRF can be used, which is computing pairwise potentials on all pairs of pixels in the image [17]. The energy function of fully connected CRF is as follows:

$$E(x) = \sum_i \Phi(x_i) + \sum_{i<j} \Psi(x_i, x_j), i, j \in \{1, 2, 3, \dots, M\} \tag{2}$$

Mean field approximation can be used to solve the optimize problem of minimizing the energy function (2) [17]. Shuai Zheng et al. [15] proposed a neural network formulated fully connected CRF, called CRF-RNN. CRF-RNN performs a mean field iteration by a stack of CNN layers, then the whole iteration steps in the mean field approximation can be formulated as Recurrent Neural Network, making it possible to integrate a CNN and CRF network as one deep network and train it with the usual back-propagation algorithm. CRF-RNN can be implemented on a GPU and has very high computational efficiency. Our CRF model refers to CRF-RNN [15], where the negative of the unary term $-\Phi(x_i)$ is directly provided by the previous segmentation network and the pairwise term $\Psi(x_i, x_j)$ is calculated by the following function:

$$\Psi(x_i, x_j) = \mu(x_i, x_j)[\omega^{(1)} exp(-\frac{|p_i - p_j|^2}{2\theta_\alpha^2} - \frac{|c_i - c_j|^2}{2\theta_\beta^2}) + \omega^{(2)} exp(-\frac{|p_i - p_j|^2}{2\theta_\gamma^2})] \tag{3}$$

In (3), μ is a label compatibility function, representing the penalty for different pixels that are assigned different labels; c_i and c_j denote the color vectors of pixels I_i and I_j; p_i and p_j denote the positions of pixels I_i and I_j; $\omega^{(k)}, k = 1, 2$ is the weight of each Gaussian kernel; θ_α, θ_β, and θ_γ are parameters that control the effect of different features (position and color). For further details about

CRF-RNN and fully connected CRF, please refer to Shuai Zheng et al. [15] and Philipp Krähenbühl et al. [17]. From (3) we can see that, when two adjacent pixels have similar color, the penalty of assigning different labels to them is large. Therefore after CRF, pixels having similar colors and positions are very likely to be assigned same label, ensuring the appearance and spatial consistency of segmentation results.

The Combination of FCNN and CRF-RNN. The proposed brain tumor segmentation network consists of FCNN and CRF-RNN. FCNN provides the preliminary probability of assigning each label to each voxel. These preliminary prediction results are considered as the negative of the unary term of CRF-RNN. CRF-RNN can globally optimize the segmentation results according to each voxel's intensity and position information shown in the pre-processed MR images. Then, the segmentation results' appearance and spatial consistency can be ensured.

In the training phase, we trained the proposed integrated network of FCNN and CRF-RNN in three steps. Firstly we used image patches to train FCNN. Then, we used image slices of the axial view to train the following CRF-RNN with parameters of the FCNN fixed. Finally, we used the image slices to fine-tune the whole network. In the testing phase, we segment brain images slice by slice. All the slices are extracted from the axial view.

2.3 Post-processing

We post-process the segmentation results by removing small 3D-connected regions and correcting some pixels' labels by a simple thresholding method. We validated the values of these thresholds by a small subset of training dataset.

3 Experiment

BRATS is a brain tumor image segmentation challenge. It is organized in conjunction with the International Conference on Medical Image Computing and Computer Assisted Intervention (MICCAI). Most of the start of art brain tumor segmentation methods have been evaluated on this benchmark. Since BRATS 2014 dataset is not available and the ranking results of BRATS 2015 testing dataset are not shown on BRATS website, we mainly evaluated our segmentation method on BRATS 2013 dataset. Also, we took part in BRATS 2016 and got satisfactory results. In BRATS 2013, the training dataset contains 20 HGG and 10 LGG. The testing dataset contains two parts. One is Challenge, containing 10 HGG. The other one is Leaderboard, containing 21 HGG and 4 LGG. In BRATS 2016, the training dataset contains 220 HGG and 54 LGG. The testing dataset contains 191 cases, including both grades. Our experiments were performed on our laboratory's server. The GPU of the server is Tesla K80, and the CPU is Intel E5-2620. As the server is public for everyone in our laboratory, we shared one GPU with other colleagues most time. We used Caffe [18] to implement our neural network.

BRATS provides four MR imaging modalities for each subject, including Flair, T1, T1c, and T2. However, we just used three of them (Flair, T1c, T2), and still achieved competitive performance. We also trained a segmentation model using all the four modalities and tested its segmentation performance. However, there is no obvious performance difference between the segmentation model trained by four modalities (Flair, T1, T1c, T2) and the segmentation model trained by three modalities (Flair, T1c, T2). We speculate that most of effective information shown in T1 is contained in T1c.

3.1 Evaluation on BRATS 2013 Dataset

On BRATS 2013 evaluation website, three metrics of Dice, Positive Predictive Value (PPV), and Sensitivity are used to evaluate a method. Each of the metrics is calculated on three kinds of tumor regions. They are complete, core, and enhancing. The complete tumor region includes necrosis, edema, non-enhancing core, and enhancing core. The core region includes necrosis, non-enhancing core, and enhancing core. The enhancing region only includes the enhancing core. Equations for calculating the three metrics are as follows:

$$Dice(P_*, T_*) = \frac{|P_* \cap T_*|}{(|P_*| + |T_*|)/2} \tag{4}$$

$$PPV(P_*, T_*) = \frac{|P_* \cap T_*|}{|P_*|} \tag{5}$$

$$Sensitivity(P_*, T_*) = \frac{|P_* \cap T_*|}{|T_*|} \tag{6}$$

where $*$ indicates complete, core, or enhancing region. T_* denotes the true region of $*$. P_* denotes the segmented $*$ region. $|P_* \cap T_*|$ denotes the overlap area between P_* and T_*. $|P_*|$ and $|T_*|$ denote the areas of P_* and T_* respectively. BRATS doesn't provide the ground truth for testing subjects. Therefore, all the metrics of testing dataset can only be calculated by BRATS evaluation website[1].

Table 1 shows the Dice scores of FCNN, FCNN+CRF and FCNN+CRF+ post-processing on BRATS 2013 Challenge dataset and Leaderboard dataset. It can be seen from Table 1 that CRF can obviously improve the segmentation accuracy, and post-processing can improve the segmentation accuracy further. FCNN+CRF+post-processing performs best on all three regions of both dataset.

Figure 4 shows some segmentation results on BRATS 2013 Challenge dataset. Figures in each row, from top to bottom, represent: Flair, T1c, T2, segmentation results of FCNN, segmentation results of FCNN+CRF, and segmentation results of FCNN+CRF+post-processing. Compared with segmentation results in Row 4 (FCNN), segmentation results in Row 5 (FCNN+CRF) are smoother and have

---

[1] https://www.virtualskeleton.ch/BRATS/Start2013.

Table 1. The Dice scores of FCNN, FCNN+CRF, and FCNN+CRF+post-processing on BRATS 2013 Challenge and Leaderboard dataset

Methods	Dice					
	Challenge			Leaderboard		
	Comp.	Core	Enh.	Comp.	Core	Enh.
FCNN	0.74	0.72	0.67	0.70	0.61	0.54
FCNN+CRF	0.85	0.80	0.70	0.83	0.66	0.57
FCNN+CRF+post-processing	**0.87**	**0.83**	**0.76**	**0.86**	**0.73**	**0.62**

more accurate boundaries, representing the effectiveness of CRF. Compared the segmentation results in Row 5 (FCNN+CRF) and Row 6 (FCNN+CRF+post-processing), we can see that, after post-processing, the number of false positives reduces further.

Comparison results with other methods are summarized in Tables 2 and 3. Nick Tustison, Raphael Meier, Syed Reza, and Liang Zhao methods' evaluation results are acquired from BRATS 2013 website[2]. Nick Tustison, Raphael Meier, Syed Reza methods obtained the top 3 positions respectively on Challenge dataset in 2013. Nick Tustison, Liang Zhao, Raphael Meier methods obtained the top 3 positions respectively on Leaderboard dataset in 2013. Sérgio Pereira method [14] ranks first on Challenge dataset and second on Leaderboard dataset right now, while our method ranks second on Challenge dataset and first on Leaderboard dataset right now. In general, the proposed method takes 2–4 min to segment one subject's imaging data, much faster than Sérgio Pereira method (average running time of 8 min). From Tables 2 and 3, we can see that our segmentation method is still competitive with Sérgio Pereira method and much better than the other methods shown in these two tables.

Table 2. Comparison with other methods on BRATS 2013 Challenge dataset

Methods	Dice			PPV			Sensitivity		
	Comp.	Core	Enh.	Comp.	Core	Enh.	Comp.	Core	Enh.
Nick Tustison et al.	0.87	0.78	0.74	0.85	0.74	0.69	0.89	**0.88**	**0.83**
Raphael Meier et al.	0.82	0.73	0.69	0.76	0.78	0.71	**0.92**	0.72	0.73
Syed Reza et al.	0.83	0.72	0.72	0.82	0.81	0.70	0.86	0.69	0.76
Mohammad Havaei et al. [12]	**0.88**	0.79	0.73	0.89	0.79	0.68	0.87	0.79	0.80
Sérgio Pereira et al. [14]	**0.88**	**0.83**	**0.77**	0.88	**0.87**	0.74	0.89	0.83	0.81
Our method	0.87	**0.83**	0.76	**0.92**	**0.87**	**0.77**	0.83	0.81	0.77

---

[2] http://martinos.org/qtim/miccai2013/results.html.

Table 3. Comparison with other methods on BRATS 2013 Leaderboard dataset

Methods	Dice			PPV			Sensitivity		
	Comp.	Core	Enh.	Comp.	Core	Enh.	Comp.	Core	Enh.
Nick Tustison et al.	0.79	0.65	0.53	0.83	0.70	0.51	0.81	0.73	0.66
Liang Zhao et al.	0.79	0.59	0.47	0.77	0.55	0.50	0.85	0.77	0.53
Raphael Meier et al.	0.72	0.60	0.53	0.65	0.62	0.48	**0.88**	0.69	0.64
Mohammad Havaei et al. [12]	0.84	0.71	0.57	0.88	0.79	0.54	0.84	0.72	**0.68**
Sérgio Pereira et al. [14]	0.84	0.72	**0.62**	0.85	**0.82**	0.60	0.86	0.76	**0.68**
Our method	**0.86**	**0.73**	**0.62**	**0.89**	0.76	**0.64**	0.84	**0.78**	**0.68**

3.2 Participation on BRATS 2016 Challenge

The testing cases in BRATS 2016 are much more challenging. Therefore, we added a manual intervention post-processing system during our participation in BRATS 2016. The manual intervention post-processing system is designed to remove some segmented tumor regions which are obvious false positives. There are two kinds of regions to remove:

① Manually determined rectangular regions.

② Regions which intensities in Flair, T1c, T2 are below three specific thresholds respectively at the same time. The threshold of Flair equals to 0.8×the mean intensity of the segmented tumor region in Flair. The threshold of T1c is a constant. The threshold of T2 equals to 0.9×the mean intensity of the segmented tumor region in T2.

In the manual intervention post-processing system, users just need to decide whether to remove those regions described in ① ② and determine the rectangular regions' sizes and locations described in ①. The manual intervention post-processing system only takes a few minutes on each subject. The regions to remove are 3D. We show an example in Fig. 5 in 2D.

There are 191 cases in BRATS 2016 testing dataset with unknown grades. During our participation on BRATS 2016, we firstly segmented the 191 cases by our proposed integrated network of FCNN and CRF-RNN on our laboratory's sever. We just used one Tesla K80 GPU and one E5-2620 CPU on the sever. It took 2–4 min to segment one case. All 191 cases were segmented in about 11.5 h. We then used the manual intervention post-processing system to post-process segmentation results with one personal computer, in which there is one Q9550 CPU and no GPU. Not every case needed to be manually post-processed. On average, the manual intervention post-processing system only took a few minutes on each case. We successfully segmented the 191 cases in BRATS 2016 testing dataset in 48 h.

There are 19 groups that took part in BRATS 2016. Our method ranked first on the multi-temporal evaluation and ranked in the top 5 on most of items in tumor segmentation. The ranking details of our method are shown in Table 4. The formulation used to calculate Dice is (3), as shown in Sect. 3.1. And the

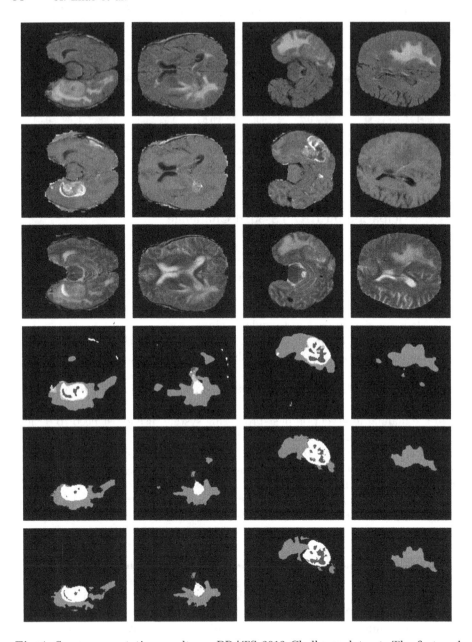

Fig. 4. Some segmentation results on BRATS 2013 Challenge dataset. The first and second columns show the segmentation results of the 50th and 80th slice of the axial view of Subject 0301. The third and fourth columns show the segmentation results of the 40th and 70th slice of the axial view of Subject 0308. Figures in each row, from top to bottom, represent: Flair, T1c, T2, segmentation results of FCNN, segmentation results of FCNN+CRF, and segmentation results of FCNN+CRF+post-processing. Each gray level in segmentation results represents a tumor class, from low to high: necrosis, edema, non-enhancing core, and enhancing core.

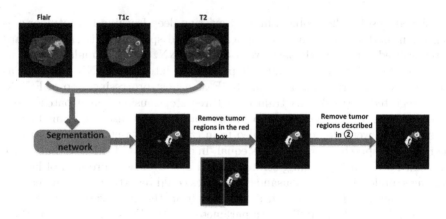

Fig. 5. A manual intervention post-processing example

Table 4. The ranking details of our method on different items on BRATS 2016 (including tie)

Items	Tumor segmentation						Multi-temporal evaluation
	Dice			Hausdorff			
	Comp.	Core	Enh.	Comp.	Core	Enh.	
Ranking	4	3	1	7	6	2	1

formulation used to calculate Hausdorff distance is as follow:

$$Haus(P_*, T_*) = max\{ \sup_{p \in \partial P_*} \inf_{t \in \partial T_*} d(p,t), \sup_{t \in \partial T_*} \inf_{p \in \partial P_*} d(t,p)\} \qquad (7)$$

The meanings of P_* and T_* have been shown in Sect. 3.1. ∂P_* denotes the surface of P_*, and ∂T_* denotes the surface of T_*. p and t denote points on ∂P_* and ∂T_* respectively. $d(p,t)$ calculates the least-square distance between points p and t. inf denotes the operation of returning the minimum value. sup and max denote the operation of returning the maximum value. Multi-temporal evaluation is designed to evaluate whether the volumetric segmentations provided by the participants are accurate enough to detect the changes indicated by the neuroradiologists[3].

4   Conclusion

Accurate automatic or semi-automatic brain tumor segmentation methods have broad application prospect. In this paper, we propose a novel brain tumor segmentation method by using an integrated model of Fully Convolutional Neural Network (FCNN) and Conditional Random Fields (CRF). This integrated model

---

[3] http://braintumorsegmentation.org/.

is designed to solve the problem in most existing deep learning brain tumor segmentation methods, by which the appearance and spatial consistency are hard to be ensured. In the CRF part, we use CRF-RNN, which formulates CRF as Recurrent Neural Network, making it possible to integrate FCNN and CRF as one deep network, rather than using CRF as a post-processing step of FCNN. Our integrated network was trained in three steps, using image patches and slices respectively. In the first step, image patches were used to train FCNN. These patches were randomly sampled from training dataset, but we controlled the number of patches for each class equal, in order to avoid the data imbalance problem. Patch-based training strategy could also avoid the problem of lacking training samples, because thousands of patches could be extracted from one subject's MR images. In the second step, slices from the axial view were used to train the following CRF-RNN, with parameters of the FCNN fixed. In the third step, slices from the axial view were used to fine-tune the whole network.

We applied a simple pre-processing strategy and a simple post-processing strategy. We pre-processed each MR image by N4ITK and intensity normalization, which normalized each MR image's intensity mainly by subtracting the gray-value of the highest frequency and dividing the revised deviation. We post-processed the segmentation results by removing small 3D-connected regions and correcting some pixels' labels by a simple thresholding method. The experimental results show that these strategies are effective.

We evaluated our method on BRATS 2013 dataset, obtaining the second position on its Challenge dataset and the first position on its Leaderboard dataset. Compared with other top ranking methods, our method could achieve competitive performance with only 3 imaging modalities (Flair, T1c, T2), rather than 4 (Flair, T1, T1c, T2). We also took part in BRATS 2016 and our method ranked first on the multi-temporal evaluation and ranked in the top 5 on most of items in tumor segmentation.

Acknowledgements. This work was supported by the National High Technology Research and Development Program of China (2015AA020504) and the National Natural Science Foundation of China under Grant No. 61572499, 61421004.

References

1. Menze, B.H., Jakab, A., Bauer, S., Kalpathy-Cramer, J., Farahani, K., Kirby, J., Burren, Y., Porz, N., Slotboom, J., Wiest, R., et al.: The multimodal brain tumor image segmentation benchmark (BRATS). IEEE Trans. Med. Imaging **34**, 1993–2024 (2015)
2. Bauer, S., Wiest, R., Nolte, L.-P., Reyes, M.: A survey of MRI-based medical image analysis for brain tumor studies. Phys. Med. Biol. **58**, 97–129 (2013)
3. Goetz, M., Weber, C., Binczyk, F., Polanska, J., Tarnawski, R., Bobek-Billewicz, B., Koethe, U., Kleesiek, J., Stieltjes, B., Maier-Hein, K.H.: DALSA: domain adaptation for supervised learning from sparsely annotated MR images. IEEE Trans. Med. Imaging **35**, 184–196 (2016)
4. Prastawa, M., Bullitt, E., Ho, S., Gerig, G.: A brain tumor segmentation framework based on outlier detection. Med. Image Anal. **8**, 275–283 (2004)

5. Cobzas, D., Birkbeck, N., Schmidt, M., Jagersand, M., Murtha, A.: 3D variational brain tumor segmentation using a high dimensional feature set. In: IEEE 11th International Conference on Computer Vision, pp. 1–8 (2007)
6. Goetz, M., Weber, C., Bloecher, J., Stieltjes, B., Meinzer, H.-P., Maier-Hein, K.: Extremely randomized trees based brain tumor segmentation. In: Proceedings MICCAI BraTS (Brain Tumor Segmentation Challenge), pp. 6–11 (2014)
7. Kleesiek, J., Biller, A., Urban, G., Kothe, U., Bendszus, M., Hamprecht, F.: Ilastik for multi-modal brain tumor segmentation. In: Proceedings MICCAI BraTS (Brain Tumor Segmentation Challenge), pp. 12–17 (2014)
8. Davy, A., Havaei, M., Warde-farley, D., Biard, A., Tran, L., Jodoin, P.-M., Courville, A., Larochelle, H., Pal, C., Bengio, Y.: Brain tumor segmentation with deep neural networks. In: Proceedings MICCAI BraTS (Brain Tumor Segmentation Challenge), pp. 1–5 (2014)
9. Urban, G., Bendszus, M., Hamprecht, F., Kleesiek, J.: Multi-modal brain tumor segmentatioin using deep convolutional neural networks. In: Proceedings MICCAI BraTS (Brain Tumor Segmentation Challenge), pp. 31–35 (2014)
10. Zikic, D., Ioannou, Y., Brown, M., Criminisi, A.: Segmentation of brain tumor tissues with convolutional neural networks. In: Proceedings MICCAI BraTS (Brain Tumor Segmentation Challenge), pp. 36–39 (2014)
11. Dvorak, P., Menze, B.H.: Structured prediction with convolutional neural networks for multimodal brain tumor segmentation. In: Proceedings MICCAI BraTS (Brain Tumor Segmentation Challenge), pp. 13–24 (2015)
12. Havaei, M., Davy, A., Warde-Farley, D., Biard, A., Courville, A., Bengio, Y., Pal, C., Jodoin, P.-M., Larochelle, H.: Brain tumor segmentation with deep neural networks. Med. Image Anal. **35**, 18–31 (2017)
13. Vaidhya, K., Thirunavukkarasu, S., Alex, V., Krishnamurthi, G.: Multi-modal brain tumor segmentation using stacked denoising autoencoders. In: Proceedings MICCAI BraTS (Brain Tumor Segmentation Challenge), pp. 60–64 (2015)
14. Pereira, S., Pinto, A., Alves, V., Silva, C.A.: Brain tumor segmentation using convolutional neural networks in MRI images. IEEE Trans. Med. Imaging **35**, 1240–1251 (2016)
15. Zheng, S., Jayasumana, S., Romera-Paredes, B., Vineet, V., Su, Z., Du, D., Huang, C., Torr, P.H.: Conditional random fields as recurrent neural networks. In: Proceedings of the IEEE International Conference on Computer Vision, pp. 1529–1537 (2015)
16. Tustison, N.J., Avants, B.B., Cook, P.A., Zheng, Y., Egan, A., Yushkevich, P.A., Gee, J.C.: N4ITK: improved N3 bias correction. IEEE Trans. Med. Imaging **29**, 1310–1320 (2010)
17. Krähenbühl, P., Koltun, V.: Efficient inference in fully connected CRFs with Gaussian edge potentials. NIPS (2011)
18. Jia, Y., Shelhamer, E., Donahue, J., Karayev, S., Long, J., Girshick, R., Guadarrama, S., Darrell, T.: Caffe: convolutional architecture for fast feature embedding. In: Proceedings of the 22nd ACM International Conference on Multimedia, pp. 675–678 (2014)

Brain Tumor Segmentation with Optimized Random Forest

László Lefkovits[1]([✉]), Szidónia Lefkovits[2], and László Szilágyi[1,3]

[1] Department of Electrical Engineering,
Sapientia University Tîrgu-Mureş, Corunca, Romania
lefkolaci@ms.sapientia.ro
[2] Department of Computer Science,
"Petru Maior" University Tîrgu-Mureş, Târgu Mureş, Romania
[3] Department of Control Engineering and Information Technology,
University of Technology and Economics Budapest, Budapest, Hungary

Abstract. In this paper we propose and tune a discriminative model based on Random Forest (RF) to accomplish brain tumor segmentation in multimodal MR images. The objective of tuning is meant to establish the optimal parameter values and the most significant constraints of the discriminative model. During the building of the RF classifier, the algorithm evaluates the importance of variables, the proximities between data instances and the generalized error. These three properties of RF are employed to optimize the segmentation framework. At the beginning the RF is tuned for variable importance evaluation, and after that it is used to optimize the segmentation framework. The framework was tested on unseen test images from BRATS. The results obtained are similar to the best ones presented in previous BRATS Challenges.

Keywords: Random forest · Feature selection · Variable importance · Statistical pattern recognition · MRI segmentation

1 Introduction

MR imaging and diagnosis is increasingly used from day to day with the worldwide spread of MR equipment. In many cases, with the help of a correct diagnosis, complicated surgery could be avoided or medical staff could be better prepared for the intervention. One part of these techniques is built around automatic image segmentation. In order to facilitate a faster diagnosis, a robust and reliable automatic segmentation system is needed. In this paper we propose a discriminative model for brain tumor segmentation in multimodal MRI. The main goal of the model is the evaluation and selection of low-level image features and the optimization of the Random Forest (RF) classifier for the segmentation task. This is achieved in two phases: first, we start with the optimization of RF considering variable importance evaluation. The second phase is the optimization of the RF structure in order to improve segmentation performance. Many discriminative segmentation models were proposed and tested in the previous

© Springer International Publishing AG 2016
A. Crimi et al. (Eds.): BrainLes 2016, LNCS 10154, pp. 88–99, 2016.
DOI: 10.1007/978-3-319-55524-9_9

four BRATS Challenges (2012–2015) [4]. The selection of the employed features was based on the intuition and experience of the authors. The exact definition and usage of the applied features in their segmentation systems remains a secret. Usually, the systems work with large sets of features having hardly any theoretical or practical analysis behind their usefulness.

In the following we will present the best-performing systems based on a discriminative model used in multimodal MR tumor segmentation.

Zikic [16] et al. and their research team from Microsoft created a discriminative model that extracts the attributes from the image intensities as well as from a generative model. In their approach, 2000 context-aware attributes are defined. As a classification ensemble, they use 40 decision trees, each having a depth of 20. Geremia et al. [7] built a discriminative model that associates a vector of 412 features to each point. The classification algorithm is an ensemble of decision trees trained on a set of images containing 20 High Grade (HG) and 10 Low Grade (LG) images. Goetz et al. [8] that uses 208 attributes; 52 attributes for each of the 4 image types. The classifier is made up of an ensemble of Extra-Randomized Trees (ERT). Reza and Iftekharuddin [14] created a discriminative model which only processes planar images that are axial sections of 3D MRI. This model uses no apriori information about the anatomical structure of the brain. The system works only with the intensity information of the pixels in multimodal images, extracting special attributes based on texton, textures and fractal dimension. The classification algorithm is again the RF. The final decision is made by weighted voting. Remarkable performance is obtained due to texture information.

A more reliable model can be built selecting the variable importance from the point of view of classification. An adequate feature set comes with the following advantages:

– increases the predictive accuracy of the classifier;
– reduces the cost of data collection;
– enhances learning efficiency;
– reduces the computational complexity of the resulting model.

The rest of this paper is structured as follows: in Sect. 2 we describe the components of our model (Sect. 2.1 Database, Sect. 2.2 Preprocessing, Sect. 2.3 Feature Extraction, Sect. 2.4 Random Forest, Sect. 2.5 Feature Selection, Sect. 2.6 Postprocessing). After the model presentation follows the fine-tuning and optimization of Random Forest parameters used in segmentation purposes, in Sect. 3. Finally, our experimental results are described and compared to other systems from the BRATS Challenge.

2   The Proposed Discriminative Model

The discriminative model proposed is similar to previously used models, but in this article we emphasize some aspects which make an important contribution to the performances reached. The performances of a segmentation model built on a discriminative function are mainly determined by three important issues: the quality of the annotated image-database, the classification algorithm applied and the feature set used.

Our model differs from the standard discriminative model by the feature selection step. In this step, the feature selection algorithm consists of the variable importance evaluation for the defined segmentation task. At the same time it allows to test new low-level features that should improve the segmentation performances or be more important than the existing features.

This paper is organized as follows: after a short introduction of the similar systems in the literature Sect. 2 describes the components of the proposed discriminative model used for brain tumor segmentation. After the model presentation follows the fine-tuning and optimization of Random Forest parameters used for segmentation purposes, presented in Sect. 3. Finally, our experimental results are described and compared to other systems from the BRATS Challenge.

2.1 Database

The most important image database for brain tumor segmentation was created during the BRATS Challenges (2012–2015), thanks to Menze and Jakab [13]. This database is expanded year after year with every challenge and has become a standard in the field. The BRATS 2015 dataset contains 220 HG and 54 LG brain images with gliomas and ensures sufficient diversity, which is a requirement for a well-performing database. All cases were acquired with similar protocols and contain four types of images: T1, T1c (with the contrast material Gadolinium), T2 and FLAIR. All images were skull stripped, resampled to 1 mm resolution in each direction and registered to the corresponding T1c image. The annotations were made by experts using an accurate protocol [10]. The annotations contain four different classes: edema, enhanced tumor, non-enhanced tumor and necrotic core.

The four classes defined by expert annotation are very hard to achieve by automatic segmentation. More realistic evaluation of segmentation results can be made by considering only three classes. It is considered that they are more representative in clinical practice. These classes are: Whole Tumor - WT (including all four tumor structures), Tumor Core - TC (including all tumor structures except for edema) and Active Tumor - AT (only the enhancing core). Of course, there are some differences between the annotations made by the same/different experts. These variations are specified in [13] and can be considered as the upper limit of the performance reachable. In this work we made the optimization considering only two classes: WT and TC (TC includes AT).

The principle of statistical pattern recognition is the assignment of some features to a well-delimited region or to every voxel. In this way the database used for statistical processing contains a large amount of instances and increases in size with each newly added feature. The database increases drastically with the increase in the number of cases. The training database, containing 274 cases, reaches a storage size of 21 GB in uncompressed format. The resulting database increases linearly with each feature added; thus, if one decides to use a set of about 1000 features, a total of 30 TB of information has to be processed. The more data can be processed and included in the training phase, the better the performance of the classifier obtained. In our work we tried to solve the issue of this huge, unmanageable dataset in two ways: (1) by reducing the irrelevant and redundant features; (2) by eliminating similar cases.

2.2 Preprocessing

In this work we have dealt with three important artifacts: inhomogeneity correction, noise filtering, and intensity standardization.

The correction of MRI inhomogeneity can be done by using the intensity information and some apriori knowledge of the anatomical tissue-structure only. In our previous work [11] we evaluated three inhomogeneity reduction methods. The best-performing and most accepted algorithm is N4 filtering [15]. For inhomogeneity reduction in MR images, we have applied the N4 filter implemented in the ITK package [2].

The most difficult task is to evaluate noise types and their levels in real images and to find the most suitable denoising method. Since we could not find a generally available method required by discriminative segmentation, we decided to use anisotropic diffusion filtering proposed in [6]. Its implementation can be found in the ITK [2] software package.

It is desirable to have the same intensity value for a given tissue in distinct images, regardless of the acquisition equipment and moment. The solution to this problem is to transform the histogram in order to match it to a predetermined shape. We extracted the quartiles points on the histogram obtained and performed linear transformations in such way that the first and third quartiles have predefined values.

In preprocessing, we filtered these three artifacts in the following order: bias field correction (ITK - N4 filtering), then noise filtering (ITK - anisotropic diffusion filtering), and finally, the proposed intensity standardization.

2.3 Feature Extraction

Image processing offers many procedures for the extraction of characteristics from images. In the field of tumor segmentation there are many studies that try to find certain characteristics with a high correlation to the brain tumor appearance in MR images. Despite these research efforts, no proper feature sets have been found yet. That is the reason for using a large feature set, with the features having little correlation to the goal of classification. In our approach we started with defining a large feature set, this is later reduced in order to eliminate the irrelevant or noisy features. For each feature, we defined many low-level characteristics that describe the intensities in the neighborhood (surrounding volume having a radius of 2–9 pixels) of the studied voxels. We have used the following features: first order operators (mean, standard deviation, max, min, median, gradient); higher order operators (Laplacian, difference of Gaussian, entropy, curvatures, kurtosis, skewness); texture features (Gabor filter); spatial context features (symmetry, projections, neighborhoods). By extracting all of these features for every voxel in all modalities, we transform the image segmentation task into a statistical pattern recognition problem. In order to deal with big amount of features it is necessary to reduce the number of used attributes. The appropriate selection of the attributes has to be done according to the goal of classification. First, we extracted 240 image features of each modality and we obtained a feature vector with 960 elements. All these features are defined in Weka Segmentation plugin form Fiji package [1].

2.4   Random Forest

RF is a powerful algorithm for segmentation purposes [5]. The RF has five important characteristics that make it applicable for segmentation tasks: manages large databases easily; handles thousands of variables; estimates the variable importance used in classification; is able to balance the error in unbalanced datasets; produces an internal unbiased estimator of generalized error.

The RF classifier is an ensemble of binary trees built on two random processes: the randomly built bootstrap set and the random feature selection in each node [5]. The creation of trees from the RF is based on two sets: the bootstrap set, containing the instances for building a tree and the OOB (out-of-bag) set, containing test instances not included in the bootstrap set. The bootstrap set is made up of the training instances by randomly sampling the training set with replacement. Each tree is trained on its own bootstrap set and evaluated on its OOB set. The maximization of the information gain is the splitting criterion applied in every node. In order to evaluate the information gain, the RF uses only a small number of variables (m_{tries}) out of all existing variables (M). These m_{tries} variables are chosen randomly and the splitting criterion is maximized only with these variables.

While the classifier is being built, the RF algorithm evaluates the so called OOB error. This error is the mean value of the classification error of each tree on its own OOB sets. The OOB error is an unbiased estimator of generalized error (GE) of the classification obtained. The relation of GE was proved by Breiman [5]:

$$GE = \rho \left(\frac{1}{s^2} - 1 \right) \tag{1}$$

where ρ is the mean value of correlation and s stands for the strength of the ensemble. The minimum of GE can be reached by decreasing the correlation between trees and by increasing the classification strength of ensemble. These two conflicting trends determine the goal of the RF parameter optimization. Determining the appropriate values of these parameters could be the objective of an experimental optimization, described in Sect. 2.6.

2.5   Feature Selection

The main part of the model is the evaluation and selection of low-level image features for the segmentation task. In the field of image segmentation, discriminative classifiers are based on several local image features. A more reliable model can be built by using a framework that selects the variable importance from the point of view of classification. In the field of statistical pattern recognition, the selection of such features is a challenging task. In order to create a well-working discriminative model, we have to select the relevant features for our application and eliminate the irrelevant ones. For this purpose we used the variable importance evaluation provided by RF. In the construction of RF classifiers there are two possibilities to evaluate variable importance: Gini importance and permuted importance [5]. In our algorithm we used only the permuted variable importance, or mean in accuracy.

Because the variable importance values depend on the forest structure, the values obtained are equivocal. The importance values obtained differ in each round; the order of importance differs only slightly. In order to increase the relevance of permuted importance; we have to evaluate it for each variable several times to determine an average importance value. The ranking of average values is relevant.

One main objective of variable selection is to find a small number of variables appropriate for a good prediction. For this task we distinguish following steps:

1. Tune RF for variable importance evaluation
2. Evaluate variable importance order
3. Eliminate the least important variables
4. Tune RF for classification
5. Evaluate classification performances
6. Accept or reject the variable reduction.

In step 3 we have to deal with many instances, each consisting of a large number of features. For this purpose we created our feature selection algorithm, presented in detail in [12]. The main idea of the algorithm is to evaluate the variable importance several times on a randomly chosen part of the training set. It eliminates the least important 20%–50% of variables in each run, ensuring that the average OOB error does not exceed the desired limit. In our experiment, after each reduction step, the RF classifiers were trained and evaluated in order to determine the segmentation performances. Further, the elimination of variables depends on the decrease of the segmentation performances. The proportion of reduction is empirical; it depends on the number of attributes used and the performances obtained. In the first step we are able to exclude a large number of attributes and in the last steps only few. It must be in correlation with the reachable performances.

We applied the proposed feature selection algorithm in order to select an important feature set for our brain tumor segmentation task. The feature vectors of a single 3D brain image require 10 GB of memory. In order to provide a good enough training set, we had to use the information from at least 50 brain volumes. Thus, the whole training database ($TDB = I \times F$) is about 500 GB in size, which is practically unmanageable. There are two ways to reduce this size: reducing the number of instances (I) and reducing the number of features (F). The number of instances can be reduced by random subsampling the database. In each image belonging to one brain there are about 1.5 million voxels from

which less than 10% are tumor voxels. Thus, in the first step, we drastically
reduced the number of instances belonging to the brain-class in order to balance
the dataset. A random subsampling reduced the number of healthy voxels in
10 : 1 ratio in the training set. The TDB size is reduced to 100 GB. The $STDB$
(sampled training database) size becomes 5 GB by randomly subsampling the
TDB 20:1. This size is still too large to be managed by our system (Intel(R)
Core(TM) i7-2600kCPU@3.40 GHz, 16 GB RAM). The training time of the RF
algorithm for a dataset of about 200 MB is 30 min, and it increases exponentially
with the increase of the training database. We used the RF implementation from
R package provided by CRAN [3]. In order to manage such a large amount of
memory, we had to reduce the number of features also. Our algorithm was created
to manage this big database and to select a set of adequate features for the given
segmentation task. We applied our algorithm several times by evaluating the
overall OOB error (Table 1). In order to determine the optimal set of attributes
(M – *number of all attributes*) used, we tested the performances of the classifier
obtained on UTI (unseen test images of 20 brain image sets). In our experiments
we analyzed in significative parameter intervals the behaviour of OOB error and
the Dice index.

Table 1. The effect of parameter M on the classification performance

M - attributes	960	480	240	120	80	60	45	30	20
OOB error		0.0501	0.0508	0.051	0.0522	0.0532	0.0551	0.058	0.0635	0.0725

M - attributes	240	120	80	60	45	30
DICE-WT	0.868	0.866	0.848	0.843	0.838	0.828
DICE-TC	0.865	0.865	0.868	0.860	0.849	0.806

The Dice coefficients obtained in segmentation are presented in Table 1. We
started the evaluation of Dice coefficient at only $M = 240$, because the training
and testing of more than 240 attributes were time consuming. Also we observed
that OOB error does not change significantly for $M \in [240, 960]$. Because there is
a relation between OOB error and Dice coefficient, we consider that the Dice coefficient, similarly, does not change in the given interval. The significant decrease
of the Dice coefficient is at $M \in [80, 120]$ attributes and differ for the analyzed
classes: $M = 120$ for WT and $M = 80$ for TC (Fig. 1). We obtained the same
interval for both TDB and UTI sets. According to the results obtained, we have
chosen $M = 120$ attributes for the final classifier.

2.6   Post-processing

In post-processing we took into consideration that the tumor is one single connected volume and the spatial relation between the different tumor classes is
$AT \subset TC \subset WT$. In this way, we were able to eliminate many small volumes
that had been interpreted as false detections.

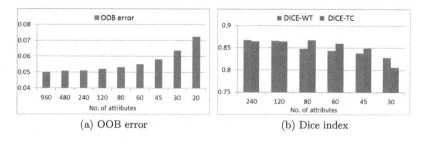

(a) OOB error   (b) Dice index

Fig. 1. OOB error and Dice coefficient against the parameter M

3 RF Optimization

The main task is to find some correlation between the OOB error and the Dice coefficient of segmentation. To achieve this task we had to optimize the RF parameters in order to obtain an efficient classifier for the segmentation task. There are three parameters that have to be tuned in RF optimization: the number of trees K_{trees}, the number of features m_{tries} and the number of nodes T_{nodes}. The minimum of generalized error (1) can be reached by decreasing the correlation between trees and by increasing the strength of the ensemble.

A binary decision tree is one of the strongest classifiers described in the literature. The overfit provided by the trees can be decreased by increasing the number of trees K_{trees} used in the forest. The rise in the number of K_{trees} will cause the GE to decrease and overfitting can be avoided. The GE has a minimum limit. Thus, further increasing the K_{trees} value, after the stabilization limit, GE remains unchanged; it is only the processing time that becomes longer without any gain in error. We analyzed the OOB error and Dice index versus the variation of K_{trees}. The OOB value decreases with the increase of K_{trees} and reaches its minimum limit at 300 trees for $M = 80$ and 400 trees for $M = 120$ (Table 2 and Fig. 2).

Table 2. The effect of number of trees K_{trees} on the classification performance

K_{trees}	20	30	40	50	100	200	300	400	500
OOB error M = 120	0.0651	0.0605	0.0581	0.0568	0.0544	0.0534	0.0533	0.0527	0.0528
OOB error M = 80	0.0655	0.0607	0.0586	0.0575	0.0549	0.0537	0.0531	0.0531	0.0531

K_{trees}	50	100	200	300
DICE-WT	0.864	0.866	0.867	0.867
DICE-TC	0.894	0.898	0.898	0.899

The Dice coefficient reaches the maximum ealier at 200 for WT and 100 for TC, thus a total of 100 trees are adequate to be used in the ensemble. Thus, our final classifier is built with a total of 100 trees.

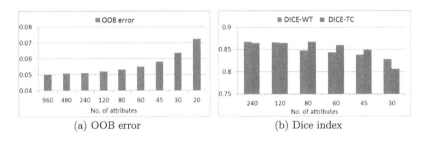

(a) OOB error   (b) Dice index

Fig. 2. OOB error and Dice coefficient against the parameter K_{trees}

The second analyzed parameter m_{tries} (the number of randomly chosen variables) used for splitting in nodes determines the uncorrelation between trees. Increasing the number m_{tries} the trees are more and more correlated, and the opposite is also true: by decreasing m_{tries}, the correlation between trees decreases. When $m_{tries} = M$ (M – the total number of variables), the RF classifier turns into bagging. When $m_{tries} = 1$, the trees are highly uncorrelated, but at the same time, they lose their strength of classification. It is recommended [9] to perform a coarse evaluation in the interval $\left(\sqrt{M/2}, 2\sqrt{M}\right)$, in order to choose the adequate value for m_{tries}. In Table 3 we can observe that the OOB error reaches its minimum at about $2\sqrt{M}$, and further increasing its value is useless ($m_{tries} = 25$ for $M = 120$, $m_{tries} = 15$ for $M = 80$). More interesting results can be obtained by analyzing the Dice coefficient versus m_{tries}. The Dice coefficient reaches the maximum at $m_{tries} = 15$ for WT and $m_{tries} = 11$ for TC in the analyzed domain (Table 3 and Fig. 3).

Table 3. The effect of m_{tries} on the classification performance

m_{tries}	5	7	9	11	15	19	25	31	43	59
OOB error M = 120	5.67	5.54	5.44	5.39	5.34	5.27	5.25	5.22	5.22	5.22
OOB error M = 80	5.65	5.54	5.49	5.44	5.33	5.33	5.33	5.33	5.33	5.33

m_{tries}	9	11	15	19	25
DICE-WT	0.850	0.850	0.852	0.849	0.846
DICE-TC	0.869	0.872	0.864	0.871	0.867

The third parameter is the number of maximal nodes of each tree T_{nodes}. Theoretically, there is no condition of limitation of the tree size (T_{nodes}), there is no generally accepted pruning condition.

In these circumstances each tree grows until every terminal node becomes a pure leaf, where no more splits are possible. This case can produce very large trees which occupy unnecessary memory space and lengthen processing time.

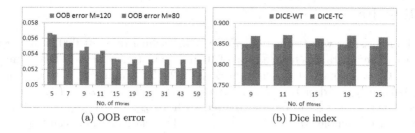

(a) OOB error   (b) Dice index

Fig. 3. OOB error and Dice coefficient against the parameter m_{tries}

Reducing the size of a tree T_{nodes} induces new diversity in the ensemble, decreases the correlation between trees and produces a smaller and more efficient classifier. The OOB error versus the T_{nodes} is given in Table 4 and Fig. 4.

We can see that the OOB error constantly decreases with the tree size and reaches its minimum for the unpruned trees. Important from the point of view of segmentation is the evolution of the Dice coefficient, it does not increase significantly for the last values. The optimal value can be determined at 2048 nodes, which is approximately 1/4 of the size of an unpruned tree.

Table 4. The effect of tree-size T_{nodes} on the classification performance

T_{nodes}	64	128	256	512	1024	2048	4096	MAX
OOBerr. M = 120	0.1246	0.1104	0.0976	0.0871	0.0768	0.0686	0.06	0.0522
OOBerr. M = 120	0.1253	0.1124	0.0986	0.0875	0.0773	0.0695	0.0612	0.0532

T_{nodes}	512	1024	2048	4096	MAX
DICE-WT	0.817	0.841	0.864	0.866	0.867
DICE-TC	0.798	0.823	0.874	0.877	0.879

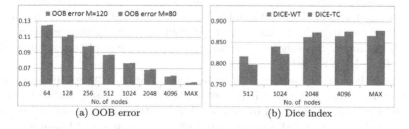

(a) OOB error   (b) Dice index

Fig. 4. OOB error and Dice coefficient against the parameter T_{nodes}

4   Results

The final classifier was trained on $STDB$ which consists of 500000 ($< 5\%$) randomly sampled instances from a total of 10 million instances of the TDB, being 50 sets of HG brain images (chosen from BRATS 2015 training set). Our optimized classifier is composed of $K_{trees} = 100$ trees, each having a size of $T_{nodes} = 2048$ nodes. The splitting criterion is evaluated with $m_{tries} = 9$ randomly chosen features from the whole $M = 120$ feature set. The classification result obtained on BRATS 2015 test set are given in Table 5 and some segmentation examples in Fig. 5. The results obtained are comparable with previously reported results described in [13].

Table 5. Compared Dice indexes

Classes	Our classifier	BRATS 2012 [13]	BRATS 2013 [13]
WT	75–91 [%]	63–78 [%]	71–87 [%]
TC	71–82 [%]	24–37 [%]	66–78 [%]

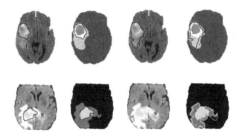

Fig. 5. Segmentation results (contour line expert annotation, gray levels segmented tumor tissues)

5   Conclusion

We are working on further optimization in order to improve segmentation performances. Analyzing the results obtained on unseen test images we can notice highly accurate. In order to increase the classification performances we have to build an optimized training set containing all appearances of tumor forms (272 images) from BRATS 2015.

This can be done by adding new instances to the training set and also measuring their proximity to the existing set. Furthermore, the segmentation framework obtained will be enlarged by new low-level features. The importance of new features could be evaluated and compared to the current set of features.

In this manner, we are able to create a better feature set for tumor segmentation. Besides, additional post-processing may lead to further improvement in segmentation performances.

References

1. Fiji Is Just ImageJ. http://fiji.sc/Fiji
2. ITK. http://www.itk.org/
3. The R project for statistical computing. https://www.r-project.org/
4. The SICAS Medical Image Repository. https://www.smir.ch/BRATS/Start2015
5. Breiman, L.: Random forests. Mach. Learn. **45**(1), 5–32 (2001)
6. Diaz, I., Boulanger, P., Greiner, R., Murtha, A.: A critical review of the effects of de-noising algorithms on MRI brain tumor segmentation. In: 2011 Annual International Conference of the IEEE Engineering in Medicine and Biology Society, EMBC, pp. 3934–3937. IEEE (2011)
7. Geremia, E., Menze, B.H., Ayache, N.: Spatial decision forests for glioma segmentation in multi-channel MR images. In: MICCAI-BRATS Challenge on Multimodal Brain Tumor Segmentation (2012)
8. Goetz, M., Weber, C., Bloecher, J., Stieltjes, B., Meinzer, H.P., Maier-Hein, M.: Extremely randomized trees based brain tumor segmentation. In: MICCAI-BRATS Challenge on Multimodal Brain Tumor Segmentation (2014)
9. Goldstein, B.A., Polley, E.C., Briggs, F.: Random forests for genetic association studies. Stat. Appl. Genet. Mol. Biol. **10**(1), 1–34 (2011)
10. Jakab, A.: Segmenting Brain Tumors with the Slicer 3D Software Manual for providing expert segmentations for the BRATS Tumor Segmentation Challenge. University of Debrecen/ETH Zürich
11. Lefkovits, L., Lefkovits, S., Vaida, M.F.: An Atlas based performance evaluation of inhomogeneity correcting effects. In: The 5th International Conference MACRO, Tîrgu-Mureş, pp. 79–90, March 2015
12. Lefkovits, L., Lefkovits, S., Vaida, M.F.: Brain Tumor Segmentation Based on Random Forest. Memoirs of the Scientific Sections of the Romanian Academy, pp. 83–93 (2016)
13. Menze, B.H., Jakab, A., Bauer, S., et al.: The multimodal brain tumor image segmentation benchmark (BRATS). IEEE Trans. Med. Imaging **34**(10), 1993–2024 (2015)
14. Reza, S., Iftekharuddin, K.M.: Multi-class abnormal brain tissue segmentation using texture features. In: MICCAI-BRATS Challenge on Multimodal Brain Tumor Segmentation (2013)
15. Tustison, N., Avants, B., Cook, P., Zheng, Y., Egan, A., Yushkevich, P., Gee, J.: N4ITK: improved N3 bias correction. IEEE Trans. Med. Imaging **29**(6), 1310–1320 (2010)
16. Zikic, D., Glocker, B., Konukoglu, E., Shotton, J., Criminisi, A., Ye, D., Demiralp, C., Thomas, O., Das, T., Jena, R., et al.: Context-sensitive classification forests for segmentation of brain tumor tissues. In: MICCAI-BRATS (2012)

CRF-Based Brain Tumor Segmentation: Alleviating the Shrinking Bias

Raphael Meier[1(✉)], Urspeter Knecht[2], Roland Wiest[2], and Mauricio Reyes[1]

[1] Institute for Surgical Technology and Biomechanics,
University of Bern, Bern, Switzerland
`raphael.meier@istb.unibe.ch`
[2] Support Center for Advanced Neuroimaging – Institute for Diagnostic and
Interventional Neuroradiology, University Hospital and
University of Bern, Bern, Switzerland

Abstract. This paper extends a previously published brain tumor segmentation method with a dense Conditional Random Field (CRF). Dense CRFs can overcome the shrinking bias inherent to many grid-structured CRFs. We focus on illustrating the impact of alleviating the shrinking bias on the performance of CRF-based brain tumor segmentation. The proposed segmentation method is evaluated using data from the MICCAI BRATS 2013 & 2015 data sets (up to 110 patient cases for testing) and compared to a baseline method using a grid-structured CRF. Improved segmentation performance for the complete and enhancing tumor was observed with respect to grid-structured CRFs.

1 Introduction

Markov or Conditional Random Fields (CRFs) have a long history in image understanding [21] and are used for a diverse range of tasks such as image segmentation or registration. In this work, we focus on image segmentation, which plays a crucial role in the analysis of medical images. Image segmentation can be used in any phase of a clinical process - from diagnosis to treatment planning to patient monitoring. The segmentation of pathological images can provide data on the spatial location and configuration as well as volumetric parameters of a disease. Graphical models such as CRFs offer a sound probabilistic framework to model spatial data contained in medical images. In the most popular type of CRF, voxels of the image correspond to nodes in a graph. Furthermore, the nodes are arranged in a grid with edges connecting the nodes, and thus establishing the neighborhood type (e.g. Moore neighborhood). Smoothness of the final segmentation is established via pairwise potentials defined for neighboring nodes. The use of a Potts prior in grid-structured pairwise CRFs is known to result in excessive smoothing of the segmentation boundary (also referred to as *shrinking bias*, illustrated in Fig. 1). Dense CRFs define pairwise potentials among all nodes in the graph modeling long-range dependencies between voxels. As a consequence, the inherent shrinking bias of grid-structured pairwise CRFs is alleviated allowing for a more detailed image segmentation. The application

A. Crimi et al. (Eds.): BrainLes 2016, LNCS 10154, pp. 100–107, 2016.
DOI: 10.1007/978-3-319-55524-9_10

of dense CRFs in medical image volumes has been prohibitive for a long time due to their huge complexity. This situation changed when Krähenbühl et al. introduced an efficient inference [8] and learning algorithm [7] for dense CRFs. In this paper, we extend our previously published methodology [10] with a dense CRF and investigate its impact on the segmentation of tumor subcompartments.

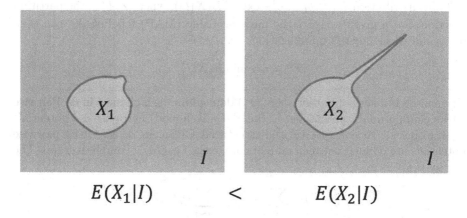

$$E(X_1|I) \qquad < \qquad E(X_2|I)$$

Fig. 1. Illustration of the shrinking bias. Grid-structured CRFs can incorporate the prior belief that segmentation boundaries are smooth via a Potts-prior used for the pairwise potentials. The limited neighborhood type in combination with such a smoothness prior encourages the generation of short object boundaries (left image). If we are given an image I, the corresponding object segmentation X_2 (right image) will be penalized making it less favorable (probable) compared to a more compact alternative segmentation X_1. This corresponds to a lower energy E for X_1 than for X_2.

2   Methodology

2.1   Brain Tumor Segmentation

We focus on the segmentation of glioblastoma, which are the most common primary malignant brain tumors [3]. A glioblastoma can be segmented into four different compartments: necrosis, edema, contrast-enhancing and non-enhancing tumor [15]. We regard segmentation as a classification problem and rely on four different MRI sequences as input data, which are T_1-, T_1 post-contrast- (T_{1c}), T_2- and FLAIR-weighted images. These sequences are part of recently proposed clinical consensus recommendations [4]. The sequences are rigidly co-registered, skull-stripped [1], bias-field corrected [20] and their intensities are normalized via histogram matching to a template image [12]. The four intensity values are stacked in a vector $\mathbf{f}_i \in \mathbb{R}^4$, which in turn is part of a vector image I. The set of voxels in I is denoted by V and the total number of voxels by N. A labeling of I is referred to by $X = \{x_i\}_{i \in V}$ with x_i being a scalar value that indicates the tissue compartment, i.e. $x_i \in \{1, \ldots, m\}$. Seven classes ($m = 7$) including three normal (csf, gray matter, white matter) and the previously mentioned four tumor tissues are defined and contained in a set $\mathcal{L}$.

2.2 Dense CRF

We model the image I as an undirected graph $G = (V, E)$, where V denotes the set of nodes and E the set of edges. Every node in G is associated with a random variable x_i. The pair (I, X) is a CRF, if for any given I the distribution $P(X|I)$ factorizes according to G. The conditional distribution corresponds to a Gibbs distribution $P(X|I) = \frac{1}{Z(I)} \exp(-E(X|I))$, where $Z(I)$ is the partition function. For a given image I the most probable (MAP) labeling $X^\star$ can then be estimated via energy minimization, i.e.

$$X^\star = \arg\min_X E(X|I). \tag{1}$$

The energy is a sum of potentials $\psi_c(x_c)$ defined for each clique c in G. Pairwise CRFs contain unary potentials ψ_u (i.e. data-likelihood) and pairwise potentials ψ_p (i.e. prior). In contrast to grid-structured CRFs, in dense CRFs pairwise potentials are defined between all pairs of voxels, i.e. G is a complete graph. The energy is given by

$$E(X|I) = \sum_i \psi_u(x_i) + \sum_{i \sim j} \psi_p(x_i, x_j). \tag{2}$$

The driving force of the shrinking bias in CRFs are the pairwise potentials $\psi_p(x_i, x_j)$ (cf. [19]). Dense CRFs model long-range interactions between voxels and thus make more consistent image labelings according to global image content more favorable during MAP-inference in Eq. (1). We define the unary potentials to take the form

$$\psi_u(x_i) = -\log(p_D(x_i|\mathbf{h}_i)), \tag{3}$$

where $\mathbf{h}$ corresponds to the feature vector proposed by Meier et al. [10] and the posterior probability p_D is estimated by a decision forest [2]. The feature vector is composed of a combination of appearance- and context-sensitive features. In the approach proposed by Krähenbühl and Koltun [8] the pairwise potentials ψ_p are restricted to correspond to a weighted mixture of Gaussian kernels. We use a combination of an appearance (using image intensities $\mathbf{f}_i$) and smoothness kernel (using voxel coordinates $\mathbf{p}_i$):

$$\psi_p(x_i, x_j) = \mu(x_i, x_j) \left\{ \exp(-\tfrac{1}{2}(\mathbf{f}_i - \mathbf{f}_j)^T \Lambda_f (\mathbf{f}_i - \mathbf{f}_j)) + \exp(-\tfrac{1}{2}(\mathbf{p}_i - \mathbf{p}_j)^T \Lambda_p (\mathbf{p}_i - \mathbf{p}_j)) \right\}. \tag{4}$$

The label compatibility function $\mu(x_i, x_j)$ is defined to be a symmetric function that takes into account interactions between all possible combinations of label pairings. The precision matrices of the two kernels are Λ_f and Λ_p.

3   Experiments and Results

In order to assess the segmentation performance of the proposed dense CRF model, we employed publicly-available data of the MICCAI BRATS 2013 & 2015 Challenges [11]. First, a comparison of the dense CRF to a grid-structured CRF was performed, for which we used 20 high-grade cases of the original BRATS 2013 data set for training (18 for training, two for validation purposes). We assessed segmentation performance of both models on the BRATS 2013 challenge set (10 patient cases), the BRATS 2013 leaderboard set (21 cases, excluding low-grade glioma), and a clinical data set of a local university hospital (25 cases). In contrast to the BRATS data sets, the clinical data set was acquired with a standardized MR acquisition protocol (all sequences except FLAIR were acquired with isotropic 1 mm resolution). A more detailed description of the clinical data set can be found in the study of Porz et al. [16]. Second, in order to facilitate future comparisons with other segmentation techniques, we evaluated the proposed approach on the BRATS 2015 data set (247 cases for training and 110 for testing). We report performance measures as tuples (median, interquartile range) for the complete tumor (all tumor labels combined), the tumor core (tumor labels except edema) and the enhancing tumor. Statistically significant differences were assessed using a paired Wilcoxon signed rank test (cf. Table 1). Statistical analysis was performed using the R software package [17].

The baseline model (G-CRF) relied on a grid-structured pairwise CRF with a Potts prior as used in [10]. Inference was performed using Fast-PD [6]. The dense CRF (D-CRF) was implemented as described in Sect. 2. To make a fair

Table 1. Evaluation results. Performance measures are given as (median, interquartile range). Left tuple: Results for BRATS 2013 Challenge set. Middle tuple: Results for Leaderboard data. Right tuple: Results for clinical data. Statistically significant differences are indicated with $^*/^{**}$ for $\alpha = 0.05/0.01$.

Region	Dice coefficient	PPV	Sensitivity
Complete tumor (G-CRF)	(0.825, 0.042)/ (0.771, 0.148)/ (0.839, 0.146)	(0.759, 0.108)/ (0.751, 0.266)/ (0.766, 0.238)	(0.943, 0.040)/ (0.969, 0.133)/ (0.922, 0.065)
Complete tumor (D-CRF)	(0.825, 0.049)/ (**0.790**, 0.168)/ (**0.856****, 0.148)	(**0.775**, 0.108)/ (**0.758***, 0.254)/ (**0.772****, 0.229)	(**0.953**, 0.040)/ (**0.979**, 0.134)/ (**0.938****, 0.067)
Tumor core (G-CRF)	(0.748, 0.075)/ (0.745, 0.200)/ (**0.693**, 0.287)	(0.802, 0.192)/ (**0.746**, 0.151)/ (**0.741****, 0.195)	(**0.715**, 0.234)/ (**0.888****, 0.372)/ (**0.713****, 0.268)
Tumor core (D-CRF)	(**0.756**, 0.086)/ (**0.746***, 0.214)/ (0.643, 0.231)	(**0.819**, 0.216)/ (0.720, 0.205)/ (0.719, 0.214)	(0.698, 0.256)/ (0.855, 0.420)/ (0.659, 0.370)
Enhancing tumor (G-CRF)	(**0.706***, 0.074)[a]/ (**0.677**, 0.218)/ (0.579, 0.140)	(0.669, 0.171)/ (**0.644**, 0.197)/ (0.508, 0.149)	(0.823, 0.205)/ (0.923, 0.403)/ (0.816, 0.224)
Enhancing tumor (D-CRF)	(0.705, 0.073)[a]/ (0.660, 0.266)/ (**0.631****, 0.161)	(**0.673**, 0.149)/ (0.626, 0.279)/ (**0.542****, 0.192)	(**0.873***, 0.257)/ (**0.944****, 0.302)/ (**0.866****, 0.163)

[a]The mean for D-CRF was 0.694 and 0.681 for G-CRF.

comparison to G-CRF, we set $\mu(x_i, x_j) = \mathbb{1}\{x_i \neq x_j\}$ (Potts prior) and set $\Lambda_f = \lambda_f I_4$ and $\Lambda_p = \lambda_p I_3$ with $I_{(.)}$ being the identity matrix and $\lambda_f, \lambda_p \in \mathbb{R}$. Note that both models employed the same unary classifier (features and decision forest as proposed in [10]). We used 100 trees, maximum depth of 18 and the number of candidate features per node was $\sqrt{n}$ with $n = 237$ features. Moreover, we did not perform a parameter learning but hand-tuned the parameter values for both CRF models using the data of the validation set. This way, we aimed at minimizing differences in segmentation performance attributed to a specific parameter learning method rather than the different degree of connectivity of each model.

The results of the comparison between G-CRF and D-CRF are shown in Table 1. In Fig. 2, an exemplary segmentation result is shown. In addition, Fig. 3

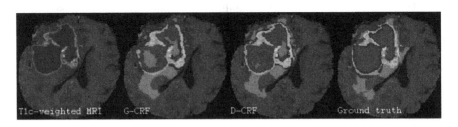

Fig. 2. Exemplary patient case (edema = green, necrosis = red, enhancing tumor = yellow, non-enhancing tumor = blue). From left to right: Contrast-enhanced T_1-weighted Magnetic Resonance sequence. Segmentation result for G-CRF. Segmentation result for D-CRF. Manual ground truth data. (Color figure online)

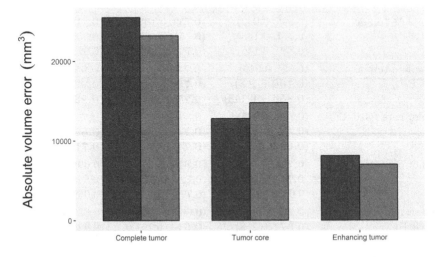

Fig. 3. Absolute volume error. The mean error in mm^3 for G-CRF (green) and D-CRF (blue) is shown for the three different tumor regions on data of 25 patients of a local university hospital. (Color figure online)

presents the volumetric error for the three tumor regions on the data of the local university hospital. The median and interquartile range of the Dice-coefficients estimated for D-CRF for the BRATS 2015 testing set are (0.847, 0.131), (0.647, 0.258) and (0.7, 0.349) for complete tumor, tumor core and enhancing tumor, respectively.

4 Discussion and Future Work

In this work, we studied the impact of the shrinking bias on brain tumor segmentation. The shrinking bias is caused by a combination of a limited neighborhood system and the usage of a Potts prior. The Potts prior encourages smooth boundaries which in grid-structured CRFs results in an oversmoothing of the object boundary. It is important to mention that different approaches have been proposed to alleviate the shrinking bias of pairwise CRFs [5,9,14,19]. They all share the goal of overcoming the limitation of grid-structured pairwise CRFs to express high-level dependencies among pixels/voxels. The proposed dense CRF model showed an improved overall performance for the complete tumor and enhancing tumor segmentation compared to a grid-structured pairwise CRF. This improvement can be attributed to the alleviation of the shrinking bias inherent to pairwise CRFs [8]. A precise delineation of tumor regions is of great importance for the emerging field of radiomics [18,22] in order to ensure the quality of extracted imaging biomarkers. The dense CRF is capable of recovering fine details (cf. Fig. 2 D-CRF, e.g. rim-enhancing tumor) as well as concave object boundaries (e.g. finger-like edematous regions) that otherwise would be smoothed out by a grid-structured pairwise CRF. The local clinical data set was acquired with a higher resolution than the BRATS data, which led to a more detailed imaging of the tumor and thus to a more significant improvement in performance for D-CRF. However, for segmenting the rather convex-shaped tumor core, oversmoothing of a grid-structured CRF can lead to better results. In case of the leaderboard data set D-CRF attained a less consistent improvement for the enhancing tumor. This can be at least partially attributed to an increased number of small false positives distant to the tumor (e.g. vessels), which in case of G-CRF were smoothed. In the future, we plan on further improving our approach by employing a richer prior combined with a parameter learning method [7,13].

Acknowledgments. This project has received funding from the European Unions Seventh Framework Programme for research, technological development and demonstration under grant agreement N°600841.

References

1. Bauer, S., Fejes, T., Reyes, M.: A skull-stripping filter for ITK. Insight J. 1–7 (2012). http://hdl.handle.net/10380/3353
2. Criminisi, A., Shotton, J.: Decision Forests for Computer Vision and Medical Image Analysis. Springer, Heidelberg (2013)

3. von Deimling, A.: Gliomas. Recent Results in Cancer Research, vol. 171. Springer, Heidelberg (2009). http://link.springer.com/10.1007/978-3-540-31206-2
4. Ellingson, B.M., Bendszus, M., Boxerman, J., Barboriak, D., Erickson, B.J., Smits, M., Nelson, S.J., Gerstner, E., Alexander, B., Goldmacher, G., Wick, W., Vogelbaum, M., Weller, M., Galanis, E., Kalpathy-Cramer, J., Shankar, L., Jacobs, P., Pope, W.B., Yang, D., Chung, C., Knopp, M.V., Cha, S., Van Den Bent, M.J., Chang, S., Al Yung, W.K., Cloughesy, T.F., Wen, P.Y., Gilbert, M.R., Whitney, A., Sandak, D., Musella, A., Haynes, C., Wallace, M., Arons, D.F., Kingston, A.: Consensus recommendations for a standardized brain tumor imaging protocol in clinical trials. Neuro Oncol. **17**(9), 1188–1198 (2015)
5. Kohli, P., Ladický, L., Torr, P.H.S.: Robust higher order potentials for enforcing label consistency. Int. J. Comput. Vis. **82**(3), 302–324 (2009)
6. Komodakis, N., Tziritas, G.: Approximate labeling via graph cuts based on linear programming. IEEE Trans. Pattern Anal. Mach. Intell. **29**(8), 1436–1453 (2007)
7. Kraehenbuehl, P., Koltun, V.: Parameter learning and convergent inference for dense random fields. In: Proceedings of the 30th International Conference on Machine Learning (ICML 2013), vol. 28, pp. 513–521 (2013). http://machinelearning.wustl.edu/mlpapers/papers/icml2013_kraehenbuehl13
8. Krähenbühl, P., Koltun, V.: Efficient inference in fully connected CRFS with Gaussian edge potentials. In: NIPS 2011, pp. 109–117 (2011). http://arxiv.org/abs/1210.5644
9. Ladick, L.U., Russell, C., Kohli, P., Torr, P.H.S.: Associative hierarchical CRFs for object class image segmentation. In: ICCV (2009). http://cms.brookes.ac.uk/research/visiongroup/, http://research.microsoft.com/en-us/um/people/pkohli/
10. Meier, R., Bauer, S., Slotboom, J., Wiest, R., Reyes, M.: Appearance-and context-sensitive features for brain tumor segmentation. In: MICCAI BRATS Challenge (2014)
11. Menze, B.H., Jakab, A., Bauer, S., Kalpathy-Cramer, J., Farahani, K., Kirby, J., Burren, Y., Porz, N., Slotboom, J., Wiest, R., Lanczi, L., Gerstner, E., Weber, M.A., Arbel, T., Avants, B.B., Ayache, N., Buendia, P., Louis Collins, D., Cordier, N., Corso, J.J., Criminisi, A., Das, T., Delingette, H., Demiralp, G., Durst, C.R., Dojat, M., Doyle, S., Festa, J., Forbes, F., Geremia, E., Glocker, B., Golland, P., Guo, X., Hamamci, A., Iftekharuddin, K.M., Jena, R., John, N.M., Konukoglu, E., Lashkari, D., António Mariz, J., Meier, R., Pereira, S., Precup, D., Price, S.J., Riklin Raviv, T., Reza, S.M., Ryan, M., Sarikaya, D., Schwartz, L., Shin, H.C., Shotton, J., Silva, C.A., Sousa, N., Subbanna, N.K., Szekely, G., Taylor, T.J., Thomas, O.M., Tustison, N.J., Unal, G., Vasseur, F., Wintermark, M., Hye Ye, D., Zhao, L., Zhao, B., Zikic, D., Prastawa, M., Reyes, M., Van Leemput, K., Golland, P., Lashkari, D., Guo, X., Schwartz, L., Zhao, B.: The multimodal brain tumor image segmentation benchmark (BRATS). TMI **34**, 1993–2024 (2015). http://www.ieee.org/publications_standards/publications/rights/index.html
12. Nyul, L.G., Udupa, J.K., Zhang, X.: New variants of a method of MRI scale standardization. IEEE Trans. Med. Imaging **19**(2), 143–150 (2000)
13. Orlando, J., Prokofyeva, E., Blaschko, M.: A discriminatively trained fully connected conditional random field model for blood vessel segmentation in fundus images. IEEE Trans. Biomed. Eng. 1 (2016). http://ieeexplore.ieee.org/lpdocs/epic03/wrapper.htm?arnumber=7420682
14. Pantofaru, C., Schmid, C., Hebert, M.: Object recognition by integrating multiple image segmentations. In: Forsyth, D., Torr, P., Zisserman, A. (eds.) ECCV 2008. LNCS, vol. 5304, pp. 481–494. Springer, Heidelberg (2008). doi:10.1007/978-3-540-88690-7_36

15. Pope, W.B., Sayre, J., Perlina, A., Villablanca, J.P., Mischel, P.S., Cloughesy, T.F.: MR imaging correlates of survival in patients with high-grade gliomas. Am. J. Neuroradiol. **26**(10), 2466–2474 (2005)
16. Porz, N., Bauer, S., Pica, A., Schucht, P., Beck, J., Verma, R.K., Slotboom, J., Reyes, M., Wiest, R.: Multi-modal glioblastoma segmentation: man versus machine. PLoS ONE **9**(5), e96873 (2014)
17. R Core Team: R: A language and environment for statistical computing (2013). http://www.r-project.org/
18. Rios Velazquez, E., Meier, R., Dunn, W., Alexander, B., Wiest, R., Bauer, S., Gutman, D., Reyes, M., Aerts, H.: Fully automatic GBM segmentation in the TCGA-GBM dataset: prognosis and correlation with VASARI features. Sci. Rep. **42**(6), 3589 (2015). http://www.ncbi.nlm.nih.gov/pubmed/26128818
19. Shelhamer, E., Jegelka, S., Darrell, T.: Communal cuts : sharing cuts across images. In: NIPS Workshop on Discrete and Combinatorial Problems in Machine Learning (DISCML), pp. 1–6 (2014)
20. Tustison, N.J., Avants, B.B.: Cook, P.A., Zheng, Y., Egan, A., Yushkevich, P.A., Gee, J.C.: N4ITK: improved N3 bias correction. IEEE Trans. Med. Imaging **29**(6), 1310–1320 (2010)
21. Wang, C., Komodakis, N., Paragios, N.: Markov random field modeling, inference & learning in computer vision & image understanding: a survey. Comput. Vis. Image Underst. **117**(11), 1610–1627 (2013). http://dx.doi.org/10.1016/j.cviu.2013.07.004
22. Yip, S.S.F., Aerts, H.J.W.L.: Applications and limitations of radiomics. Phys. Med. Biol. **61**(13), R150–R166 (2016). http://stacks.iop.org/0031-9155/61/i=13/a=R150?key=crossref.134478778713970aff90f16abe110608/, http://www.ncbi.nlm.nih.gov/pubmed/27269645/, http://www.pubmedcentral.nih.gov/articlerender.fcgi?artid=PMC4927328

Fully Convolutional Deep Residual Neural Networks for Brain Tumor Segmentation

Peter D. Chang[✉]

Department of Radiology, Columbia University Medical Center,
New York City, NY, USA
pdc9002@nyp.org

Abstract. In this paper, a fully convolutional residual neural network (FCR-NN) based on linear identity mappings is implemented for medical image segmentation, employed here in the setting of brain tumors. Inspired by deep residual networks which won the ImageNet ILSVRC 2015 classification challenge, the FCR-NN combines optimization gains from residual identity mappings with a fully convolutional architecture for image segmentation that efficiently accounts for both low- and high-level image features. After training two separate networks, one for the task of whole tumor segmentation and a second for tissue sub-region segmentation, the serial FCR-NN architecture exceeds state-of-the art with complete tumor, core tumor and enhancing tumor validation Dice scores of 0.87, 0.81 and 0.72 respectively. Despite each FCR-NN comprising a complex 22 layer architecture, the fully convolutional design allows for complete segmentation of a tumor volume within 2 s.

1 Introduction

In recent years, convolutional neural networks (CNN) have become the technique of choice for state-of-the-art implementations in various image classification tasks [1–5]. In this study a novel fully convolutional residual neural network (FCR-NN) architecture is proposed for medical image segmentation synthesizing several recently described techniques including: (1) deep residual learning; (2) multi-resolution recursive topology; and (3) fully convolutional neural network architecture.

1.1 Deep Residual Learning

Deep residual learning [4] posits that any traditional neural network layer may be reformulated as a residual function by means of a linear transformation identity mapping with respect to the layer input:

$$x_L = W x_l + f(x_l) \qquad (1)$$

Here the output layer, x_L, is the sum of x_l, the input layer, and $f(x_l)$, a residual change from the original input represented by an arbitrary sequence of non-linear

© Springer International Publishing AG 2016
A. Crimi et al. (Eds.): BrainLes 2016, LNCS 10154, pp. 108–118, 2016.
DOI: 10.1007/978-3-319-55524-9_11

functions. The projection matrix, W, is an optional term to match input and output layer dimensions. By preserving a linear relationship between the input and output layers, residual neural networks are able to stabilize gradients during backpropagation, leading to improved optimization and facilitating greater network depth. Networks based on this residual architecture have achieved top results in the ImageNet ILSVRC 2015 international challenge.

Image Segmentation Adaptation. In this study we hypothesize that the image segmentation problem can be similarly reformulated as a residual function, such that the final classification labels can be derived from a simple linear combination between the original input image, x_l, and some arbitrary residual, $f(x_l)$. In addition to the advantages for optimization and network depth described above, this architecture benefits from using the original input image directly in the final classification task. This latter proposition may be counterintuitive at first; in fact a widely help assumption is that the raw image inputs contain too much inherent noise and variation to be useful directly for classification. However unique to medical image segmentation is that after accounting for high-level contextual anatomic cues, final segmentation is heavily influenced by low-level features of the original image, namely the signal intensity of any given voxel. For this reason we hypothesize that a deep residual architecture may be optimally suited for the medical image segmentation task.

1.2   Residual Functions for Multi-resolution Features

It is well-established that for the task of object localization a synthesis of contextual cues at multiple spatial resolutions is required for optimal performance [3,6,7]. For neural networks this has been implemented by combining feature maps from various layers, with the convolutional transpose operation used to upsample high-order deep layer activations to match those of more superficial layers [8]. Ronneberger et al. [9] further elaborated on this technique by proposing a symmetric contracting and expanding topology that efficiently combines low- and high-level features.

This study reformulates the latter strategy in the form of residual functions. Specifically, from Eq. (1) above, an explicit definition is made such that the residual function, f_l, represents some arbitrary nonlinear transformation performed on the original image, x_l, that captures its higher-level features and which is subsequently combined with its original lower-level properties. A more precise formulation of the higher-level feature map, x_{l+1}, is given by:

$$x_{l+1} = \sigma_l(x_l) \tag{2}$$

Here $\sigma_l(x_l)$ represents a sequence of convolutions and nonlinear activation functions which act to transform the original image, x_l, to its higher-level feature map, x_{l+1}. As a result, the original function f_l in Eq. (1) which was defined in the previous paragraph as the residua arising from the influence of higher-level features can be written as:

$$f_l(x_l) = x_{l+1} + f_{l+1}(x_{l+1}) = \sigma_l(x_l) + f_{l+1}(\sigma_l(x_l)) \tag{3}$$

Here f_{l+1} is a new residual function which like its predecessor represents an incremental change arising from the influence of even higher-level features from the first feature map x_{l+1}. Expanding Eq. (1) recursively allows us to formulate the neural network for image segmentation as a simple series of residual functions, each term of which represents the additional incremental change of gradually higher-level spatial features:

$$x_L = Wx_l + f_l(x_l) = Wx_l + \sigma_l(x_l) + \sigma_{l+1}(\sigma_l(x_l)) + ... \tag{4}$$

The formulations as described by Eqs. (3) and (4) are visually demonstrated in Fig. 1.

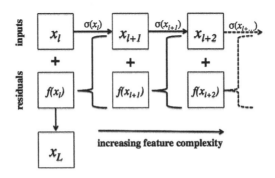

Fig. 1. Recursive series of residual functions for image segmentation.

1.3 Fully Convolutional Neural Networks

Originally introduced by Long et al. [8] fully convolutional neural networks are implemented by a series of upsampling convolutional transpose operators performed on the deepest network layers, resulting in a final dense classification matrix equal in dimension to the original image size for each forward pass. In contradistinction to the typical sliding window CNN approach for image segmentation [10–12], a fully convolutional architecture is highly efficient. In the proposed FCR-NN where an entire axial MR slice is used as the input image, the number of required forward passes for classification of each patient is equal only to the number of slices in the MR volume, a task that can be achieved in less than a few seconds on a GPU optimized workstation.

Several additional less apparent benefits from fully convolutional neural networks include: (1) increased inherent regularization; and (2) influence of per voxel classification from a larger field-of-view. The first effect relating to increased regularization arises from observation that the loss function for each forward/backward pass is derived from contributions at each voxel within the input image. In this specific example with an input image size of 240×240 voxels, the loss function is thus driven by 240^2 derivatives per slice. Furthermore the ratio of different tissue classes is reflected accurately by the conglomerate of axial slices in each mini-batch, and thus there is no requirement for multiphase training to account for class imbalances as is typically the case for non-fully convolutional designs [10].

Secondly, compared to a sliding scale CNN design whereby classification is limited to a small input patch, a fully convolutional network allows voxel-wise prediction to be influenced by a larger field-of-view proportional to the network depth. This effect is further complemented by the fact that residual networks allow for relatively deep architectures. In the proposed FCR-NN, convolution of the deepest 15×15 feature map with a series of three 3×3 kernels results in an effective receptive field that covers nearly one quarter (7×7) of the feature map.

2   Related Work

Despite significant research over the past several decades, brain tumor segmentation remains a challenging task. Common strategies cited in the literature include: edge-based methods including active contours [13]; region-based methods [14]; classification or clustering methods with constraints based on atlases [15,16], deformable models [17] or neighborhood regularization [18]; or hybrid generative-discriminative frameworks [19–24]. However these traditional methods are limited to a priori assumptions about a set of rules or features that best model the segmentation mask.

Convolutional neural networks are an emerging technique in computer vision increasingly recognized as the state-of-the-art approach for various image recognition tasks [25]. The power of neural networks arises from its unique capacity for unsupervised feature extraction, independently learning a high-order representation of the data that best approximates any given problem. In recent years, CNN-based algorithms have been adopted for various medical image segmentation tasks [1–5,9]. In the BRaTS 2015 challenge, the 2nd [26] and 4th [10] ranked submissions were based on CNN architectures.

3   Network Architecture

A fully convolutional residual neural network (FCR-NN) is proposed for medical image segmentation. The network is composed by a series of recursive residual identity mapping blocks, the prototype of which is shown in Fig. 1.

The network comprises a total of 22 layers (18 regular convolutional kernels and 4 upsampling convolutional transpose kernels) and 661,700 parameters. The entire network architecture for a given single FCR-NN is diagrammed in Fig. 2.

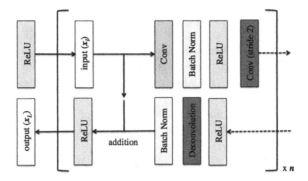

Fig. 2. Residual identity mapping blocks for image segmentation.

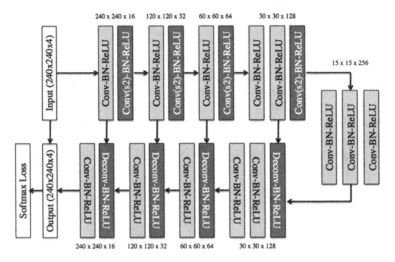

Fig. 3. Fully convolutional residual neural network (FCR-NN) architecture for image segmentation. Abbreviations: Conv = 3×3 convolution; Conv(s2) = 3×3 convolution with stride 2 (downsample); Deconv = 2×2 deconvolution (upsample); BN = batch normalization; ReLU = rectified linear unit

3.1 Fully Convolutional Residual Neural Networks

Convolutional Neural Networks. CNNs are an adaptation of the traditional artificial neural network architecture whereby stacks of 4D convolutional kernels and nonlinear activation functions act to transform a multidimensional input image into progressively higher-order feature representations [27]. The proposed CNN is implemented completely by 3×3 convolutional kernels to prevent overfitting as described by [2]. No pooling layers are used; instead downsampling is implemented simply by means of a 3×3 convolutional kernel with stride length of 2 to decrease the feature maps by 75% in size. All nonlinear functions are modeled by the rectified linear unit (ReLU) [28]. Batch normalization is used between the convolutional and ReLU layers to limit drift of layer activations during train- ing [29]. In successively deeper layers the number of feature channels gradually increases from 16, 32, 64, 128 and 256, reflecting increasing representational complexity.

Deconvolutions. To upsample each high-level feature map, a deconvolutional or convolutional transpose operator is implemented by means of a 2×2 kernel with a stride length of 2, resulting in an increase in feature map by 75%. At the same time, the number of feature channels is reduced by 50% to match the corresponding activation layer in the mirror image pathway (Figs. 2 and 3).

Residual Connections. As shown in Fig. 2 residual identity mappings are imple- mented by means of a channel-wise addition operation between an input and its corresponding deconvoluted feature map with the same activation layer size. The addition operation is performed after batch normalization of the deconvoluted output but before the nonlinear ReLU activation as suggested by [4].

3.2   Serial Architecture

The task of brain tumor segmentation as defined in the BRATS challenge can be divided into two corresponding goals. The first task is in differentiating between normal and abnormal brain tissue (whole tumor segmentation). Subsequently, using this result as an input, the second task is differentiate between various brain tumor tissue types. This process is diagrammed in Fig. 4.

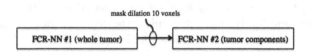

Fig. 4. Implementation of serial fully convolutional residual neural networks (FCR-NN) for the two-part segmentation task.

As shown in the figure, these tasks are learned independently by two separate FCR-NNs. During test time, the segmentation mask generated from the first FCR-NN is dilated by 10 voxels; all voxels outside of this mask are set to 0 and the resulting masked image is used as an input for the second FCR-NN. By separating out these tasks explicitly, the two separate neural networks can be independently optimized for the highest performance for each respective goal.

3.3   Training Details

Image Preprocessing. Each MR volume was normalized simply to a mean signal intensity of 0.5 and standard deviation of 1/6 such that the range [0, 1] con- tains three standard deviations in each direction from the mean. No other image preprocessing was necessary.

Data Augmentation. Given the relatively limited training dataset available for the BRATS 2016 challenge, and more generally in the realm of medical imaging where annotated datasets are rare, judicious use of data augmentation is critical for successful CNN implementation. In this study two primary forms of data augmentation are employed. First, a separate cohort of IRB-approved patients at our institution with annotations by a board-certified radiologist were included to increase the breadth of data available for training. Importantly, these included a large number of patients with suboptimal brain extraction and/or significant imaging artifact. In addition, this institutional dataset was predominantly acquired at 3-Tesla MR imaging which, although yields higher sensitivity to pathology, also results in increased image noise and decreased contrast resolution particularly on T2-FLAIR sequences. It is important to point out that upon visual inspection, the test set for the 2016 BRaTS challenge compromised of a disproportionate of 3-Tesla MR imaging relative to the training data available online.

The second type of data augmentation employed by this study involves a number of real-time modifications to the source images at the time of training. Specifically, 50% of all images in a mini-batch were modified randomly by means of: (1) addition across all voxels of a scalar between $[-0.1, 0.1]$; (2) rotation of the image at an angle between $45°$ to $45°$; (3) addition of a bias field gradient of strength between $[0, 0.4]$ at a random angle between $0°$ and $360°$.

Training Parameters. Training is implemented using standard stochastic gradient descent technique with Nesterov momentum [30]. Parameters are initialized using the heuristic described by He et al. [31]. L2 regularization is implemented to prevent over-fitting of data by limiting the squared magnitude of the kernel weights. To account for training dynamics, the learning rate is annealed and the mini-batch size is increased whenever training loss plateaus. Furthermore a normalized gradient algorithm is employed to allow for locally adaptive learning rates that adjust according to changes in the input signal [32].

Implementation. Software code for this study was written in Matlab (R2016a), and benefited greatly from the MatConvNet toolbox [33]. Experiments were performed on a GPU-optimized workstation with a single NVIDIA GeForce GTX Titan X (12 GB). The combined software and hardware configurations allowed for test time (forward pass only) classification of approximately 155.1 images per second. An entire brain volume with 151 axial slices could be classified in approximately 1.94 s (two cumulative forward passes for serial FCR-NNs).

4   Experiments and Results

All 274 cases of gliomas (220 high-grade gliomas; 54 low-grade gliomas) in the BRaTS 2016 training set were included in this study. An additional 150 institutional cases with high-grade gliomas were included to augment the available training data, all acquired on 3T MR scanners. A total of 186 cases in the

BRaTS 2016 database (132/220 high-grade gliomas; 54/54 low-grade gliomas) and 84 institutional cases represented treatment naive (preoperative) tumors. The remaining cases were obtained at various postoperative time points.

Eighty percent of the cases (n = 339) were randomly assigned to the training data set, with the remaining 20% of the cases (n = 85) used as an independent validation set. All four channels (FLAIR, T1-precontrast, T1-postcontrast, T2) across an entire axial cross-sectional image slice ($240 \times 240 \times 4$ voxels) were used as inputs into the FCR-NN.

Dice scores and Hausdorff distances (mean and range) for the validation set data are reported in Table 1. The results are competitive with historic trends, and finished overall tied for the top two in the BRaTS 2016 challenge.

Table 1. Validation set dice score and Hausdorff distances.

	Complete tumor	Core tumor	Enhancing tumor
Dice	0.89(0.76–0.95)	0.83(0.68–0.91)	0.78(0.41–0.89)
Hausdorff(mm)	8.0(3.0–27)	10.0(4.2–27)	5.9(3.3–21)

Acknowledging limitations in direct comparison with the top four performing algorithms in the BRaTS 2015 challenge due to differences in validation data cited in published results (2013 BRaTS training set in [10, 34]; partial 2015 BRaTS training set in [23]; full 2015 BRaTS training set in [26] which is identical to the 2016 BRaTS training set used in this study), several general patterns can nonetheless be seen. With regards to complete tumor segmentation, the FCR-NN Dice of 0.89 is only marginally better than the previous top four algorithms (0.86–0.88). However given that expert human rater agreement for complete tumor segmentation is reported to be between 0.85–0.91 [35] this metric is likely approaching a plateau for theoretical upper limits of accuracy. By contrast, the much more visually challenging task of separating tumor subcomponents remains to be fully solved. In this case the FCR-NN approach yields a more significant improvement both in Dice score for core tumor (0.83 vs. 0.73–0.79 for previous top performing algorithms) and enhancing tumor (0.78 vs. 0.59–0.73). This is likely in part secondary to a serial architecture which dedicates an entire separate CNN to identification of tumor subcomponents (thus isolating the task from a second CNN that is responsible just for identifying tumor margins).

5   Conclusion

The proposed serial FCR-NN architecture implemented here in the setting of brain tumors is a robust method for medical image segmentation incorporating contextual cues from multiple spatial resolutions. The residual linear transformation identity mappings facilitate optimization and allow for direct contributions from the original input images for final classification. The fully convolutional architecture results in an efficient classifier which can segment an entire tumor volume in less than 3 s with state-of-the-art accuracy.

Acknowledgments. The author of this paper gratefully acknowledges the support of NVIDIA Corporation with the donation of GeForce GTX Titan X (12 GB) GPU used for this research.

References

1. Krizhevsky, A., Sutskever, I., Hinton, G.E.: ImageNet classification with deep convolutional neural networks (2012)
2. Simonyan, K., Vedaldi, A., Zisserman, A.: Networks, deep inside convolutional: visualising image classification models and saliency maps. In: ICLR, p. 1 (2014)
3. Szegedy, C., Liu, W., Jia, Y., Sermanet, P., Reed, S., Anguelov, D., Erhan, D., Vanhoucke, V., Rabinovich, A.: Going deeper with convolutions. In: Proceedings of the IEEE Computer Society Conference on Computer Vision and Pattern Recognition, 07–12 June, 1–9 Sep 2015 (2015)
4. He, K., Zhang, X., Ren, S., Sun, J.: Deep residual learning for image recognition. **7**(3), 171–180 (2015). Arxiv.Org
5. Ciresan, D., Giusti, A.: Deep neural networks segment neuronal membranes in electron microscopy images. In: Advances in Neural Information Processing Systems, pp. 1–9 (2012)
6. Yang, S., Ramanan, D.: Multi-scale recognition with DAG-CNNs (2015)
7. Girshick, R., Donahue, J., Darrell, T., Malik, J.: Rich feature hierarchies for accurate object detection and semantic segmentation (2014)
8. Long, J., Shelhamer, E., Darrell, T.: Fully convolutional networks for semantic segmentation. In: 2015 IEEE Conference on Computer Vision and Pattern Recognition (CVPR), pp. 3431–3440 (2014)
9. Ronneberger, O., Fischer, P., Brox, T.: U-Net: convolutional networks for biomedical image segmentation. In: Navab, N., Hornegger, J., Wells, W.M., Frangi, A.F. (eds.) MICCAI 2015. LNCS, vol. 9351, pp. 234–241. Springer, Cham (2015). doi:10.1007/978-3-319-24574-4_28
10. Havaei, M., Davy, A., Warde-Farley, D., Biard, A., Courville, A., Bengio, Y., Pal, C., Jodoin, P.-M., Larochelle, H.: Brain tumor segmentation with deep neural networks. In: Proceedings of MICCAI-BRATS (Multimodal Brain Tumor Segmentation Challenge), pp. 29–33 (2015)
11. Kleesiek, J., Urban, G., Hubert, A., Schwarz, D., Maier-hein, K., Bendszus, M., Biller, A.: NeuroImage deep MRI brain extraction: a 3D convolutional neural network for skull stripping. NeuroImage **129**, 460–469 (2016)
12. Chen, H., Dou, Q., Yu, L., Heng, P.-A.: VoxResNet: deep voxelwise residual networks for volumetric brain segmentation, pp. 1–9 (2016). arXiv:1608.05895v1
13. Sachdeva, J., Kumar, V., Gupta, I., Khandelwal, N., Ahuja, C.K.: A novel content-based active contour model for brain tumor segmentation. Magn. Reson. Imaging **30**(5), 694–715 (2012)
14. Harati, V., Khayati, R., Farzan, A.: Fully automated tumor segmentation based on improved fuzzy connectedness algorithm in brain MR images. Comput. Biol. Med. **41**(7), 483–492 (2011)
15. Prastawa, M., Bullitt, E., Gerig, G.: Simulation of brain tumors in MR images for evaluation of segmentation efficacy. Med. Image Anal. **13**(2), 297–311 (2009)

16. Menze, B.H., Leemput, K., Lashkari, D., Weber, M.-A., Ayache, N., Golland, P.: A generative model for brain tumor segmentation in multi-modal images. In: Jiang, T., Navab, N., Pluim, J.P.W., Viergever, M.A. (eds.) MICCAI 2010. LNCS, vol. 6362, pp. 151–159. Springer, Heidelberg (2010). doi:10.1007/978-3-642-15745-5_19

17. Hamamci, A., Kucuk, N., Karaman, K., Engin, K., Unal, G.: Tumor - cut: segmentation of brain tumors on contrast enhanced MR images for radiosurgery applications. IEEE Trans. Med. Imaging **31**(3), 790–804 (2012)

18. Zhu, Y., Young, G.S., Xue, Z., Huang, R.Y., You, H., Setayesh, K., Hatabu, H., Cao, F., Wong, S.T.: Semi-automatic segmentation software for quantitative clinical brain glioblastoma evaluation. Acad. Radiol. **19**(8), 977–85 (2012)

19. Menze, B.H., Geremia, E., Ayache, N., Szekely, G.: Segmenting glioma in multimodal images using a generative-discriminative model for brain lesion segmentation. In: Proceedings of MICCAI-BRATS (Multimodal Brain Tumor Segmentation Challenge), p. 7 (2012)

20. Meier, R., Reyes, M., Bauer, S., Slotboom, J., Wiest, R.: A hybrid model for multimodal brain tumor segmentation. In: Proceedings of NCI-MICCAI BRATS (Multimodal Brain Tumor Segmentation Challenge), pp. 31–37 (2013)

21. Bakas, S., Zeng, K., Sotiras, A., Rathore, S., Akbari, H., Gaonkar, B., Rozycki, M., Pati, S., Davatzikos, C.: Segmentation of gliomas in multimodal magnetic resonance imaging volumes based on a hybrid generative - discriminative framework. In: Proceedings of MICCAI-BRATS (Multimodal Brain Tumor Segmentation Challenge), pp. 5–12 (2015)

22. Menze, B.H., Van Leemput, K., Lashkari, D., Riklin-Raviv, T., Geremia, E., Alberts, E., Gruber, P., Wegener, S., Weber, M.-A., Szekely, G., Ayache, N., Golland, P.: A generative probabilistic model and discriminative extensions for brain lesion segmentation with application to tumor and stroke. IEEE Trans. Med. Imaging **35**(4), 933–946 (2016)

23. Bakas, S., et al.: GLISTRboost: combining multimodal MRI segmentation, registration, and biophysical tumor growth modeling with gradient boosting machines for glioma segmentation. In: Crimi, A., Menze, B., Maier, O., Reyes, M., Handels, H. (eds.) BrainLes 2015. LNCS, vol. 9556, pp. 144–155. Springer, Cham (2016). doi:10.1007/978-3-319-30858-6_13

24. Zeng, J., See, A.P., Phallen, J., Jackson, C.M., Belcaid, Z., Ruzevick, J., Durham, N., Meyer, C., Harris, T.J., Albesiano, E., Pradilla, G., Ford, E., Wong, J., Hammers, H.-J., Mathios, D., Tyler, B., Brem, H., Tran, P.T., Pardoll, D., Drake, C.G., Lim, M.: Anti-PD-1 blockade and stereotactic radiation produce long-term survival in mice with intracranial gliomas. Int. J. Rad. Oncol. Biol. Phys. **86**(2), 343–349 (2013)

25. LeCun, Y., Bengio, Y., Hinton, G.: Deep learning. Nature **521**(7553), 436–444 (2015)

26. Pereira, S., Pinto, A., Alves, V., Silva, C.A.: Deep convolutional neural networks for the segmentation of gliomas in multi-sequence MRI. In: Crimi, A., Menze, B., Maier, O., Reyes, M., Handels, H. (eds.) BrainLes 2015. LNCS, vol. 9556, pp. 131–143. Springer, Cham (2016). doi:10.1007/978-3-319-30858-6_12

27. Lecun, Y., Bengio, Y.: Convolutional networks for images, speech, and time-series (1995)

28. Nair, V., Hinton, G.E.: Rectified linear units improve restricted boltzmann machines (2010)

29. Ioffe, S., Szegedy, C.: Batch normalization: accelerating deep network training by reducing internal covariate shift, pp. 1–11 (2015). arXiv:1502.03167

30. Bengio, Y., Boulanger-Lewandowski, N., Pascanu, R.: Advances in optimizing recurrent networks. In: ICASSP, IEEE International Conference on Acoustics, Speech and Signal Processing - Proceedings, pp. 8624–8628 (2013)
31. He, K., Zhang, X., Ren, S., Sun, J.: Delving deep into rectifiers: surpassing human-level performance on imagenet classification (2015)
32. Mandic, D.P.: A generalized normalized gradient descent algorithm. IEEE Signal Process. Lett. **11**(2), 115–118 (2004)
33. Vedaldi, A., Lenc, K.: MatConvNet. In: Proceedings of the 23rd ACM International Conference on Multimedia - MM 2015, pp. 689–692 (2015)
34. Agn, M., Puonti, O., Rosenschöld, P.M., Law, I., Leemput, K.: Brain tumor segmentation using a generative model with an RBM prior on tumor shape. In: Crimi, A., Menze, B., Maier, O., Reyes, M., Handels, H. (eds.) BrainLes 2015. LNCS, vol. 9556, pp. 168–180. Springer, Cham (2016). doi:10.1007/978-3-319-30858-6_15
35. Menze, B.H., Jakab, A., Bauer, S., Kalpathy-Cramer, J., Farahani, K., Kirby, J., Burren, Y., Porz, N., Slotboom, J., Wiest, R., Lanczi, L., Gerstner, E., Weber, M.A., Arbel, T., Avants, B.B., Ayache, N., Buendia, P., Collins, D.L., Cordier, N., Corso, J.J., Criminisi, A., Das, T., Delingette, H., Demiralp, Ç., Durst, C.R., Dojat, M., Doyle, S., Festa, J., Forbes, F., Geremia, E., Glocker, B., Golland, P., Guo, X., Hamamci, A., Iftekharuddin, K.M., Jena, R., John, N.M., Konukoglu, E., Lashkari, D., Mariz, J.A., Meier, R., Pereira, S., Precup, D., Price, S.J., Raviv, T.R., Reza, S.M.S., Ryan, M., Sarikaya, D., Schwartz, L., Shin, H.C., Shotton, J., Silva, C.A., Sousa, N., Subbanna, N.K., Szekely, G., Taylor, T.J., Thomas, O.M., Tustison, N.J., Unal, G., Vasseur, F., Wintermark, M., Ye, D.H., Zhao, L., Zhao, B., Zikic, D., Prastawa, M., Reyes, M., Leemput, K.V.: The multimodal brain tumor image segmentation benchmark (BRATS). IEEE Trans. Med. Imaging **34**(10), 1993–2024 (2015)

Nabla-net: A Deep Dag-Like Convolutional Architecture for Biomedical Image Segmentation

Richard McKinley[1]([✉]), Rik Wepfer[1], Tom Gundersen[2], Franca Wagner[1], Andrew Chan[3], Roland Wiest[1], and Mauricio Reyes[4]

[1] Department of Diagnostic and Interventional Neuroradiology, Inselspital,
University of Bern, Bern, Switzerland
richard.mcKinley@gmail.com
[2] Red Hat AB, Oslo, Norway
[3] University Clinic for Neurology, Inselspital, University of Bern, Bern, Switzerland
[4] Institute for Surgical Technology and Biomechanics,
University of Bern, Bern, Switzerland

Abstract. Biomedical image segmentation requires both voxel-level information and global context. We report on a deep convolutional architecture which combines a fully-convolutional network for local features and an encoder-decoder network in which convolutional layers and max-pooling compute high-level features, which are then upsampled to the resolution of the initial image using further convolutional layers and tied unpooling. We apply the method to segmenting multiple sclerosis lesions and gliomas.

1 Introduction

Medical image segmentation is a fundamental problem in biomedical image computing. Manual segmentation of medical images is both time-consuming and prone to substantial inter-rater error: automated techniques offer the potential for robust, repeatable and fast image segmentation.

In the past few years, neural networks have returned to the fore as the most promising technique for supervised machine learning (LeCun et al. 2015). In particular, convolutional neural networks have dominated the field of image recognition. More recently, techniques for image recognition have been reworked to object location and segmentation. One recurring theme is that segmentation requires a combination of low-level and high-level features, with several techniques and architectures having been suggested for upscaling and incorporating high-level with low-level features (Hariharan et al. 2015; Long et al. 2015; Ronneberger et al. 2015; Brosch et al. 2016).

In this paper, we introduce an architecture, called nabla net, for image segmentation, with application in the medical image segmentation domain. Nabla net is a dag-like deep neural network architecture, combining a fully-convolutional pathway learning low-level features and an encoder-decoder network learning high-level features. We describe the general features of nabla-net, its application to the segmentation of multiple sclerosis lesions, and its application to segmenting low- and high-grade gliomas.

© Springer International Publishing AG 2016
A. Crimi et al. (Eds.): BrainLes 2016, LNCS 10154, pp. 119–128, 2016.
DOI: 10.1007/978-3-319-55524-9_12

2   Method

2.1   Summary

The fundamental basis of nabla net is a deep encoder/decoder network, as described by Badrinarayanan et al. (2015). Such a network comprises a series of encoder layers, each of which reduces feature maps with higher spatial dimensions to feature maps with lower spatial dimension, followed by a series of decoder layers, which expand features with low spatial dimensions to features with high spatial dimensions. The goal of such an encoder-decoder pathway is to learn long-scale, global features of an image, and then reconstruct those features at the same resolution as the orinial image, to allow segmentation.

Concretely, the encoder-decoder pathway of the nabla net applied to a 256 * 256 image would compute in the first encoder layer a block of 256 * 256 feature maps, which are then reduced to 128 * 128 feature maps by maxpooling. This is repeated in encoder layer two, yielding 64 * 64 feature maps, and then one further time, yielding 32 * 32 feature maps.

These feature maps are then upscaled by decoder layers, yielding subsequently 64 * 64 feature maps, 64 128 * 128 feature maps, and finally 256 * 256 feature maps. The upscaling is performed by using "tied unpooling", as described below.

Such an encoder-decoder network can be trained to reconstruct the input image: in this case, the network would be called a "convolutional autoencoder". Autoencoders have been popular in the past as a method of unsupervised pretraining for image classification, but have largely fallen out of favour, as better methods of assigning network weights have emerged. In this case, we instead train the network to reproduce the MS lesion or Glioma segmentation.

The results of training a pure encoder-decoder network, as proposed by Badrinarayanan et al., on MS lesion data is shown in Fig. 1. The output provides a good localisation of the lesions, but is unable to provide crisp boundaries.

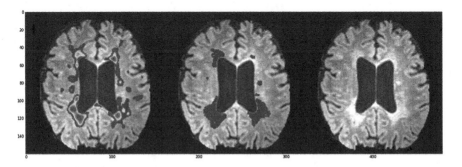

Fig. 1. Example raw output of the pure encoder-decoder network (Segnet), showing good localisation of the lesions but poor delineation. Left, posterior of the classifier, centre, manual delineation, right, FLAIR

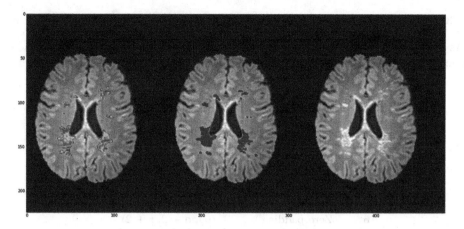

Fig. 2. Example raw output of Nabla net trained on axial FLAIR slices, showing improved lesion outline detection Left, posterior of the classifier, centre, manual delineation, right, FLAIR

Our hypothesis is that information regarding the boundaries of the lesions can be found in the initial block of 256 * 256 features, and for that reason, the final prediction of a nabla net is produced by combining the 256 * 256 layer arising from the first layer encoder layer with the 256 * 256 output of the final decoder layer. These feature maps are then processed by a final fully convolutional layer, before the final prediction of the lesion map is made. This ensures that a combination of low-level and high-level features are available for the prediction.

2.2 Techniques Used

To downscale feature maps, we make use of maxpooling (Jarrett et al. 2009), with non-overlapping pool size 2, in which the feature map is scaled by a factor of two in both dimensions, by replacing 2 by 2 patches with the maximum intensity in that patch. To scale up the feature maps, we use "tied unpooling" (Zeiler et al. 2011; Badrinarayanan et al. 2015). In tied unpooling an upscaling layer is linked with a maxpooling layer: for each feature to be upscaled, we associate a feature which was downscaled in the maxpooling layer, and the feature map is upscaled by filling only the positions of the maximums of the corresponding maxpooling layer. We use make use of batch normalization (Ioffe and Szegedy 2015) to accelerate the learning process. The architecture of the nabla net is fully convolutional, making no use of fully-connected layers, and as such it can be applied to any image with dimensions divisible by eight, this being enforced by the number of maxpooling steps.

2.3   The Nabla Net Architecture for MS Lesion Segmentation

As stated above, the nabla net is built from encode and decode layers. Each encode layer has the following structure:

Layer	Name	Dimension of output
1	Input	(p, q, r)
2	Zero padding	(64, q + 2, r + 2)
3	3 by 3 convolutional	(64, q, r)
4	Batch normalization	(64, q, r)
5	ReLu	(64, q, r)
6	Zero padding	(64, q + 2, r + 2)
7	3 by 3 convolutional	(64, q, r)
8	Batch normalization	(64, q, r)
9	ReLu	(64, q, r)

Each decode layer has the following structure

Layer	Name	Dimension of output
1	Input	(p, q, r)
2	Zero padding	(64, q + 2, r + 2)
3	3 by 3 convolutional	(64, q, r)
4	Batch normalization	(64, q, r)
5	Zero padding	(64, q + 2, r + 2)
6	3 by 3 convolutional	(64, q, r)
7	Batch normalization	(64, q, r)

The whole networks differed for the different application domains (MS and brain tumor) and will be described in the subsequent sections. In all cases, the networks were built using the Keras framework (https://github.com/fchollet/keras), and trained using Theano (http://deeplearning.net/software/theano) as a backend, using an Adadelta optimizer.

3   Multiple Sclerosis Lesion Segmentation (MSSEG Challenge)

MSSEG (https://portal.fli-iam.irisa.fr/msseg-challenge/overview) was a grand challenge at MICCAI 2016, the goal of which was to segment white-matter brain lesions in patients with multiple sclerosis. Fifteen training cases were made available, from three different scanner models. We developed a pipeline based on nabla net for addressing this problem.

The pipeline developed segments white-matter brain lesions from a skull-stripped 1 mm isovoxel FLAIR volume. The pipeline integrates three nabla net models: one segmenting lesions from axial slices, one segmenting from coronal slices, and one from saggital slices. This ensures that the segmentation given makes sense in three dimensions, without sacrificing the efficiency of 2d vs 3d convolutions. The "beliefs" (output of the logistic function in the final layer) of the three networks are averaged, and a final lesion mask extracted by a random walk segmentation starting from seeds with high belief (>0.5)

3.1 Architecture

Each network used on the MS dataset had the following architecture:

Layer	Name	Dimension of output	Comments
1	Input	(5, n * 8, m * 8)	Five slices, dimensions (n * 8, m * 8)
2	Encode 1	(64, n * 8, m * 8)	
3	Maxpool 1	(64, n * 4, m * 4)	
4	Encode 2	(64, n * 4, m * 4)	
5	Maxpool 2	(64, n * 2, m * 2)	
6	Encode 3	(64, n * 2, m * 2)	
7	Maxpool 3	(64, n, m)	
8	Encode 4	(64, n, m)	
9	Decode 4	(64, n, m)	
10	Unpool 3	(64, n * 2, m * 2)	Tied to maxpool 3
11	Decode 3	(64, n * 2, m * 2)	
12	Unpool 2	(64, n * 4, m * 4)	Tied to maxpool 2
13	Decode 2	(64, n * 4, m * 4)	
14	Unpool 1	(64, n * 8, m * 8)	Tied to maxpool 1
15	Merge	(128, n * 8, m * 8)	Concatenate the outputs of layers 2 and 14
16	Encode final	(64, n * 8, m * 8)	
17	1 * 1 convolutional	(1, n * 8, m * 8)	
18	Sigmoid	(1, n * 8, m * 8)	Loss = binary crossentropy

3.2 Experiments

Nabla Net Trained on Locally Sourced Data. As a first experiment to test generalisability of the method, a version of Nabla net was trained on skull-stripped 45 FLAIR images from the Inselspital. Segmentations of these cases were prepared by a medical student under supervision and revision of a neuro-radiologist with more than 15 years of experience in multiple sclerosis imaging (R.W.). Lesions were identified if appearing hyper-intense compared to the sur-rounding normal-appearing white matter on T2w and FLAIR. was applied to the MSSEG training cases, and achieved a mean Dice score of 0.67, and a standard deviation of 0.11.

Nabla Nets for the MSSEG Challenge. For the purposes of the MSSEG challenge, a new classifier was trained, only on the training data from that challenge. This was a substantially smaller training set (15 patients) and more heterogeneous than the Insel dataset (data from 3 scanner types, a mix of 1.5 and 3T and two different vendors, varying voxel sizes). To account for differences in scanner and sequence, we opted to train models not on raw data but on a set of pre-processed data provided by the competition organisers which had been skull-stripped and smoothed. To account for differences in voxel dimensions, all training examples were resampled to have 1 mm isovoxels using bicubic spline interpolation.

We trained three copies of nabla net, one for each of the three directions {axial, saggital, coronal}. The networks were trained on the unprocessed FLAIR data, resampled to isotropic 1 mm voxel spacing. Each training case comprised the data from five consecutive {axial, saggital, coronal} slices, with such a set of slices being included as training data if the middle slice contained voxels within the brain mask. Ground truth for such a set of slices was given by the lesion mask of the central slice: thus, the lesion mask of a slice was predicted from the slice itself and the four slices surrounding it. For each of the three models trained, one example from each scanner type was randomly selected, and the data from those cases used as validation data, to monitor for overfitting.

There was a substantial data imbalance between lesion and non-lesion pixels in the training data, owing not only to the size of the lesions, but also to the presence of pixels outside of the brain mask in the image. Since sampling the training data was not an option (as nabla net operates on whole slices), instead the individual voxels were weighted according to their importance to the model. Rather than simply weighting all lesion voxels (which typically has the effect of moving the optimal decision boundary, but not improving the classifier) we instead calculated, for each case, the 25th percentile of the scaled intensity within the lesion mask, and weighted the loss function from voxels above that intensity ten times more than other voxels. The models were trained with the Adadelta method. Models were trained until no improvement in loss was seen in the validation set over five epochs (early stopping) and the model with best performance (binary crossentropy) on the validation set was selected for the final model.

Applying to New MSSEG Cases. Given a new case, the lesion mask was predicted, using only the processed FLAIR maps, as follows.

Given a case from the MSSEG training data, the pipeline for lesion segmentation was as follows: resample the processed FLAIR volume to 1 mm isovoxels. Apply the saggital, coronal and axial models to the resampled volume (padding the image to ensure that the slice dimensions are divisible by eight). The final lesion heatmap is given by averaging the heatmaps arising from the three models. This heatmap is then resampled to the native voxel spacing of the original volume. An initial segmentation is made by setting all voxels with posterior >0.5 as lesion voxels, and all voxels with posterior <0.1 as non lesion: the final segmentation is derived by using a random walk segmentation (beta = 10) as implemented in the python scikit-image package (http://scikit-image.org/).

Processing a single case, on a laptop with an 8 Gb NVIDIA GTX980M GPU, took an average of 210 s.

Validation on Local Data. We validated the models trained on the MSSEG data on 129 cases from the Inselspital, segmented by a masters student as for our initial experiments. An indication of the volumetric performance can be seen in Fig. 4. An example case is shown in Fig. 3, where it can be seen that the automated procedure can in some cases provide a more accurate segmentation than the human rater (in particular in the posterior, where the manual rater's delineation does not follow the contours of the lesion as visible in the sagittal FLAIR). This can be explained by observing that all cases in our dataset were segmented in the axial direction (the rater may of course refer to the sagittal and coronal view, but in practice this is too time consuming to be done thoroughly). Lesions with small axial cross-section were likely to be missed by the human rater, but detected by the automated system, since it segments also in the sagittal and coronal planes.

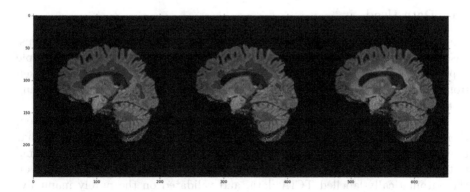

Fig. 3. Right: Sagittal slice of a Flair acquisition. Centre: Manual segmentation. Left: segmentation by Nabla net.

4   Brain Tumor

We subsequently adapted the nabla net architecture to segment low- and high-grade gliomas.

The initial portion of the network consists of four small encode layers (with 32, rather than 64 feature maps), each working on a separate modality from {T1, T1c, T2, FLAIR}. The output of these four encode layers is then fed into the encoder-decoder network:

Layer	Name	Dimension of output	Comments
1	Input	(4 * 32, n * 8, m * 8)	Five slices, dimensions (n * 8, m * 8)
2	Encode 1	(64, n * 8, m * 8)	
3	Maxpool 1	(64, n * 4, m * 4)	
4	Encode 2	(64, n * 4, m * 4)	
5	Maxpool 2	(64, n * 2, m * 2)	
6	Encode 3	(64, n * 2, m * 2)	
7	Maxpool 3	(64, n, m)	
8	Encode 4	(64, n, m)	
9	Decode 4	(64, n, m)	
10	Unpool 3	(64, n * 2, m * 2)	Tied to maxpool 3
11	Decode 3	(64, n * 2, m * 2)	
12	Unpool 2	(64, n * 4, m * 4)	Tied to maxpool 2
13	Decode 2	(64, n * 4, m * 4)	
14	Unpool 1	(64, n * 8, m * 8)	Tied to maxpool 1
15	Merge	(128, n * 8, m * 8)	Concatenate the outputs of layers 2 and 14
16	Encode final	(64, n * 8, m * 8)	
17	1 * 1 convolutional	(4, n * 8, m * 8)	
18	Sigmoid	(4, n * 8, m * 8)	Loss = binary crossentropy

4.1 Data Used

The training data in the BRATS challenges can be divided into two groups, based on how they are labelled. An initial thirty cases were labelled by multiple expert raters, and the resulting label masks fused. A further 240 cases, taken from the NIH TCIA database, were segmented using a fusion of top-performing methods from the 2012 and 2013 BRATS challenges.

While the automatically labelled TCIA cases have been manually inspected, there remain numerous false identifications. For this reason, we considered that they were not suitable for validating our algorithm. However, restricting training to the thirty well-labelled cases led to overfitting. For this reason, we trained on the automatically-labelled TCIA data, and validated on the purely manually-labelled data.

4.2 Label Sets

The label set for the BRATS challenge has four labels: edema, non-enhancing tumor, enhancing tumor, and necrosis. However, the manual segmentation proceeds as follows: identify whole tumor (on FLAIR/T2 imaging), then within that identify the gross tumor. Finally, identify the contrast-enhancing and necrotic parts of the whole tumor. In this work, we attempt to reproduce the segmentation steps produced by a radiologist, in particular to improve performance on the gross tumour segmentation.

The output of the model has four channels, each corresponding to one of the four classes {Whole Tumour, Gross Tumour, Contrast enhancing, Necrosis}. Since these label sets overlap (i.e., Gross Tumor is contained within whole

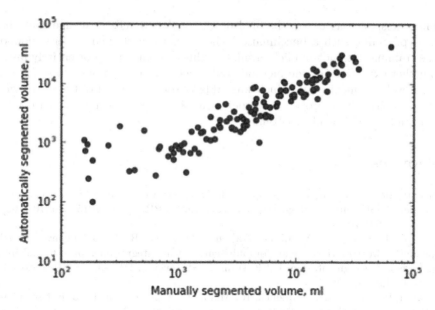

Fig. 4. Volumetric comparison of manual (masters student) and automated (nabla net) segmentation on 129 cases from the Inselspital, Bern, Switzerland. Log scale on both axes.

tumor), we again use Binary Crossentropy applied to each of the output channels separately as a loss function. As for MS lesion segmentation, the we trained three models to segment in the saggital, coronal and axial directions, and ensembled them for the final challenge segmentation.

The pipeline for lesion segmentation was as follows: apply the network to obtain heatmaps for the whole tumour, gross tumour, contrast-enhancing tumour and necrosis. The final lesion maps are extracted from the heatmaps using a random walk segmentation, as implemented in the python scikit-image package, for each of the four classes. All voxels outside the whole tumour are labelled as non-tumour: voxels inside the gross tumour but not inside the contrast-enhancing or necrosis are labelled as noncontrast-enhancing, and voxels outside the gross tumour but in the whole tumour are labelled as edema.

When applied to the 30 BRATS 2012 training cases (which were not used for training), the method achieved a mean Dice score of 0.87 for the whole tumour, 0.69 for the tumour core, and 0.56 for contrast-enhancing tumour.

5   Conclusions

The current paper reports on a method, applied in two recent biomedical volume segmentation challenges. The method performed well in both challenges, in particular performing best in terms of DICE coefficient in the MSSEG challenge. It would of course, be beneficial to benchmark the method against other architectures, such as U-net: the final results of the BRATS challenge could be seen as providing such a benchmark, although since participants were allowed to use training data not publicly available, this comparison is not entirely fair.

Further extensions of the method could include, for example, replacing the random walk segmentation (which was added close to the end of the challenge, since it empirically improved Dice coefficient scores) with a more usual conditional random field regularisation.

References

Badrinarayanan, V., Kendall, A., Cipolla, R.: SegNet: a deep convolutional encoder-decoder architecture for image segmentation. In: CVPR, vol. 5 (2015). doi:10.1103/PhysRevX.5.041024

Brosch, T., Tang, L., Yoo, Y., Li, D., Traboulsee, A., Tam, R.: Deep 3D convolutional encoder networks with shortcuts for multiscale feature integration applied to multiple sclerosis lesion segmentation. IEEE Trans. Med. Imaging **PP**(99), 1 (2016). doi:10.1109/TMI.2016.2528821

Hariharan, B., Arbeláez, P., Girshick, R., Malik, J.: Hypercolumns for object segmentation and fine-grained localization. In: Proceedings of the IEEE Computer Society Conference on Computer Vision and Pattern Recognition, pp. 447–456, 07–12 June 2015. doi:10.1109/CVPR.2015.7298642

Ioffe, S., Szegedy, C.: Batch normalization: accelerating deep network training by reducing internal covariate shift, pp. 1–11. ArXiv:1502.03167 (2015). doi:10.1007/s13398-014-0173-7.2

Jarrett, K., Kavukcuoglu, K., Ranzato, M., LeCun, Y.: What is the best multi-stage architecture for object recognition? In: Proceedings of the IEEE International Conference on Computer Vision, pp. 2146–2153 (2009). doi:10.1109/ICCV.2009.5459469

LeCun, Y., Bengio, Y., Hinton, G.: Deep learning. Nature **521**(7553), 436–444 (2015). doi:10.1038/nature14539

Long, J., Shelhamer, E., Darrell, T.: Fully convolutional networks for semantic segmentation. In: Proceedings of the IEEE Computer Society Conference on Computer Vision and Pattern Recognition, pp. 3431–3440, 07–12 June-2015. doi:10.1109/CVPR.2015.7298965

Ronneberger, O., Fischer, P., Brox, T.: U-net: convolutional networks for biomedical image segmentation. In: Navab, N., Hornegger, J., Wells, W.M., Frangi, A.F. (eds.) MICCAI 2015. LNCS, vol. 9351, pp. 234–241. Springer, Cham (2015). doi:10.1007/978-3-319-24574-4_28

Zeiler, M.D., Taylor, G.W., Fergus, R.: Adaptive deconvolutional networks for mid and high level feature learning. In: Proceedings of the IEEE International Conference on Computer Vision, pp. 2018–2025 (2011). doi:10.1109/ICCV.2011.6126474

Brain Tumor Segmantation Using Random Forest Trained on Iteratively Selected Patients

Abdelrahman Ellwaa$^{(\boxtimes)}$, Ahmed Hussein, Essam AlNaggar, Mahmoud Zidan, Michael Zaki, Mohamed A. Ismail, and Nagia M. Ghanem

Faculty of Engineering, Alexandria University, Alexandria, Egypt
abdelrahmanellwaa@gmail.com, michaelzaki1212@gmail.com

Abstract. This paper extends a previously published brain tumor segmentation methods based on Random Decision Forest (RDF). An iterative approach is used in training the RDF in each iteration some patients are added to the training data using some heuristics approach instead of randomly selected training dataset. Feature extraction and selection were applied to select the most discriminative features for training our Random Decision forest on. The post-processing phase has a morphological filter to deal with misclassification errors. Our method is capable of detecting the tumor and segmenting the different tumorous tissues of the glioma achieving competitive results.

Keywords: Brain tumor segmentation · Random forests

1 Introduction

Gliomas are the most frequent primary brain tumors in adults. They are originated from glial cells and infiltrate the surrounding tissues. Gliomas can be divided into Low Grade Gliomas (LGG) and High Grade Gliomas (HGG). Although the former are less aggressive, the later can be very deadly [8,9]. Despite considerable advances in glioma research, patient diagnosis remains poor. Segmentation of brain tumors from MR images is important in cancer treatment planning as well as for cancer research. In current clinical practice, the analysis of brain tumor images is mostly done manually. Apart from being time-consuming, this has the additional drawback of significant intra- and inter-rater variability. Accurate brain tumour segmentation is difficult, because in MR images, brain tumors may have the same appearance with gliosis and stroke, have a variety of shapes, appearances and sizes, and may appear in any position in the brain, invade the surrounding tissue rather than displacing it, causing fuzzy boundaries and also there exists intensity inhomogeneity in MR images. The main goal of brain tumor segmentation is to identify areas of the brain whose configuration deviates from normal tissues. Segmentation methods typically look for active tumorous tissues, necrotic tissues, and edema by exploiting several Magnetic resonance imaging (MRI) modalities, such as T1, T2, T1-Contrasted (T1C) and Flair.

© Springer International Publishing AG 2016
A. Crimi et al. (Eds.): BrainLes 2016, LNCS 10154, pp. 129–137, 2016.
DOI: 10.1007/978-3-319-55524-9_13

In this paper, we introduce a random forest approach which chooses the patients to be used in training according to a cost function instead of randomly selecting them from our dataset (BRATS 2016 dataset), training is iterative at each iteration some patients are added to the training set to be used in the next iteration, this approach tries to prevent over fitted random forest by choosing patients that get the worst results, patients with brain tumors having various shapes, appearances, and sizes, and may appear in any position in the brain, in the previous iteration. Through the paper, we will illustrate in details the approach and the parameters of the approach.

In the past years there are many approaches that used the random forest in brain tumor segmentation those approaches varies in the features selected and the training approach: five class random forest classifier [4] or cascaded random forest that classifies each voxel on two stages the first is two class classifier tumorous or not and the second classifies tumorous voxels to four tumor classes, so this approach tries to balance the training data in each classifier [5].

The paper is organized in the following way, Sect. 2 contains a description of the training pipeline of the random forest. Section 3 refers to different models used in experiments and the obtained results. Finally, Sect. 4 presents the main conclusions.

2   Training Pipeline

The training pipeline consists of four main steps: pre-processing, feature extraction and selection, training random forest, and post-processing step. In the following, we will introduce each step in details respectively. Figure 1 shows the training pipeline of the random forest.

2.1   Preprocessing

– Bias field signal is a low-frequency and very smooth signal that corrupts MRI images, especially those produced by old MRI machines. Image processing algorithms such as segmentation, texture analysis or classification that use the gray level values of image pixels will not produce satisfactory results. A pre-processing step is needed to correct for the bias field signal. Bias field correction on the MR images is applied using open source code N4ITK [1].
– The second step in pre-processing is histogram matching [2,3] which is proposed to correct the variations in scanners sensitivity. This is because quantitative comparisons of abnormalities in MRI scans between patients or within patients serially are affected by variations in MR scanners performance.

2.2   Feature Extraction and Selection

In this phase, we extracted 328 features from the MR images after being preprocessed. Mainly, three categories of features were extracted: gradient features, appearance features, and context aware features. Most of them were from other

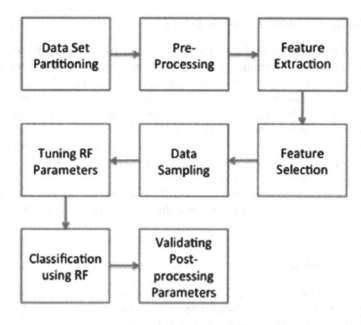

Fig. 1. Random forest training pipeline

published papers from BRATS challenge [4–6]. The first type of features is gradient features which include gradient filter at different Sigma values of 0.5, 1, 2, 3 in each of the three directions x, y, and z and their resultant, difference gradient features, Laplace features, and Recursive Gaussian features. The second type of features is Appearance features which include the voxels intensities, its logarithmic and exponential transformations. The last type of features is the context aware features, which is intensity based, it includes features extracted from the neighbouring voxels, the surrounding cube of the voxel, as most similar, most different, Minimum, Maximum, Range, Kurtosis, Skewness, Standard deviation, and Entropy for all modalities, as well as the local histogram of the cube surrounding the voxel and partitioned into eleven bins, all the previous features were extracted for all modalities Flair, T1, T1c, and T2.

Random forest was used in feature selection using mean decrease impurity, as when training a tree, it can be computed how much each feature decreases the weighted impurity in a tree. For a forest, the impurity decrease from each feature can be averaged and the features are ranked according to this measure.

After feature extraction and selection, each patient will consist of a set of tuples, where each tuple consists of some features which correspond to a voxel in the four modalities of the brain. On average each patient has 1,500,000 tuples. Random sampling is used without replacement, since the health voxels are dominating, to balance healthy and unhealthy tuples. 60,000 health voxels and 15,000 from each other tumor label are randomly sampled from each patient. Each patient finally will contain 100,000 voxels.

2.3 Training Random Decision Forest

Before training the random forest there are some parameters of the random forest that should be determined to be used in training, as the number of trees and number of attributes to split on at each node. So we trained a model by the validation dataset and determined the best values for those parameters based on the k-fold cross validation error, which turns out to be using a random forest with number of trees equals to 45 and number of attributes to split on equals to the square root of the number of features, as we found that the gain in the accuracy is negligible compared to the huge computation it takes when increasing the Random forest parameters values.

Random forest implementation on H2O [7] was used as it is fast, distributed, using the full processing power of the machine, and work on different platforms like python and R.

2.4 Post Processing

The post-processing step is applying binary morphology filter to the output image of the classifier, three binary morphology filters were applied to reduce misclassification errors by connecting large tumorous regions and removing small isolated regions.

The radii used in binary morphology were validated using the validation dataset and they were found to be 8, 8, 0 for complete, core, and enhanced tumors respectively for high-grade gliomas and 1, 8, 2 for complete, core, and enhanced tumors respectively for low-grade gliomas.

3 Experiment and Results

3.1 Experiment

This section explains the models used in classification. BRATS 2016 dataset was used and partitioned into training (70%), testing (20%), and validation (10%) datasets.

Iterative Model. The iterative model mainly addresses the problem of choosing a subset of training patients to train the random forest, so the model is trained through number of iterations, in each iteration the number of patients increases according to a cost function so that the worst N patients are added, there is also a maximum number of patients that is selected according to the hardware resources available. The flowchart in Fig. 2 explains how the iterative model works.

There are many parameters that must be specified first as the number of patients added in each iteration that is set to 5 patients per iteration, initial set of patients that are 30 patients (BRATS 2013 dataset 20 HGG and 10 LGG), maximum number of LGG patients to prevent overfitting LGG patients which

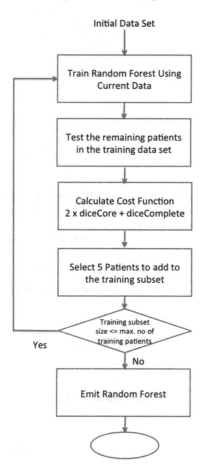

Fig. 2. Flowchart of selecting patients for training the iterative model

is set to 18 patients, the maximum number of patients which is limited to 50 patients, and the cost function which is equal to

$$costFunction = 2 * coreDice + completeDice$$

Cascaded Model. This model consists of two random forests, the first random forest classifies only health voxels (label 0) and non-health voxels (all non-health labels are merged into one representative label for non-health labels), then the second random forest takes the output results from the first random forest and tries to classify the non-health voxels. This approach mainly tries to enhance non-health voxels classification. Firstly, by making a dedicated classifier for health versus non-health voxels which will have many advantages as by merging all non-health labels into one label, this will increase the balancing of the dataset input to the random forest to train on, which is supposed to decrease the number

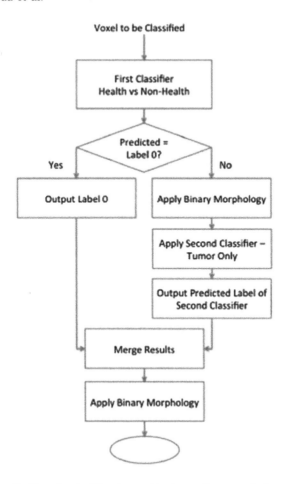

Fig. 3. Flowchart of testing patients on the cascaded model

of non-health voxels classified as health voxels. Secondly, by making a dedicated classifier for non-health labels.

This model was trained on 50 randomly chosen patients from the training data set, the random forest consists of 100 trees each of depth 45. The flowchart in Fig. 3 explains the testing of patients on the cascaded model.

One-Phase Model. This model was trained on 50 randomly chosen patients from the training data set, the random forest consists of 100 trees each of depth 45.

3.2   Results

Those models are tested on 20 (15 HGG and 5 LGG) randomly unseen patients, the results are shown in Table 1 by the dice, specificity and sensitivity scores.

Table 1. The table contains the dice, specificity and sensitivity scores of testing 20 (15 HGG and 5 LGG) randomly unseen patients on our different models.

Model	Complete			Core			Enhancing		
	Dice	Sens	Spec	Dice	Sens	Spec	Dice	Sens	Spec
One-phase HGG	0.81 ± 0.09	0.84 ± 0.10	0.98 ± 0.01	0.62 ± 0.23	0.83 ± 0.16	0.98 ± 0.01	0.75 ± 0.15	0.81 ± 0.12	1.00 ± 0.00
One-phase LGG	0.80 ± 0.06	0.76 ± 0.14	0.99 ± 0.01	0.53 ± 0.17	0.74 ± 0.20	0.99 ± 0.01	0.36 ± 0.32	0.62 ± 0.43	1.00 ± 0.00
Cascaded HGG	0.78 ± 0.10	0.89 ± 0.08	0.97 ± 0.02	0.63 ± 0.23	0.88 ± 0.11	0.98 ± 0.02	0.71 ± 0.18	0.83 ± 0.10	1.00 ± 0.00
Cascaded LGG	0.76 ± 0.11	0.91 ± 0.06	0.98 ± 0.01	0.55 ± 0.20	0.79 ± 0.22	0.99 ± 0.01	0.24 ± 0.31	0.57 ± 0.48	1.00 ± 0.00
Iterative HGG	0.80 ± 0.10	0.84 ± 0.11	0.98 ± 0.01	0.72 ± 0.19	0.79 ± 0.18	0.99 ± 0.01	0.73 ± 0.15	0.75 ± 0.12	1.00 ± 0.00
Iterative LGG	0.84 ± 0.02	0.83 ± 0.09	0.99 ± 0.01	0.72 ± 0.12	0.82 ± 0.14	0.99 ± 0.01	0.39 ± 0.33	0.51 ± 0.42	1.00 ± 0.00

From our results, We found that our one phase model which was trained on 50 random patients including patients with high-grade gliomas and low-grade gliomas, with depth 45 performs well in case of Complete tumor and enhanced

Table 2. The table contains the random forest parameters and training datasets descriptions of our different models used in experiments

Model id	Maximum depth	Mtries	Ntrees	Dataset description
Model 1	45	13	100	50 patients are HGG (20 from 2013 BraTS dataset (subset of 2016 BraTS data set) and 30 randomly sampled from the rest of HGG)
Model 2	45	13	100	50 patient from both HGG and LGG (20 HGG, and 10 LGG from 2013 BraTS dataset (subset of 2016 BraTS data set), and 20 random sampled patients from the rest of patients)
Model 3	30	13	100	50 patient from both HGG and LGG (20 HGG, and 10 LGG from 2013 BraTS dataset (subset of 2016 BraTS data set), and 20 random sampled patients from the rest of patients)
Cascade	45	13	100	50 patient from both HGG and LGG (20 HGG, and 10 LGG from 2013 BraTS dataset (subset of 2016 BraTS data set), and 20 random sampled patients from the rest of patients)
Iterative 1	45	13	100	The initial dataset is 2013 BraTS data set (subset of 2016 BraTS data set), maximum number of patients is limited to 50 patient
Iterative 2	45	13	100	The initial dataset is subset of 2013 BraTS data set (15 HGG and 5 LGG) to give the model more flexibility to select more patients, maximum number of patients is limited to 50 patient

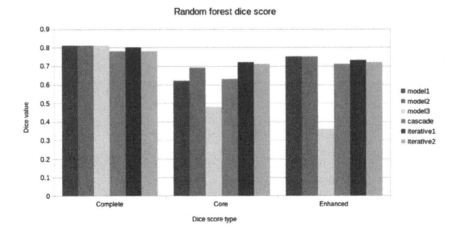

Fig. 4. The figure shows the dice scores of our different models described in Table 2

tumour hitting 81% and 74% respectively for high graded glioma, while our iterative model performs well in case of core tumor by passing 70% which was because the dataset of that model was mainly selected to include patients having different cases for core tumors. Also, we found that training a random forest at depth 30 on the same data on a depth of 45 performed very bad for core and enhanced tumors. Actually, we tried many other approaches like using all our data set as patients with high-grade gliomas and using cascaded approach by classifying first health and non-health voxels, then applying binary morphology and finally classifying the non-health voxels but it turns out that all the previous approaches don't out perform the iterative model.

The Graph in Fig. 4 shows the dice scores of our different models described in Table 2.

4   Conclusion

In this paper, we proposed an approach based on Random Forest that differs from past years' submissions as we mainly tried to extract as much information as we can from our large dataset (BRATS 2016 dataset). We achieved this by applying our iterative selection method to choose the best patients to train our Random Forest with them and then by extracting as much information as we can then applying feature selection, and our proposed method improves the performance over the cascaded method and over training the RF using randomly selected patients.

References

1. Tustison, N., Gee, J.: N4ITK: Nicks N3 ITK implementation for MRI bias field correction. Insight J. (2009)
2. Nyu, L.G., Udupa, J.K.: On standardizing the MR image intensity scale image, vol. 1081 (1999)
3. Nyu, L.G., Udupa, J.K.: New variants of a method of MRI scale standardization. IEEE Trans. Med. Imaging **19**(2), 143–150 (2000)
4. Dinis, H., Pinto, A., Pereira, S., Silva, C.A.: Random decision forests for automatic brain tumor segmentation in multi-modal MRI images
5. Peyrat, J.-M., Abinahed, J., Malmi, E., Parambath, S., Chawla, S.: CaBS: a cascaded brain tumor segmentation approach
6. Wilms, M., Maier, O., Handels, H.: Highly discriminative features for glioma segmentation in MR volumes with random forests
7. http://www.h2o.ai/
8. Bauer, S., Wiest, R., Nolte, L.P., Reyes, M.: A survey of MRI-based medical image analysis for brain tumor studies. Phys. Med. Biol. **58**(13), R97 (2013)
9. Menze, B., et al.: The multimodal brain tumor image segmentation benchmark (BRATS). IEEE Trans. Med. Imaging (2014)

DeepMedic for Brain Tumor Segmentation

Konstantinos Kamnitsas[1,2(✉)], Enzo Ferrante[1], Sarah Parisot[1],
Christian Ledig[1], Aditya V. Nori[2], Antonio Criminisi[2],
Daniel Rueckert[1], and Ben Glocker[1]

[1] Biomedical Image Analysis Group, Imperial College London, London, UK
[2] Microsoft Research, Cambridge, UK
konstantinos.kamnitsas12@imperial.ac.uk

Abstract. Accurate automatic algorithms for the segmentation of brain tumours have the potential of improving disease diagnosis, treatment planning, as well as enabling large-scale studies of the pathology. In this work we employ DeepMedic [1], a 3D CNN architecture previously presented for lesion segmentation, which we further improve by adding residual connections. We also present a series of experiments on the BRATS 2015 training database for evaluating the robustness of the network when less training data are available or less filters are used, aiming to shed some light on requirements for employing such a system. Our method was further benchmarked on the BRATS 2016 Challenge, where it achieved very good performance despite the simplicity of the pipeline.

1 Introduction

Accurate estimation of the relative volume of the subcomponents of a brain tumour is critical for monitoring progression, radiotherapy planning, outcome assessment and follow-up studies. For this, accurate delineation of the tumour is required. Manual segmentation poses significant challenges for human experts, both because of the variability of tumour appearance but also because of the need to consult multiple images from different MRI sequences in order to classify tissue type correctly. This laborious effort is not only time consuming but prone to human error and results in significant intra- and inter-rater variability [2].

Automatic segmentation systems aim to provide a cheap and scalable solution. Over the years, automatic methods for brain tumour segmentation have attracted significant attention. Representative early work is the atlas-based outlier detection method [3]. Segmentation was later solved jointly with the registration of a healthy atlas to a pathological brain [4], making use of a tumour growth model and the Expectation Maximization algorithm. In [5] the problem was tackled as the joint optimization of two Markov Random Fields (MRFs). The state of the art was raised further by supervised learning methods, initially represented mainly by Random Forests, coupled with models such as Gaussian Mixtures for the extraction of tissue type priors [6], MRFs for spatial regularisation and a variety of engineered features [7].

K. Kamnitsas—Part of this work was carried on when KK was an intern at Microsoft.

© Springer International Publishing AG 2016
A. Crimi et al. (Eds.): BrainLes 2016, LNCS 10154, pp. 138–149, 2016.
DOI: 10.1007/978-3-319-55524-9_14

Recent years saw the success of deep learning, with the methods in [8,9] being the top performing automatic approaches in BRATS 2014 and 2015 [10], using 3D and 2D Convolutional Neural Networks (CNNs) respectively. The latter approached the accuracy of the winning semi-automatic method [11]. The fact that the employed models are rather simple in design reveals the high potential of CNNs. The method presented in [12] also exhibited good performance, based on a 3-layers deep 2D network that separately processes each axial slice. The authors empirically showed that the class bias introduced to a network when training with patches extracted equiprobably from the task's classes can be partially alleviated with a second training stage using patches uniformly extracted from the image. In [13] an ensemble of 2D networks is used to process three orthogonal slices of a brain MR image. Finally, in [1] we showed that multi-scale 3D CNNs of larger size can accomplish high performance while remaining computationally efficient. In that work we also analysed how the size of the input segments relates to the captured class distribution by the training samples. It was shown that this meta-parameter can be exploited for capturing a partially adaptive distribution of training samples that in practice leads to good performance in a variety of segmentation tasks. Our segmentation system exhibited excellent performance on stroke lesion segmentation, winning the first position in the SISS-ISLES 2015 challenge [14,15], brain tumours and traumatic brain injuries [1]. It's generic architecture and processing of 3D content also allow its use on diverse problems, such as the segmentation of the placenta from motion corrupted MR images [16], where it achieved very promising results.

In this work we further extend our network, the DeepMedic [1], with residual connections [20] and evaluate their effect. We then investigate the behaviour of our system when trained with less data or when its capacity is reduced to explore requirements for employing such a segmentation method. Finally, we discuss its performance on the BRATS 2016 challenge where it was further benchmarked.

2   Method

DeepMedic is the 11-layers deep, multi-scale 3D CNN we presented in [1] for brain lesion segmentation. The architecture consists of two parallel convolutional pathways that process the input at different scales to achieve a large receptive field for the final classification while keeping the computational cost low. Inspired by VGG [19], the use of small convolutional kernels is adopted. This design choice was shown [19] to be effective in building deeper CNNs without increasing the number of trainable parameters, and we showed it allows building high performing yet efficient 3D CNNs thanks to the much less computation required for convolutions with small 3^3 kernels [1]. The CNN is employed in a fully convolutional fashion on image segments in both training and testing stage[1].

We extend the DeepMedic with residual connections in order to examine their effect on segmentation. Residual connections were recently shown to facilitate preservation of the flowing signal and as such have enabled training of

---

[1] Code publicly available at: https://github.com/Kamnitsask/deepmedic.

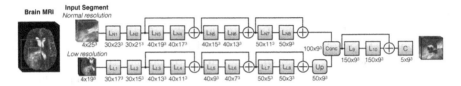

Fig. 1. The DeepMedic [1] extended with residual connections. The operations within each layer block are applied in the order: Batch-Normalization [17], non-linearity and convolution. [18] empirically showed this format leads to better performance. *Up* and *C* represent an upsampling and classification layer respectively. Number of filters and their size depicted as (*Number* × *Size*). Other hyper-parameters as in [1].

very deep neural networks [18,20]. In [20] the authors did not observe a performance improvement when a 18-layers deep network was employed, but only in experiments with architectures deeper than 34-layers. The networks employed on biomedical applications tend to consist of less layers than modern architectures in computer vision. However, the problem of preserving the forward and backwards propagated signal as well as the difficulty of optimization can be substantial in 3D CNNs due to the large number of trainable parameters in 3D kernels, as previously discussed in [1]. For this reason we set off to investigate such an architecture.

We extended the network by adding residual connections between the outputs of every two layers, except for the first two of each pathway to enforce abstracting away from raw intensity values. The architecture is depicted in Fig. 1. In our work, a residual connection after layer l performs the element-wise addition $\oplus$ between corresponding channels of the output out_l of layer l and the input in_{l-1} to the previous layer. This choice follows the investigation in [18] that found identity mappings on the residual path to perform best. More formally:

$$in_{l+1}^m = \begin{cases} out_l^m \oplus \hat{in}_{l-1}^m, & \text{if } m \leq M^{l-1} \\ out_l^m, & \text{otherwise} \end{cases} \quad (1)$$

where l denotes any layer after which a residual connection is added, the superscript m is the m-th channel and M^l is the number of feature maps in the l-th layer. $\hat{in}_l$ is the input of the previous layer after padding in the (x, y, z) dimensions with reflection in order to match the dimensions of out_l.

3   Evaluation

3.1   Data

The training database of BRATS 2015 (common with BRATS 2016) includes 220 multi-modal scans of patients with high (HGG) and 54 with low grade glioma (LGG). Scans include pre- and post-operative scans. T1-weighted, contrast enhanced T1c, T2-weighted and FLAIR sequences are available. The images were registered to a common space, resampled to isotropic 1 mm × 1 mm × 1 mm resolution with image dimensions 240 × 240 × 155 and were skull stripped by the organisers. Annotations are provided that include four labels: (1) Necrosis (NC), (2) oedema (OE), (3) non-enhancing (NE) and (4) enhancing tumor (ET). The annotations for the training database were obtained semi-automatically, fusing the predictions of multiple automatic algorithms, followed by expert review. The official evaluation is performed by merging the predicted labels into three sets: whole tumor (all 4 labels), core (1, 3, 4) and enhancing tumor (4).

The testing database of BRATS 2016 consists of 191 datasets. They are scans of 94 subjects, with 1–3 time points, including both pre- and post-operative scans. The scans were acquired in multiple clinical centers, some of which are distinct from those centers that provided the data for the training database. MRI modalities are the same as the training database. Ground truth annotations have been made manually by experts but were kept private for the evaluation. The MRI images have been preprocessed similarly to the training data and then provided to the participating teams. Interesting to note is that skull stripping had significant flaws in many cases, leaving behind portions of skull and extra-cerebral tissue at a significantly greater extent that what is observed in the training database. Such heterogeneity between testing and training data poses a significant challenge for automated machine learning methods that try to model the distribution of the training data. Yet they reflect a realistic scenario and an interesting benchmark for fully automated systems, which ideally should perform adequately even after inaccuracies introduced by individual blocks in the processing pipeline.

3.2 Evaluation on the BRATS 2015 Training Database

Preprocessing and Augmentation: Each scan was further individually normalized by subtracting the mean and dividing by the standard deviation of the intensities within the brain. Training data were augmented via reflection with respect to the mid-sagittal plane.

Effect of Residual Connections: To evaluate the effect of the residual connections we performed 5-fold cross validation on the mixed HGG and LGG data, while ensuring that all pre- and post-operative scans of a subject are within the same fold. First we reproduced results similar to what was reported in [1] for the original version of DeepMedic. The extension with residual connections gave a modest but consistent improvement over all classes of the task, as shown in Table 1. Important is that performance increases even on small challenging substructures like the necrosis and non-enhancing tumor, which may not be individually evaluated for the challenge but is interesting from an optimization perspective. The improvement seems mainly due to an increase in sensitivity,

Table 1. Performance of the original *DeepMedic* and its extension with residual connections *DMRes*, evaluated with a 5-fold validation over the whole BRATS 2015 training database. For consistency with the online evaluation platform, cases that do not present enhancing tumor in the provided annotations are still considered for the calculation of the average, as zeros, thus lowering the upper bound of accuracy for the class. Bold numbers indicate significant difference, according to a two-sided, paired t-test on the DSC metric ($p < 5 \cdot 10^{-2}$).

	DSC			Precision			Sensitivity			DSC			
	Whole	Core	Enh.	Whole	Core	Enh.	Whole	Core	Enh.	NC	OE	NE	ET
DeepMedic	89.6	75.4	71.8	89.7	84.5	74.3	90.3	73.0	73.0	38.7	78.0	36.7	71.8
DMRes	89.6	**76.3**	**72.4**	87.6	82.4	72.5	92.2	75.4	76.3	**39.6**	78.1	**38.1**	**72.4**

however at the cost of a lower precision. This is a positive side-effect as in practice it can prove easier to clear false positives in a post-processing step, for instance with a Conditional Random Field as performed in [1,14], rather than capturing areas previously missed by the CNN.

Behaviour of the Network with Less Training Data and Filters: CNNs have shown promising accuracy when trained either on the extensive database of BRATS 2015 or on the rather limited of BRATS 2013. However, qualitative differences of the two databases do not allow estimating the influence of the database's size. Additionally, although various architectures were previously suggested, no work has investigated the required capacity of a network for the task. This factor is significant in practice, as it defines the computational resources and inference time required.

We evaluate the behaviour of our network on the tumour segmentation task with respect to the two above factors. To avoid bias towards subjects scanned at more than one time-point, only the earliest dataset was used from each subject. Out of the 198 remaining datasets, we randomly chose 40 (29 HGG, 11 LGG) as a validation fold. The same validation fold was used in all experiments of this section. We then trained the original version of DeepMedic on the remaining 158 datasets, as well as on a reduced number of training data. Finally, versions of the network where all layers had their filters reduced to 50% and 33% were trained on the whole training fold of 158 datasets.

It can be observed on Table 2 that although accuracy is negatively affected, the network still retains most of its performance for the three merged classes of the challenge even when trained with little data or its capacity is significantly reduced. A more thorough look in the accuracy achieved for the 4 non-merged classes of the task shows that the greatest decline is observed for the challenging necrotic (NC) and non-enhancing (NE) classes, which however does not influence the segmentation of the overall core as severely. Even though the exact quantitative results can be affected by randomness in training, the observed trends suggest that both a large training database and large number of network filters

Table 2. Behaviour of *DeepMedic* with reduced training data or number of filters at each layer. Note that the difference of the top row in comparison to the entry *DeepMedic* in Table 1 is due to the use of a subset of data here (see text). Bold numbers indicate significant difference in comparison to the top row, according to a two-sided, paired t-test on the DSC metric ($p < 5 \cdot 10^{-2}$).

	DSC			Precision			Sensitivity			DSC			
	Whole	Core	Enh.	Whole	Core	Enh.	Whole	Core	Enh.	NC	OE	NE	ET
DM, all data	91.4	83.1	79.4	89.2	87.7	82.8	94.1	80.8	79.5	50.0	79.6	35.1	79.4
75% data	91.2	82.5	79.6	89.0	84.4	82.4	93.9	80.4	79.7	**45.9**	79.0	35.1	79.6
50% data	91.4	82.6	78.8	91.0	85.3	81.7	92.3	82.3	78.5	**44.7**	79.2	36.8	78.8
33% data	90.5	**79.7**	**77.7**	90.6	86.5	82.8	91.0	77.1	77.1	**45.8**	**77.9**	**31.8**	**77.7**
20% data	**89.8**	**80.5**	**77.6**	91.1	83.9	81.8	89.7	80.5	76.5	**41.3**	**76.9**	34.1	**77.6**
50% filters	91.4	**80.8**	79.8	92.2	89.0	82.5	91.3	76.3	80.2	49.0	79.2	**29.4**	79.8
33% filters	90.8	81.7	79.4	90.0	91.9	78.2	92.1	76.6	83.0	**44.4**	79.3	**27.9**	79.4

to learn fine and detailed patterns are important for the segmentation of small and challenging structures[2].

3.3   Evaluation on the BRATS 2016 Testing Database

Our team participated in the BRATS 2016 Challenge in order to further benchmark our system. In the testing stage of the challenge, each team is given 48 h after they are provided the data, to apply their systems and submit predicted segmentations.

Preprocessing: Similarly to the preprocessing of the training data, we normalized each image individually by subtracting the mean and dividing by the standard deviation of the intensities of the brain. Additionally, for the subjects that had multiple scans acquired at different time-points, since the brains have been co-registered, we tried to mitigate the problem of the failed brain extraction by fusing with majority voting the brain masks from different time-points, hoping that the errors are not consistent at all time-points. Unfortunately this step did not resolve the issue. We decided not to apply ourselves an additional brain extraction step, since this is not guaranteed to work on the already (well or partially) stripped data and would require case-by-case visual inspection and intervention, which is against our interest in a fully automatic pipeline.

Network Configuration and Training: Prior to the testing stage of the challenge we had trained three models with identical architecture as shown in Fig. 1. They were trained on the whole BRATS 2015 Training database, without distinction of HGG from LGG cases, or pre- from post-operative scans. Training

---

[2] Although these experiments were performed with the original version of the network, we expect the trends to continue after the extension with residual connections.

of a single model required approximately a day when using an NVIDIA GTX Titan X GPU. Our network can then segment a multi-modal dataset in less than 35 s when using CuDNN v5.0. The probability maps of the three models were then fused by averaging before the post-processing.

Post-processing with a 3D Fully Connected CRF: In previous work [1,14] we had implemented and evaluated a 3D fully connected Conditional Random Field (CRF) [21] for the segmentation of multi-sequence volumetric scans. Our evaluation had shown that the model consistently offers beneficial regularisation in a variety of lesion segmentation tasks. The CRF was found to be particularly beneficial in cases where the main segmenter underperforms. We employ the CRF in the same fashion. We provide as the CRF's unary term the whole-tumor probability map, constructed by merging the multi-class predictions of the CNN. This way the CRF regularizes the overall size of the tumor and clears small spurious false positives. The whole-tumor segmentation mask produced by the CRF is used to mask the segmentation produced by the CNNs, leaving the internal structure of the tumor mostly intact[3]. The CRF's parameters were configured via random search on subset of the training database. Finally, any left out connected-components smaller than 1000 voxels were removed.

Results: In the testing stage of the challenge 19 teams participated. To evaluate the quality of their segmentations, the teams were ranked according to the statistically significant differences in the achieved DSC scores and Haussdorf distances with respect to each other. Additionally, they were assessed and ranked for their capability in following shrinkage or growth of the tumor between different time-points. The exact quantitative results on the testing database have not been made public by the organizers yet.

Our system achieved a place among the top ranking methods, performing well on the DSC metric. The high performing methods were rather close in terms of the DSC metric for the segmentation of the Whole Tumor. Greater were the differences for the Tumor Core and Enhancing Tumor. Our system achieved the top rank for the segmentation of the tumor core. The position was shared with another CNN-based approach [22], the overall most accurate model in the challenge. Note that in order to generalize, this model was trained on external data from a private brain tumor database with manual annotations, in addition to the BRATS 2015 data, and thus direct comparison may not be completely fair. Notice that out of the three main tumor classes, the core was found to be the one most influenced by the amount of training data in our experiments (Table 2), which explains the high DSC for this class achieved by the competing method. Moreover, since the testing data appear to have a significantly different distribution from the training data, the influence of additional external data should be significantly stronger than what was found in our experiments, where we only explored the effect of the amount of data when training and testing distributions are the same. Our system also achieved the top rank for the segmentation

---

[3] Code of the 3D CRF available at: https://github.com/Kamnitsask/dense3dCrf/.

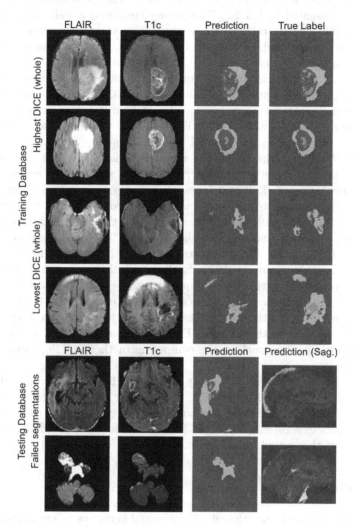

Fig. 2. Cases with the highest (two top rows) and lowest (third and forth rows) DICE for the whole tumor segmentation from the 5-fold validation on the training database. Note that the semi-automatically generated training labels also contain mistakes. (Two bottom rows) Two examples of the most common type of failed segmentation observed in the predictions on the testing data. Subset of the data provided in the testing stage of the challenge show significantly more remnants of skull and extra-cerebral tissue left behind from the brain extraction than what observed in the training database. The network fails to handle tissues that it has rarely seen during training. Colors represent: cyan: necrotic core, green: oedema, orange: non enhancing core, red: enhancing core. Cases from top to bottom row: tcia_242_01, tcia_479_01, tcia_164_01, tcia_222_304, cbica_ABH_341, cbica_AAM_285 (Color figure online)

of enhancing tumor in terms of the DSC measure. This position was shared with the systems presented in [23,24]. The former employed a well engineered cascade of Random Forests tailored for segmentation of brain tumors, trained on a selected high quality subset of the training data to avoid learning from errors within the semi-automatically generated annotations (Fig. 2). The latter applied a CNN and a CRF similar to ours, but with the two jointly trained. Interestingly, we achieved higher performance in terms of DSC for the core and enhancing tumor and comparable accuracy for the whole tumor in comparison to [25], who employed an extended version of GLISTRboost [11], the semi-automatic method that won the first place in the BRATS 2015 challenge.

Less satisfying was the Haussdorf distance achieved by our method, with respect to which it achieved average ranking. We speculate a reason for this is false segmentation of skull and extra-cerebral tissue, portions of which were observed in many of the testing cases where the provided brain extraction was inaccurate (Fig. 2). Such tissues were not present in the training database to this extent, so our system never learnt to classify them. The resulting false positives decrease the DSC metric, but influence even more the Haussdorf distance since they lie well outside the brain. With further careful brain extraction we could alleviate the problem but this would require case-by-case inspection as it is prone to fail on the already (successfully or not) stripped testing cases, thus render the pipeline not fully automatic. At the time of writing it has not been reported yet how other teams dealt with this issue. Finally, semi-automatic systems that rely on manual initialization, such as the competing method in [25], should be less prone to this issue.

Finally, our system performed very well in predicting the temporal change of the volumes of whole and enhancing tumor, with its average performance for these classes achieving the third position. Interestingly, the two overall winners of this category [24,26] employed a CRF similar to ours, which indicates the effectiveness of this model for this task.

4   Conclusion

This paper has investigated the effect of residual connections on a recently presented 3D CNN model on the task of brain tumour segmentation, where their incorporation led to a small but consistent improvement. Our work reveals that an 11-layers 3D CNN gains from such an extension, mostly thanks to increased sensitivity, unlike the observation in [20] where benefits were found only for significantly deeper 2D networks.

In an attempt to explore the generalization and efficiency of CNNs for a task such as brain tumor segmentation, we also investigated the behaviour of DeepMedic when trained with smaller number of data or when less filters are used. Our experiments show that segmentation accuracy for the whole, core and enhancing tumour, even though affected, it is not severely hindered by the two factors to an extent that would render the system impractical. However, they are very important for segmenting challenging, fine substructures such as necrosis and non-enhancing tumour. On the other hand, in applications where segmentation of such substructures is not required, small networks can be a suitable option, thanks to lower computational requirements and shorter inference times (35 s versus 8 s per multi-modal scan for the original and smallest model in Table 2 respectively). Note that in our experiments we only explored the effect of the amount of data when training and testing distributions are the same. Networks, similarly to most machine learning algorithms, face generalization problems when the two differ significantly, such as in cases shown in Fig. 2. In this case, additional training data from new distributions should amplify generalization to an heterogeneous testing database more effectively. This is supported by the high performance of the rather small model of [22], overall winner of BRATS 2016 challenge, which was trained on an external private database along with the BRATS 2015 training set, as well as reports by the respective team that their incorporation amplified performance. It would be interesting to explore how much data is needed from a new source in order for a network to also generalize satisfyingly to the new distribution. Additionally, it would be worth investigating a relation between ideal network capacity versus the amount of available training data, as well as explore these factors on other segmentation tasks.

Finally, the version of DeepMedic with residual connections was further benchmarked on the BRATS 2016 challenge among 19 teams. It exhibited very good performance, achieving top ranking for the Core and Enhancing tumour classes in terms of DICE. Our system also performed very well in assessing the longitudinal change of the whole and enhancing tumor volume, ranking third for its average performance on these classes. Less satisfying was the achieved Haussdorf distance, which we mostly attribute to false segmentation of parts of the skull and extra-cerebral tissue that were left behind from incomplete skull stripping of the testing data. This performance is particularly satisfying considering the minimal preprocessing and the generic architecture of our system. Its performance is likely to benefit from a more extensive pre-processing pipeline, such as from careful skull stripping, bias field correction, as well as from careful selection of high quality training data. Finally, an interesting trend is that histogram matching to a common template has been a part of top performing pipelines in BRATS 2015 and 2016 challenges [9,11,22], even though the technique is often criticized as not well suited for the problem of tumour segmentation.

Acknowledgements. This work is supported by the EPSRC (grant No: EP/N023668/1) and partially funded under the 7th Framework Programme by the European Commission (TBIcare: http://www.tbicare.eu/; CENTER-TBI: https://www.center-tbi.eu/). Part of this work was carried on when KK was an intern at Microsoft Research Cambridge. KK is also supported by the President's PhD Scholarship of Imperial College London. We gratefully acknowledge the support of NVIDIA Corporation with the donation of two Titan X GPUs for our research.

References

1. Kamnitsas, K., Ledig, C., Newcombe, V.F., Simpson, J.P., Kane, A.D., Menon, D.K., Rueckert, D., Glocker, B.: Efficient multi-scale 3D CNN with fully connected CRF for accurate brain lesion segmentation. Med. Image Anal. **36**, 61–78 (2016)

2. Mazzara, G.P., Velthuizen, R.P., Pearlman, J.L., Greenberg, H.M., Wagner, H.: Brain tumor target volume determination for radiation treatment planning through automated MRI segmentation. Int. J. Radiat. Oncol. Biol. Phys. **59**(1), 300–312 (2004)

3. Prastawa, M., Bullitt, E., Ho, S., Gerig, G.: A brain tumor segmentation framework based on outlier detection. Med. Image Anal. **8**(3), 275–283 (2004)

4. Gooya, A., Pohl, K.M., Bilello, M., Biros, G., Davatzikos, C.: Joint segmentation and deformable registration of brain scans guided by a tumor growth model. In: Fichtinger, G., Martel, A., Peters, T. (eds.) MICCAI 2011. LNCS, vol. 6892, pp. 532–540. Springer, Heidelberg (2011). doi:10.1007/978-3-642-23629-7_65

5. Parisot, S., Duffau, H., Chemouny, S., Paragios, N.: Joint tumor segmentation and dense deformable registration of brain MR images. In: Ayache, N., Delingette, H., Golland, P., Mori, K. (eds.) MICCAI 2012. LNCS, vol. 7511, pp. 651–658. Springer, Heidelberg (2012). doi:10.1007/978-3-642-33418-4_80

6. Zikic, D., et al.: Decision forests for tissue-specific segmentation of high-grade gliomas in multi-channel MR. In: Ayache, N., Delingette, H., Golland, P., Mori, K. (eds.) MICCAI 2012. LNCS, vol. 7512, pp. 369–376. Springer, Heidelberg (2012). doi:10.1007/978-3-642-33454-2_46

7. Tustison, N., Wintermark, M., Durst, C., Brian, A.: ANTs and arboles. In: Proceedings of BRATS-MICCAI (2013)

8. Urban, G., Bendszus, M., Hamprecht, F., Kleesiek, J.: Multi-modal brain tumor segmentation using deep convolutional neural networks. In: Proceedings of BRATS-MICCAI (2014)

9. Pereira, S., Pinto, A., Alves, V., Silva, C.A.: Brain tumor segmentation using convolutional neural networks in MRI images. IEEE Trans. Med. Imaging **35**(5), 1240–1251 (2016)

10. Menze, B.H., Jakab, A., Bauer, S., Kalpathy-Cramer, J., Farahani, K., Kirby, J., Burren, Y., Porz, N., Slotboom, J., Wiest, R., et al.: The multimodal brain tumor image segmentation benchmark (BRATS). IEEE Trans. Med. Imaging **34**(10), 1993–2024 (2015)

11. Bakas, S., et al.: GLISTRboost: combining multimodal MRI segmentation, registration, and biophysical tumor growth modeling with gradient boosting machines for glioma segmentation. In: Crimi, A., Menze, B., Maier, O., Reyes, M., Handels, H. (eds.) BrainLes 2015. LNCS, vol. 9556, pp. 144–155. Springer, Cham (2016). doi:10.1007/978-3-319-30858-6_13

12. Havaei, M., Davy, A., Warde-Farley, D., Biard, A., Courville, A., Bengio, Y., Pal, C., Jodoin, P.M., Larochelle, H.: Brain tumor segmentation with deep neural networks. arXiv preprint arXiv:1505.03540 (2015)

13. Lyksborg, M., Puonti, O., Agn, M., Larsen, R.: An ensemble of 2D convolutional neural networks for tumor segmentation. In: Paulsen, R.R., Pedersen, K.S. (eds.) SCIA 2015. LNCS, vol. 9127, pp. 201–211. Springer, Cham (2015). doi:10.1007/978-3-319-19665-7_17

14. Kamnitsas, K., Chen, L., Ledig, C., Rueckert, D., Glocker, B.: Multi-scale 3D convolutional neural networks for lesion segmentation in brain MRI. Ischemic Stroke Lesion Segm., 13–16 (2015)

15. Maier, O., Menze, B.H., von der Gablentz, J., Häni, L., Heinrich, M.P., Liebrand, M., Winzeck, S., Basit, A., Bentley, P., Chen, L., et al.: ISLES 2015-a public evaluation benchmark for ischemic stroke lesion segmentation from multispectral MRI. Med. Image Anal. **35**, 250–269 (2017)

16. Alansary, A., et al.: Fast fully automatic segmentation of the human placenta from motion corrupted MRI. In: Ourselin, S., Joskowicz, L., Sabuncu, M.R., Unal, G., Wells, W. (eds.) MICCAI 2016. LNCS, vol. 9901, pp. 589–597. Springer, Cham (2016). doi:10.1007/978-3-319-46723-8_68

17. Ioffe, S., Szegedy, C.: Batch normalization: accelerating deep network training by reducing internal covariate shift. arXiv preprint arXiv:1502.03167 (2015)

18. He, K., Zhang, X., Ren, S., Sun, J.: Identity mappings in deep residual networks. arXiv preprint arXiv:1603.05027 (2016)

19. Simonyan, K., Zisserman, A.: Very deep convolutional networks for large-scale image recognition. arXiv preprint arXiv:1409.1556 (2014)

20. He, K., Zhang, X., Ren, S., Sun, J.: Deep residual learning for image recognition. arXiv preprint arXiv:1512.03385 (2015)

21. Krähenbühl, P., Koltun, V.: Efficient inference in fully connected CRFs with Gaussian edge potentials. Adv. Neural Inf. Process. Syst. **24**, 109–117 (2011)

22. Chang, P.D.: Fully convolutional neural networks with hyperlocal features for brain tumor segmentation. In: Proceedings of BRATS-MICCAI (2016)

23. Le Folgoc, L., Nori, A.V., Alvarez-Valle, J., Lowe, R., Criminisi, A.: Segmentation of brain tumors via cascades of lifted decision forests. In: Proceedings of BRATS-MICCAI (2016)

24. Zhao, X., Wu, Y., Song, G., Li, Z., Fan, Y., Zhang, Y.: Brain tumor segmentation using a fully convolutional neural network with conditional random field. In: Proceedings of BRATS-MICCAI (2016)

25. Zeng, K., Bakas, S., Sotiras, A., Akbari, H., Rozycki, M., Rathore, S., Pati, S., Davatzikos, C.: Segmentation of gliomas in pre-operative and post-operative multimodal magnetic resonance imaging volumes based on a hybrid generative-discriminative framework. In: Proceedings of BRATS-MICCAI (2016)

26. Meier, R., Knecht, U., Wiest, R., Reyes, M.: CRF-based brain tumor segmentation: alleviating the shrinking bias. In: Proceedings of BRATS-MICCAI (2016)

3D Convolutional Neural Networks for Brain Tumor Segmentation: A Comparison of Multi-resolution Architectures

Adrià Casamitjana$^{(\boxtimes)}$, Santi Puch, Asier Aduriz, and Verónica Vilaplana

Signal Theory and Communications Department,
Universitat Politècnica de Catalunya. BarcelonaTech, Barcelona, Spain
{adria.casamitjana,veronica.vilaplana}@upc.edu

Abstract. This paper analyzes the use of 3D Convolutional Neural Networks for brain tumor segmentation in MR images. We address the problem using three different architectures that combine fine and coarse features to obtain the final segmentation. We compare three different networks that use multi-resolution features in terms of both design and performance and we show that they improve their single-resolution counterparts.

1 Introduction

Gliomas are the most common type of brain tumors, and their segmentation and assessment provide relevant information for further evaluation, treatment planning and follow up. Patients' life expectancy greatly vary depending on the tumor grade, ranging from 15 months to 10 years in median, requiring immediate treatment in its more aggressive stages.

The main goal of brain tumor segmentation is to detect and localize tumor regions by identifying abnormal areas when compared to normal tissue. This distinction is rather challenging as borders are often fuzzy, and also because tumors vary across patients in size, location and extent. Several imaging modalities can be used to solve this task, individually or combined, including T1, T1-contrasted, T2 and FLAIR, each one providing different biological information.

Automatic brain tumor segmentation methods are usually categorized in two broad groups: generative models, which rely on prior knowledge about the appearance and distribution of different tissue types and discriminative models, which directly learn the relationship between image features and segmentation labels. Within the second group, the early approaches used hand-crafted features in a machine-learning pipeline (e.g. random forest [5,12]). However, in the last two years there has been an increasing use of deep learning methods (and specifically convolutional neural networks CNN) to tackle the problem, motivated

This work has been partially supported by the project BIGGRAPH-TEC2013-43935-R, financed by the Spanish Ministerio de Economía y Competitividad and the European Regional Development Fund (ERDF). Adrià Casamitjana is supported by the Spanish "Ministerio de Educación, Cultura y Deporte" FPU Research Fellowship.

© Springer International Publishing AG 2016
A. Crimi et al. (Eds.): BrainLes 2016, LNCS 10154, pp. 150–161, 2016.
DOI: 10.1007/978-3-319-55524-9_15

by the state of the art performance of deep learning models in several computer vision tasks. As opposed to classical discriminative models based on feature engineering, deep learning models learn a hierarchy of increasingly complex features directly from data, by applying several layers of trainable filters and optional pooling operations. Most of these methods do not completely exploit the available volumetric information but use two-dimensional CNN, processing 2D slices independently or using three orthogonal 2D patches to incorporate contextual information [1,3,4]. A fully 3D approach is proposed in [2], consisting of a 3D CNN that produces soft segmentation maps, followed by a fully connected 3D CRF that imposes generalization constraints and obtains the final labels.

In this paper we explore the use of 3D CNN for automatic brain segmentation using the BRATS dataset [1]. We train different CNN architectures that gather both local and contextual information comparing their design, quantitative and qualitative performance. The paper is organized as follows: in Sect. 2, we describe the 3D CNN framework as well the training scheme employed. Section 3 introduces three different architectures that combine multi-scale features. In Sect. 4 we perform several experiments to assess the performance of the three architectures and we compare them to their single-resolution counterparts. Finally, Sect. 5 draws some conclusions.

2   3D CNN Framework

We employ a fully convolutional [8] 3D approach. The extension of 2D-CNN to 3D introduces significant challenges: an increased number of parameters and important memory and computational requirements. In this section we discuss these and other critical design issues like the depth of the network, the sampling strategy used for training and the fully convolutional approach adopted to achieve dense inference.

2.1   Deep 3D CNN

Network depth is a crucial parameter of the system, yielding greater discriminative power for deeper networks. Although deep networks may be harder to train than shallow ones, the use of more layers boosts the performance as shown empirically in [10]. However, the use of pooling layers in deeper networks provide coarse, contextual features and, for segmentation tasks, it limits the scale of detail in the upsampled outputs. To address this problem, finer resolution features should as well be included in the final segmentation. For brain tumor segmentation task, we aim at combining coarse features that are useful for detection and localization with fine-grained information that is required to capture local intensity changes of the tumor tissue relative to the non-tumor tissue. In Sects. 3 and 4 we present and compare three different models that combine low detail and fine-grained features.

One of the limitations of 3D architectures is the demanding memory requirements. The use of pooling layers to reduce intermediate layer sizes is common to deal with memory constraints when using deep networks. Another key hyperparameter constrained by memory requirements is the number of filters per layer, especially in the first layers where the features have higher dimensionality. Finally, input and batch sizes need also to be designed to properly fit the hardware memory. For training, we use image patches of size 64^3 and we build batches of 10–20 images per batch, depending on the architecture, in a TITAN X GPU. Another limitation of 3D networks is that 3D convolutions are computationally expensive and increase exponentially the number of parameters. Thus, employing 3D kernels in a rather deep network makes the overall system prone to over-fitting. This problem can be alleviated by using small filter sizes ($k = 3$) in every convolutional layer and a sufficiently large training set.

For training, we use the scheme presented in [2], which is an hybrid between the dense-training procedure presented in [8], where the whole image is input and segmented in a single forward pass, and the classic approach of classifying the central voxel of each input patch. Dense-training was considered but rapidly discarded due to memory constraints. Similarly, the hybrid training strategy exploits the dense inference technique on image patches of smaller size, relaxing memory constraints. Hence, this efficient strategy reduces the computation time compared with the classical approach. In addition, the fully convolutional nature of the networks analysed allow employing dense-inference during test time.

2.2 Non-uniform Sampling

High class imbalance data, as seen in Fig. 1, may drive the networks to predict the most common class in the training set and thus, the final segmentation will not be able to detect any tumor tissue. A simple approach to tackle this problem consists in weighting the loss function with higher weights for less common classes and lower weights for more common classes. However, empirical results show a rather large bias to detect healthy tissue, the most probable class. In this case, it seems that the training distribution is too skewed and the problem cannot be solved by simply weighting the loss function. Instead, a non-uniform sampling scheme has to be applied to create training patches. One possible solution consists in creating training patches with equiprobable classes. However, it failed to predict the whole volume since the resulting training distribution strongly differs from the true distribution and many false positives appeared in the final segmentation.

Instead, the approach proposed in [2] is used in this work: we construct training patches by sampling the central-voxel with the same probability of belonging to background or foreground (gross-tumor). When employing this scheme, as analysed in [2], the relative distribution between the foreground voxels is closely preserved and the imbalance in comparison to healthy tissue is alleviated.

Patch size becomes an important hyperparameter and a trade-off between different factors is considered. From above, patch size is limited by memory

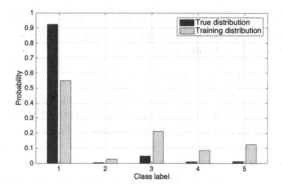

Fig. 1. Class distribution. The true dataset distribution (blue) and the training samples distribution used in this paper (yellow). (Color figure online)

constraints and class imbalance: in the limit, when the patch size is equal to the image size, it will recover the true distribution just as uniform sampling does. On the other side, small patch sizes is limited by the contextual information of each patch and tend to overrepresent rare classes in the final segmentation.

3 Architectures

We propose two fully convolutional 3D CNN architectures inspired in two well known 2D models used for generic image segmentation. We also train a third model which is a variant of the two-pathway DeepMedic network proposed in [2]. Networks are build upon the following block:

– $Conv + ReLU + BN$: the main layer is built as the concatenation of a convolutional layer (Conv) with ReLU activation and batch normalization (BN). Kernel size is 3^3.
– Convolutional block: it is built as a concatenation of several $Conv + ReLU + BN$ layers.
– Pooling layer: it uses max-pooling to downsample the feature maps. Pooling sizes are always 2^3.
– Prediction block: it uses a convolutional layer with kernel size 1^3
– Upsampling layer: it concatenates a repetition layer with a $Conv + ReLU + BN$ layer with kernel size 3^3. Upsampling factor is always 2^3. To get higher upsampling factors, a concatenation of upsampling layers is used.

3.1   3DNet_1

The first model, 3DNet_1, is a 3D fully convolutional network based on the VGG architecture [9] with skip connections that combine coarse, high scale information with fine, low scale information. The configuration of the network is inspired by [8] and it is illustrated in Fig. 2. Given the characteristic large number of parameters of 3D networks, a reduction in the number and dimensions of the filters with respect to its 2D analog was necessary in order to ensure that the model could be trained with the available resources.

Skip connections are built by taking the output of a certain layer and adding a $1 \times 1 \times 1$ convolutional layer on top of it to produce additional class predictions. 3DNet_1 adds those multi-scale predictions up and upscales the final result to the input size. The higher resolution predictions in the architecture provide the local information that helps to define the contours while the lower ones help to detect and localize the gross-tumor. The use of this architecture is motivated by the finer segmentation output provided by the multi-scale network compared with a network that uses only the low resolution information (see Sect. 4.2). The receptive field of the network is 212^3 voxels combined with predictions at receptive fields of 40^3 and 92^3 voxels.

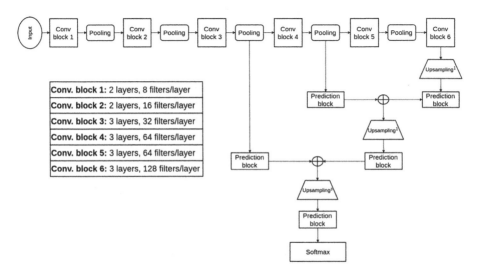

Fig. 2. Schematic representation of 3DNet_1. Upsampling^m represents m upsampling layers concatenated.

3.2   3DNet_2

The second model, 3DNet_2, is the 3D version of U-net, the network proposed in [6]. It is based on the architecture presented in [7], where on top of a VGG-like net (contracting/analysis path) there is a multilayer deconvolution network (expanding/synthesis path). The model is illustrated in Fig. 3. It is worth mentioning that a 3D U-net-type architecture appeared in the literature by the time we were working on this model, [11], using a shallower network than us and, thus, a much smaller receptive field. In contrast, [11] employ twice more filters for each convolutional layer. For comparison reasons, we kept the same number of filters for layers of the same dimensionality in all architectures, even though current hardware allows using more filter per layer.

The way 3DNet_2 combines multi-scale features is by concatenating all features maps from corresponding resolutions in the contracting path to the expanding path. Thus, the networks tries to synthesize information at each scale fusing local and contextual information. The receptive field of the network is 140^3 voxels and the concatenating paths are at receptive fields of 5^3, 14^3, 32^3 and 68^3 voxels.

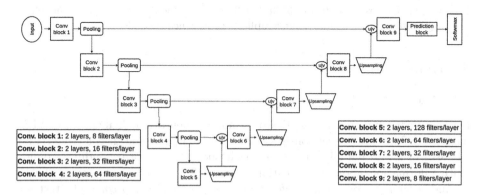

Fig. 3. Schematic representation of 3DNet_2. The $u|v$ operator stands for concatenation.

3.3   3DNet_3

The third architecture, 3DNet_3, is a modification of DeepMedic network [2] and it is illustrated in Fig. 4. The aim of using two paths is, again, gathering both low and high resolution features from the input image. The network proposed in [2] combines multi-scale information by using different input sizes for each path and thus, relaxing memory requirements. In contrast, we employ the same input size for both paths but different receptive fields to focus onto different information. In our implementation, the shorter path has a receptive field of 17^3 voxels while the longer one has a receptive field of 136^3 voxels. Like the other architectures, this scheme allows us to input the same image to both paths and fully segment each subject in a single forward pass during test-time.

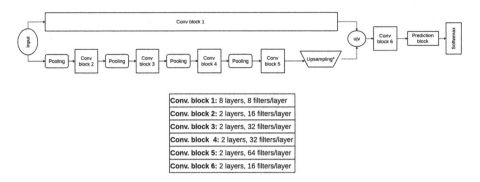

Fig. 4. Schematic representation of 3DNet_3. The $u|v$ operator stands for concatenation. Upsampling^m represents m upsampling layers concatenated

4 Experiments

4.1 Data

For the experiments we use the Brain Tumor Segmentation Challenge (BRATS) dataset [1]. The training set consists of 220 cases of high-grade glioma (HGG) and 54 cases of low-grade glioma (LGG), each one with its corresponding ground-truth information about the location of the different tumor structures: background, *necrotic core, edema, enhancing core, non-enhancing core*. The test set for the challenge comprises 191 cases, either LGG or HGG, with longitudinal measurements among some subjects. For each subject, 4 different MRI modalities are available: T1, T1-contrast, T2 and FLAIR. The dataset is preprocessed and MR images are provided skull-stripped. For each subject, all modalities are resampled to $1\,\mathrm{mm}^3$ resolution and registered to the T1 modality and normalized to zero mean and unit variance. Normalization is performed independently for each modality.

To evaluate the performance of the segmentation methods, the predicted labels are grouped into three tumor regions that better represent the clinical application tasks:

- The *whole* tumor region, which comprises all four tumor structures
- The *core* region, including all tumor regions except *edema*
- The *enhancing core* region.

For each tumor region, *Dice* similarity coefficient, *Precision* and *Recall* are computed:

$$Dice(P,T) = \frac{P_1 \wedge T_1}{(|P_1| + |T_1|)/2} \tag{1}$$

$$Precision(P,T) = \frac{P_1}{(|P_1| + |T_1|)} \tag{2}$$

$$Recall(P,T) = \frac{P_1 \wedge T_1}{|T_1|} \tag{3}$$

where $P \in \{0,1\}$ is the predicted segmentation and $T \in \{0,1\}$ is the ground truth. Thus, P_1 and T_1 represent the set of voxels where $P = 1, T = 1$.

In all experiments, we split the BRATS15 dataset into training set (60%) and validation set (40%), leaving some subjects to asses the segmentation performance. Experiments were set to compare the single- and multi-resolution schemes and to compare between the different multi-resolution architectures.

4.2   Single- vs. Multi-resolution Architectures

The first experiments that we carried out were focused on comparing the contribution of multi-resolution features on the final tumor segmentation. We trained a reduced, single-scale network equivalent for each architecture. For the 3DNet_1, we delete the lower level predictions (i.e. skip connections) leaving only the core network (upper path in Fig. 2). The resulting network has a huge receptive field (212^3 voxels). For the 3DNet_2, we cut the connections between contracting and expanding paths in Fig. 3. The receptive field of this architecture is also high (140^3 voxels). Finally, for the 3DNet_3, we build another network by just using the upper path in Fig. 4 that corresponds to the high-resolution features with small receptive field (17^3 voxels).

In Fig. 5 we analyze the evolution of training and validation loss for all the single- and multi-resolution architectures. The first thing that we observe is that the training error plateaus in a slightly greater value in the simple networks than in the multi-resolution ones, but without showing large difference in terms of convergence rates. More interestingly, we find that the multi-scale networks generalize much better to unseen data compared to single-scale networks.

In Table 1, we compare the different networks in terms of accuracy and Dice scores. 3DNet_1 and 3DNet_2, in their single-resolution forms, fail in their overall segmentations mainly due to using only coarse information. In contrast, 3DNet_3 single-resolution architecture uses a smaller receptive field that helps to outperform the others. Besides, we empirically show that multi-scale architectures outperform their single-scale counterparts.

Table 1. Results for our validation set from BRATS2015 training set.

Single-res	Accuracy	Dice score			Multi-res	Accuracy	Dice score		
		Whole	Core	Active			Whole	Core	Active
3DNet_1	99.09	38.88	29.00	23.94	3DNet_1	99.69	89.64	76.87	63.12
3DNet_2	97.33	48.09	24.16	44.69	3DNet_2	99.71	91.59	69.90	73.89
3DNet_3	99.55	84.19	71.38	69.09	3DNet_3	99.71	91.74	83.61	76.82

Finally, a visual investigation of the final segmentation is shown in Fig. 6. We observe that 3DNet_1 in its single-resolution form completely fails to predict the tumor region, even for large structures, such as edema. On the contrary, 3DNet_3

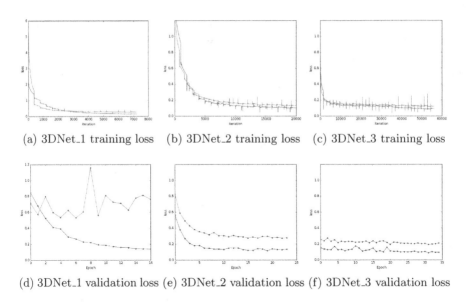

(a) 3DNet_1 training loss   (b) 3DNet_2 training loss   (c) 3DNet_3 training loss

(d) 3DNet_1 validation loss (e) 3DNet_2 validation loss (f) 3DNet_3 validation loss

Fig. 5. Train and validation loss curves comparing the convergence rate of multi-resolution architectures (blue) and their corresponding single-resolution approaches (red). (Color figure online)

in its single-path implementation shows overall good segmentation results. Even though detecting false tumor substructures inside and outside the gross-tumor, this model correctly predicts tumor boundaries and accounts for higher variability in intra-tumoral regions. Finally, 3DNet_2, is able to detect tumoral and intra-tumoral substructures but with rather low resolution. More interestingly, we observe many false-positives in the final segmentation, both in brain and non-brain tissue. In this case, the network fails in identifying general brain features, such as brain/non-brain tissue, grey matter or white matter tissue that is shown to significantly improve the segmentation performance [12].

4.3   A Comparison of the Multi-resolution Architectures

The second set of experiments compares the three different multi-scale architectures in terms of their design parameters. 3DNet_3 is by far the one with more memory constraints due to its local path without pooling layers. It requires employing small batch sizes ($\sim$10) and using few filters per layer and thus, becoming the network with less number of parameters. At the same time, it is the most costly in terms of computation, being slower to train but making almost no difference in inference time. On the other hand, 3DNet_1 and 3DNet_2 have a much larger number of parameters due to using more filters per layer, especially the latter, that also concatenates several feature maps in the synthesis path. Its decreasing computation time is due to a reduced number of convolutions. Each architecture was trained using the same sampling scheme which provides 2.1M

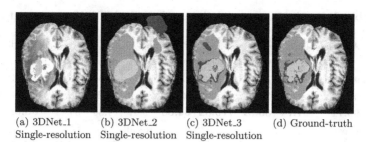

(a) 3DNet_1   (b) 3DNet_2   (c) 3DNet_3   (d) Ground-truth
Single-resolution Single-resolution Single-resolution

Fig. 6. Segmentation results of the three single-resolution networks. We distinguish intra-tumoral regions by color-code: edema (green), necrotic core (light blue), enhancing core (yellow) and non-enhancing core (dark blue) (Color figure online)

voxels/epoch to classify, although not all input voxels are different. In training samples, we have some redundancy, especially in tumor regions, were several patches may partially overlap. However, the number of different voxels provided at each epoch is still greater than the number of parameters, what makes the overall system well-conditioned (Table 2).

Table 2. Network characteristics comparison.

	Train time [s]	Voxels/epoch[a]	Test time [s]	N. parameters	GPU [MB/image][b]
3DNet_1	5–7 k	2.1 M	6–7	994469	76
3DNet_2	6–8 k	2.1 M	7–8	1473655	167
3DNet_3	9–12 k	2.1 M	8–10	386429	256

[a] Patches are selected with overlap, so effective number of voxels is much lower.
[b] GPU memory is counted in a forward pass.

Comparing the performance of the three networks, we show relevant metrics on our validation set in Table 3. We can see that even though 3DNet_3 performs better according to many metrics (especially Dice coefficients), we can not categorically state which network is significantly better. The slightly better performance of 3DNet_3 compared with the others is neither gained in terms of capacity nor in network depth, since 3DNet_1 and 3DNet_2 have deeper paths. Instead, we think the local path with low receptive field and without using pooling layers helps the final segmentation. Besides, the use of pooling layers is useful to provide contextual information but it looses finer details. In addition, since it uses less parameters, it might be easier to optimize. However, 3DNet_3 is the one with highest computational cost, yielding larger training and inference times.

Table 3. Results for our validation set from BRATS2015 training set.

	Accuracy	Dice score			Precision			Recall		
		Whole	Core	Active	Whole	Core	Active	Whole	Core	Active
3DNet_1	99.69	89.64	76.87	63.12	93.92	85.71	74.03	86.19	73.53	66.94
3DNet_2	**99.71**	91.59	69.90	73.89	92.99	**87.08**	**82.65**	**90.68**	65.63	73.37
3DNet_3	**99.71**	**91.74**	**83.61**	**76.82**	**94.60**	85.47	74.06	89.43	**83.08**	**87.29**

	Precision					Recall				
	1-Nec	2-Edm	3-NEnh	4-Enh	0-Else	1-Nec	2-Edm	3-NEnh	4-Enh	0-Else
3DNet_1	65.33	81.49	28.40	66.94	**99.95**	44.71	74.09	28.40	66.94	**99.95**
3DNet_2	**75.21**	79.07	43.57	**82.65**	99.92	41.10	**84.16**	32.35	73.38	99.93
3DNet_3	67.45	**85.06**	**49.44**	74.06	99.90	**51.29**	77.50	**37.61**	**87.29**	**99.95**

In Fig. 7 we see that for rather big and smooth tumor subregions, our three architectures perform well. On the other hand, they fail to capture high variability in small tumor sub-regions, but still being able to segment the gross tumor with good performance.

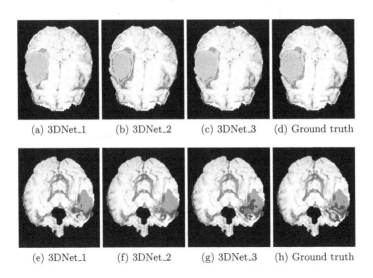

(a) 3DNet_1   (b) 3DNet_2   (c) 3DNet_3   (d) Ground truth

(e) 3DNet_1   (f) 3DNet_2   (g) 3DNet_3   (h) Ground truth

Fig. 7. Qualitative analysis in the axial plane. In the first row, we show examples with large and smooth tumor regions, while in the bottom row we show an example of high variability within intra-tumoral regions. We distinguish intra-tumoral regions by color-code: edema (green), necrotic core (light blue), enhancing core (yellow) and non-enhancing core (dark blue). (Color figure online)

5   Conclusions

In this paper we present several methods for the automatic brain segmentation task, using 3D convolutional neural networks. We compare and analyze three different multi-resolution architecture implementations that combine local and global information in the final segmentation. This combination is shown to be crucial to boost the performance of the system. We compared these three multi-resolution architectures with its single-resolution counterparts, in terms of performance and visual inspection. Furthermore we trained and assess the three different architectures in order to participate in BRATS challenge 2016, reaching competitive results, being the 3DNet_3 the better ranked among the three presented methods.

References

1. Menze, B.H., Jakab, A., et al.: The multimodal brain tumor image segmentation benchmark (BRATS). IEEE Trans. Med. Imaging **34**(10), 1993–2024 (2015)
2. Kamnitsas, K., Ledig, C., et al.: Efficient multi-scale 3D CNN with fully connected CRF for accurate brain lesion segmentation. Medical Image Analysis **36**, 61–78 (2017)
3. Pereira, S., Pinto, A., Alves, V., Silva, C.A.: Deep convolutional neural networks for the segmentation of gliomas in multi-sequence MRI. In: Crimi, A., Menze, B., Maier, O., Reyes, M., Handels, H. (eds.) BrainLes 2015. LNCS, vol. 9556, pp. 131–143. Springer, Cham (2016). doi:10.1007/978-3-319-30858-6_12
4. Havaei, M., Davy, A., et al.: Brain tumor segmentation with deep neural networks. Med. Image Anal. (2016)
5. Maier, O., Wilms, M., Handels, H.: Image features for brain lesion segmentation using random forests. In: Crimi, A., Menze, B., Maier, O., Reyes, M., Handels, H. (eds.) BrainLes 2015. LNCS, vol. 9556, pp. 119–130. Springer, Cham (2016). doi:10.1007/978-3-319-30858-6_11
6. Ronneberger, O., Fischer, P., Brox, T.: U-Net: convolutional networks for biomedical image segmentation. In: Navab, N., Hornegger, J., Wells, W.M., Frangi, A.F. (eds.) MICCAI 2015. LNCS, vol. 9351, pp. 234–241. Springer, Cham (2015). doi:10.1007/978-3-319-24574-4_28
7. Noh, H., Hong, S., Han, B.: Learning deconvolution network for semantic segmentation. In: ICCV, Santiago, Chile (2015)
8. Long, J., Shelhamer, E., Darrel, T.: Fully convolutional networks for semantic segmentation. In: CVPR, Boston, USA (2015)
9. Simonyan, K., Zisserman, A.: Very Deep Convolutional Networks for Large-Scale Image Recognition. arXiv:1409.1556v6 (2015)
10. He, K., et al.: Deep residual learning for image recognition. In: The IEEE Conference on Computer Vision and Pattern Recognition (CVPR) (2016)
11. Çiçek, Ö., Abdulkadir, A., Lienkamp, S.S., Brox, T., Ronneberger, O.: 3D U-Net: learning dense volumetric segmentation from sparse annotation. In: Ourselin, S., Joskowicz, L., Sabuncu, M.R., Unal, G., Wells, W. (eds.) MICCAI 2016. LNCS, vol. 9901, pp. 424–432. Springer, Cham (2016). doi:10.1007/978-3-319-46723-8_49
12. Zikic, D., et al.: Decision forests for tissue-specific segmentation of high-grade gliomas in multi-channel MR. In: Ayache, N., Delingette, H., Golland, P., Mori, K. (eds.) MICCAI 2012. LNCS, vol. 7512, pp. 369–376. Springer, Heidelberg (2012). doi:10.1007/978-3-642-33454-2_46

Anatomy-Guided Brain Tumor Segmentation and Classification

Bi Song$^{(\boxtimes)}$, Chen-Rui Chou, Xiaojing Chen, Albert Huang,
and Ming-Chang Liu

US Research Center, Sony Electronics Inc., San Jose, USA
bi.song@am.sony.com

Abstract. In this paper, we consider the problem of fully automatic brain tumor segmentation in multimodal magnetic resonance images. In contrast to applying classification on entire volume data, which requires heavy load of both computation and memory, we propose a two-stage approach. We first normalize image intensity and segment the whole tumor by utilizing the anatomy structure information. By dilating the initial segmented tumor as the region of interest (ROI), we then employ the random forest classifier on the voxels, which lie in the ROI, for multi-class tumor segmentation. Followed by a novel pathology-guided refinement, some mislabels of random forest can be corrected. We report promising results obtained using BraTS 2015 training dataset.

1 Introduction

Segmentation of brain tumor from medical images is of high interest in surgical planning, treatment monitoring and is gaining popularity with the advance of image guided surgery. The goal of segmentation is to delineate different tumor structures, such as active tumorous core, necrosis and edema. Typically, this process requires several hours of a clinician's time to manually contour the tumor structures. As manual processing is so labor intensive, automated approaches are being sought. Automatic brain tumor segmentation is challenging due to the large variation in appearance and shape across patients.

Most state-of-the-art methods sample the entire MRI volume data to build classifier for multi-class tumor segmentation, which involve high demand of computation and memory. In this paper, we propose a two-stage automatic segmentation method. We first segment the whole tumor by utilizing anatomy structure information for data intensity normalization and tumor separation from non-tumor tissues. Using this initially segmented tumor as a ROI, we then employ a random forest classifier followed by a novel pathology based refinement to distinguish between different tumor structures. As we only apply classification on the voxels within a ROI, our algorithm is more efficient in terms of both time and memory. The workflow of proposed method is shown in Fig. 1.

We provide an empirical evaluation of our method on publicly available BraTS [11] 2015/2016 training set, and compare with the top performing algorithms. The results demonstrate that the proposed method performs the best

A. Crimi et al. (Eds.): BrainLes 2016, LNCS 10154, pp. 162–170, 2016.
DOI: 10.1007/978-3-319-55524-9_16

in segmentation of active tumor core, and comparably to the top performing algorithms in the other tumor structures.

2   Method

In this section, we present the technical details of our proposed methods, as shown in Fig. 1, including data normalization, initial segmentation, feature extraction, voxel classification and refinement.

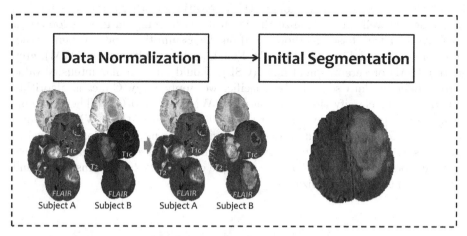

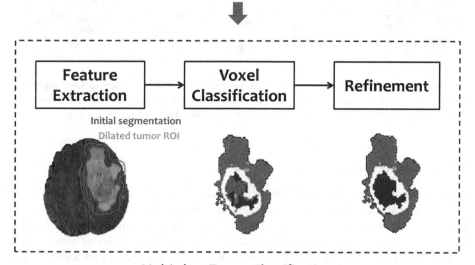

Fig. 1. The proposed two-stage brain tumor segmentation workflow.

2.1 Data Normalization

Intensity inhomogeneities appearing in MRI produce spatial intensity variations of the same tissue over the image domain. To correct the bias field, we applied the N4ITK approach [12]. However, there are large intensity variations across brain tumor MRI data sets and intensity ranges are not standardized; bias correction is not enough to ensure that the intensity of a tissue type across different subjects or even different scans of same subject lie in a similar scale. In [9], a cerebrospinal fuid (CSF) normalization technique is proposed to normalize each individual modality with the mean value of the CSF. However, just utilizing CSF information is not enough, the intensities of other structures need to be aligned as well. To normalize the intensity of imaging data, we propose an anatomy-structure-based method based on the assumption that the same structures of same modality (T1, T1c, T2, Flair), such as white matter (WM), grey matter (GM) or cerebrospinal fluid (CSF), should have similar intensity value across different data sets. To be specific, we apply fuzzy C-means algorithm (FCM) [2,5] to classify the input data into WM, GM and CSF. Then the normalization is performed by aligning the median values of these WM, GM, and CSF classes for each modality and do piecewise linear normalization in between. Thus ensure these tissue types have similar intensity across the image datasets of same modality. Figure 2 shows an example of intensity histograms before and after data intensity normalization.

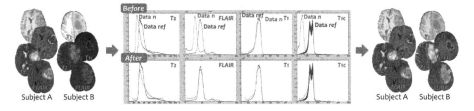

Fig. 2. An example of data normalization results. Note that contrary to just applying histogram matching, the proposed data normalization scheme provides similar intensity scale across subjects and meanwhile keeps the specific structure of each subject's data.

2.2 Initial Segmentation

Among different modalities of MRI, Flair and T2 provide better boundary contrast of the whole tumor. In [13], symmetric template difference is used as a feature in their supervised segmentation framework. In our method, we also explore symmetric information. By assuming tumor rarely happens completely symmetrically, symmetric differences of Flair and T2 are calculated for locating the initial seeds of tumors. After thresholding and union of the symmetric differences of Flair and T2, we remove the connected components whose size is too small, to reduce the false positive introduced by noise. By selecting the center of the initial seeds as the target seeds and a bounding box as the background seeds, the GrowCut algorithm [14] is employed on the linear combination of Flair and T2, $\alpha \cdot I_{Flair} + (1 - \alpha) \cdot I_{T2}$, for segmenting the whole tumor. An illustration of initial segmentation is shown in Fig. 3.

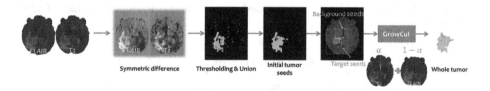

Fig. 3. An illustration of initial tumor segmentation.

2.3 Feature Extraction

The initial segmentation results are dilated to provide a ROI for further multi-class segmentation. The features are extracted from the ROI. Our features include voxel-wise and context-wise features. The voxel-wise features are composed of appearance features, texture features and location features. The context-wise features [7] aim to capture the neighborhood information.

– *Appearance*: Voxel's intensity value of smoothed T1, T1c, T2 and FLAIR. Gaussian kernel is applied to suppress the data noise.
– *Texture*: Variance of T2 and Laplacian of Gaussian (LoG) on T2, which represent local inhomogeneity.
– *Location*: Initial segmentation results indicating the prior information about the location of tumor.
– *Context*: Multiscale local mean intensity within a box of different size centered on each voxel to catch neighborhood information. Context features are combined from T1c and T2.

An illustration of extracted features is shown in Fig. 4.

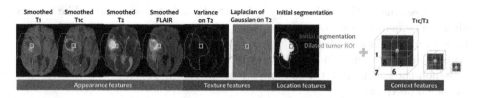

Fig. 4. An illustration of extracted features. The voxel-wise features are shown on the left, and the context-wise features are shown on the right.

2.4 Voxel Classification

A random forest classifier [3] is used for multi-class classification of pixels into five classes: (i) label 1 for necrosis (ii) label 2 for edema (iii) label 3 for non-enhancing tumor, (iv) label 4 for enhancing tumor and (v) label 0 for all other tissues. As illustrated in Fig. 5, each tree outputs a probability of tumor class. The final label of each voxel is decided based on the majority voting of the probabilities.

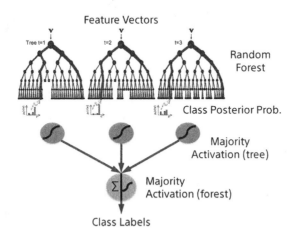

Fig. 5. An illustration of voxel classification using random forest.

2.5 Refinement

Pixel misclassification error might occur in the random forest classification results due to overlapping intensity ranges. For example, necrosis and non-enhancing cores may be mislabeled as edema. We propose a pathology-guided refinement scheme to correct the mislabels based on pathology rules, such as edema is usually not inside the active cores, and non-enhancing cores often sur-round active cores. Figure 6 shows example results before and after refinement. In Fig. 6(a), the output of random forest classification is shown in the middle, the necrosis inside the active cores is incorrectly labeled as edema. The results after refinement are shown on the right, these errors are corrected based on the pathology-guided rules. In Fig. 6(b), middle shows the output of random forest classification. The non-enhancing core is mislabeled as edema. By identifying core/non-core seeds from the random forest results, these errors can be corrected as shown on the right.

3 Experimental Results

To evaluate the performance of our method, we show results on the BraTS 2015 training data set (identical to BraTS 2016 training data set) [11], which contains

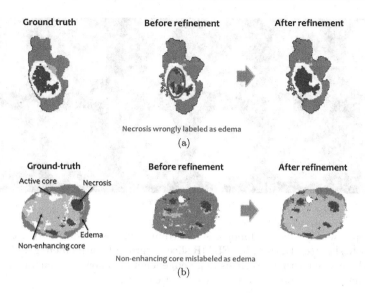

Fig. 6. Example of results before and after refinement. (a) Left: Ground truth, Middle: Random forest output, necrosis inside the active cores is wrongly labeled as edema. Right: Results after refinement. (b) Left: Ground truth, Middle: Random forest output, non-enhancing core is mislabeled as edema. Right: Results after refinement.

220 high-grade and 54 low-grade glioma cases. The dataset include MRI with four different sequences: T1, T1 after gadolinium enhancement (i.e., T1c), T2 and FLAIR. The data volumes are already skull-stripped and registered intra-patient. The volumes include four tumor labels: necrosis, edema, non-enhancing core and tumor active core. The result of our classification framework is a label at every voxel in the 3D MRI volumes. The accuracy measures employed are Dice's coefficient and Hausdorff distance. Similar to the Virtual Skeleton Database (VSD) [1] online evaluation system for BraTS, the metrics are evaluated on three structures: the "whole" tumor (i.e., all four tumor structures), the tumor "core" (i.e., all tumor structures except "edema") and the "active" tumor (i.e., only the tumor active core). We perform a leave-one-out cross validation. Note that we do not take high-grade or low-grade as a prior knowledge during training and testing.

3.1   Qualitative Results

Examples of our tumor classification results are shown in Fig. 7. The results are shown on one high grade tumor case and one low grade tumor case alone with the corresponding T1, T1c, T2 and FLAIR slices. In both cases, it can be seen that visually our results are comparable to the ground truth labeling. The Dice scores (%) for these two cases are: Case 1 (HGG) Necrosis 85.22, edema 91.45, non-enhancing core 9.19 and tumor active core 94.79; Case 2 (LGG) Necrosis 80.17, edema 66.62, non-enhancing core 56.31 and tumor active core 65.90.

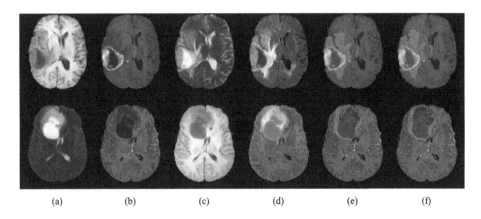

Fig. 7. Top row: high grade tumor case. Bottom row: low grade tumor case. (a) T1 slice, (b) T1c slice, (c) T2 slice, (d) FLAIR slice, (e)ground truth labeling and (f) labels produced by our algorithm (Necrosis in green, edema in yellow, non-enhancing core in red and tumor active core in cyan). (Color figure online)

3.2   Quantitative Results

Table 1 shows the average Dice and Hausdorff distance obtained using our method on a total of 274 cases. The boxplots of Dice and Hausdorff distance are shown in Fig. 8.

Table 1. Results obtained on BraTS 2015 Training dataset, reporting average Dice coefficient and Hausdorff distance. Dice scores for active tumor are calculated for high-grade cases only.

	Whole	Core	Active
Dice (%)	87.0	72.2	75.4
Hausdorff distance (mm)	9.3	9.1	6.5

We compare our results on BraTS 2016 training data set with top performing algorithms in testing phase of the BraTS 2016 Challenge in Table 2. The results show that the proposed method performs the best in segmentation of active tumor core, and comparably to the top performing algorithms in the other tumor structures.

Run time. The run time of training using 254 cases on a computer with 2.67 G Hz GPU, 24 G memory is about 15 min and run time of testing one case is about 1 min.

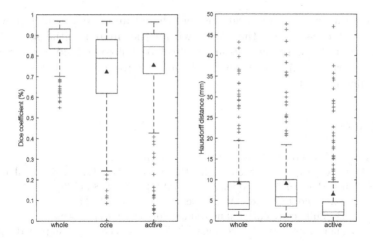

Fig. 8. Boxplots of Dice and Hausdorff distance on 274 cases. The blue triangle shows the mean and red line shows the median. (Color figure online)

Table 2. Comparison of the average dice scores of proposed method and top performing algorithms in BraTS 2016 Challenge. Note that not all the top performing algorithms report their results on all the 274 cases.

	Whole	Core	Active	Data
Chang [4]	87	81	72	29 HGG, No LGG
Kamnitsas [8]	89.6	76.3	72.4	All 220 HGG, 54 LGG
Zeng [15]	89	77	65	176 HGG, 54 LGG
Le Folgoc [6]	82	73	75	176 HGG, no LGG
Meier [10]	84.7	64.7	70	MEDIAN on the BRATS-2015 TESTING database
Our	87.0	72.2	75.4	Whole+Core 220 HGG, 54 LGG. "Active" on HGG

2016 Testing Phase. We apply our model trained with BraTS 2016 training data set on the BraTS 2016 testing data set (291 cases). The results on testing data set are not as good as the ones we get on the training data set. One possible reason is that the cases of the training data set are all of 1.5 T while testing data set contains many 3 T cases.

4   Conclusion

In this paper, we considered the problem of fully automatic multimodal brain tumor segmentation. We proposed a two-stage approach for efficiency in terms of both time and memory. We first utilized anatomy structure information to normalize data intensity and segment the whole tumor. Next, we employed the random forest classifier on the voxels within the dilated initial segmentation for multi-class tumor segmentation. A novel pathology-guided refinement was applied to further improve accuracy. Promising results are shown on BraTS 2015 training dataset.

References

1. The Virtual Skeleton Database (VSD). www.virtualskeleton.ch
2. Bezdek, J.: A convergence theorem for the fuzzy ISODATA clustering algorithms. IEEE Trans. Pattern Anal. Mach. Intell. PAMI **2**(1), 1–8 (1980)
3. Breiman, L.: Random forests. Mach. Learn. **45**(1), 5–32 (2001)
4. Chang, P.D.: Fully convolutional neural networks with hyperlocal features for brain tumor segmentation. In: Proceedings MICCAI-BRATS Workshop 2016, pp. 4–9 (2016)
5. Dunn, J.: A fuzzy relative of the isodata process and its use in detecting compact well-separated clusters. J. Cybern. **3**(3), 32–57 (1973)
6. Folgoc, L.L., Nori, A.V., Alvarez-Valle, J., Lowe, R., Criminisi, A.: Segmentation of brain tumors via cascades of lifted decision forests. In: Proceedings MICCAI-BRATS Workshop 2016, pp. 26–30 (2016)
7. Geremia, E., Clatz, O., Menze, B.H., Konukoglu, E., Criminisi, A., Ayache, N.: Spatial decision forests for MS lesion segmentation in multi-channel magnetic resonance images. In: Proceedings of MICCAI (2011)
8. Kamnitsas, K., Ferrante, E., Parisot, S., Ledig, C., Nori, A., Criminisi, A., Rueckert, D., Glocker, B.: DeepMedic on brain tumor segmentation. In: Proceedings MICCAI-BRATS Workshop 2016, pp. 18–22 (2016)
9. Kleesiek, J., Biller, A., Urban, G., Köthe, U
10. Meier, R., Knecht, U., Wiest, R., Reyes, M.: CRF-based brain tumor segmentation: alleviating the shrinking bias. In: Proceedings MICCAI-BRATS Workshop 2016, pp. 35–39 (2016)
11. Menze, B.: The multimodal brain tumor image segmentation benchmark (brats). IEEE Trans. Med. Imaging **34**(10), 1993–2024 (2015)
12. Tustison, N.J., Avants, B.B., Cook, P.A., Zheng, Y., Egab, A., Yushkevich, P.A., Gee, J.C.: N4ITK: Improved N3 bias correction. IEEE Trans. Med. Imaging **29**(6), 1310–1320 (2010)
13. Tustison, N., Wintermark, M., Durst, C., Avants, B.: ANTs and Árboles. In: Proceedings MICCAI-BRATS Workshop 2013, pp. 47–50 (2013)
14. Vezhnevets, V., Konouchine, V.: "GrowCut" - interactive multi-label N-D image segmentation by cellular automata. In: Proceedings of GraphiCon, pp. 150–156 (2005)
15. Zeng, K., Bakas, S., Sotiras, A., Akbari, H., Rozycki, M., Rathore, S., Pati, S., Davatzikos, C.: Segmentation of gliomas in pre-operative and post-operative multimodal magnetic resonance imaging volumes based on a hybrid generative-discriminative framework. In: Proceedings MICCAI-BRATS Workshop 2016, pp. 60–67 (2016)

Lifted Auto-Context Forests for Brain Tumour Segmentation

Loic Le Folgoc$^{(\boxtimes)}$, Aditya V. Nori, Siddharth Ancha, and Antonio Criminisi

Microsoft Research Cambridge, Cambridge, UK
t-lolefo@microsoft.com

Abstract. We revisit Auto-Context Forests for brain tumour segmentation in multi-channel magnetic resonance images, where semantic context
is progressively built and refined via successive layers of Decision Forests
(DFs). Specifically, we make the following contributions: (1) *improved
generalization* via an efficient node-splitting criterion based on hold-
out estimates, (2) *increased compactness* at a tree-level, thereby yielding
shallow discriminative ensembles trained orders of magnitude faster, and
(3) *guided semantic bagging* that exposes latent data-space semantics
captured by forest pathways. The proposed framework is practical: the
per-layer training is fast, modular and robust. It was a top performer in
the MICCAI 2016 BRATS (Brain Tumour Segmentation) challenge, and
this paper aims to discuss and provide details about the challenge entry.

1 Introduction

The past few years have witnessed a vast body of machine learning (ML)
techniques for the automatic segmentation of medical images. Decision forests
(DFs) [18,21], and more recently, deep neural networks [11] have yielded state-
of-the-art results at MICCAI BRATS (Brain Tumour Segmentation) challenges.

In this paper, we describe an approach that builds upon the framework of
DFs, departing from the usual hand-crafting of powerful features based on *e.g.*
texture, elastic registration, supervoxels [6,17] with a complementary scheme
that is entirely generic and free of additional computations. More specifically, we
introduce an efficient node-splitting criterion based on cross-validation estimates
that improves the feature *selection* during the training stage. Consequently,
learnt features are more discriminative and generalize better to unseen data:
we refer to this process as *lifting* (see Sect. 4). Furthermore, the proposed cost
function induces a natural stopping condition to grow or prune decision trees,
resulting in an *Occam's razor*-like, principled trade-off between tree complexity
and training accuracy. We show that lifted DFs can outperform standard DFs
using compact, shallow tree architectures (several dozens or hundreds of nodes).

We exploit the resulting computational gains to revisit *auto-context* [13–
15] segmentation forests. In particular, we extend the approach with a meta-
architecture of cascaded DFs that naturally intertwine high-level *semantic* reasoning with *intensity*-based low-level reasoning (described in Sect. 5). The framework aims to be practical: the per-layer training is simple, modular and robust.

© Springer International Publishing AG 2016
A. Crimi et al. (Eds.): BrainLes 2016, LNCS 10154, pp. 171–183, 2016.
DOI: 10.1007/978-3-319-55524-9_17

Furthermore, this sequential design enables the decomposition of complex segmentation tasks into series of simpler subtasks that, for instance, exploit the hierarchical structure between labels (*e.g.*, whole tumour, tumour core, enhancing tumour parts). Beyond auto-context, another contribution is a clustering mechanism (see Sect. 5.2) that exposes the latent data-space semantics encoded within DF pathways. The learnt semantics are exploited to automatically guide classification in subsequent layers. Finally, in Sect. 7, we discuss results and details of our BRATS challenge entry.

2   Background: Random Forests for Image Segmentation

Let $I = \{I_j\}_{j=1...J}$ be the set of input channels in a multichannel image, x be a voxel, and $c \in \mathcal{C} = \{1 ... K\}$ be the class to predict for x. We define $\mathbf{x} = \{x, I\} \in \mathcal{X}$ as the feature vector of x. DF classifiers predict the probability $p(c|\mathbf{x})$ that a voxel x belongs to class c given its feature representation $\mathbf{x}$. This is done by aggregating predictions of an ensemble of $\mathcal{T}$ decision trees. Simple averaging is typically used, so that:

$$p(c|\mathbf{x}) = 1/|\mathcal{T}| \cdot \sum_{t=1}^{|\mathcal{T}|} p_t(c|\mathbf{x}),$$

where $p_t(c|\mathbf{x})$ denotes the prediction by tree $t \in \mathcal{T}$. The class with maximum probability is then returned (maximum a posteriori probability) as the prediction. Tree predictions are obtained as follows: a feature vector $\mathbf{x}$ is routed along a path in the tree from the root node by evaluating it at every internal (*split*) node n w.r.t. a routing function $h_n(\mathbf{x}) \triangleq [f(\mathbf{x}, \boldsymbol{\theta}_n) \leq \tau_n] \in \{0, 1\}$, and taking the left child n_L if $h_n(\mathbf{x}) = 1$, and the right child n_R otherwise, until a leaf node $n(\mathbf{x})$ is reached. Here $f : \mathcal{X} \times \Theta \mapsto \mathbb{R}$ is a weak learner parameterized by a node-specific feature $\boldsymbol{\theta}_n \in \Theta$, and $\tau_n \in \mathbb{R}$ a node-specific threshold. Examples of weak learners are given in Sect. 3. Each terminal (*leaf*) node $n \in \mathcal{L}$ is paired with a class predictor $p_n(c|\mathbf{x}) \triangleq p_n(c)$ such that $0 \leq p_n(c) \leq 1$, $\sum_{c=1}^{K} p_n(c) = 1$. The tree then predicts class c with probability $p_{n(\mathbf{x})}(c)$.

Decision trees are trained in a supervised manner from training data $D = \{\mathbf{x}_i, c_i\}_{i=1}^{N}$ with known class labels c_i, greedily and recursively, starting from a single root node. Training a node n entails finding the optimal feature $\boldsymbol{\theta}_n^*$ and threshold τ_n^* such that the node training data $D_n = \{\mathbf{x}_i, c_i\}_{i \in \mathcal{I}_n}$ is split between left and right children n_L and n_R in a way that maximizes class purity. Specifically, $\psi^* = (\boldsymbol{\theta}_n^*, \tau_n^*)$ and the resulting split $D_n = D_{n_L}(\psi) \coprod D_{n_R}(\psi)$ maximizes the Information Gain G$(\psi; D_n)$, which is defined as follows:

$$G(\psi; D_n) \triangleq \sum_{\epsilon = \{L, R\}} \frac{|D_{n_\epsilon}(\psi)|}{|D_n|} \sum_{c \in \mathcal{C}} p_{n_\epsilon}(c; \psi) \log p_{n_\epsilon}(c; \psi) - \sum_{c \in \mathcal{C}} p_n^*(c) \log p_n^*(c),$$

$$(1)$$

where $p_{n_\epsilon}(c; \psi) \triangleq |\{i \in \mathcal{I}_{n_\epsilon}(\psi) | c_i = c\}| / |D_{n_\epsilon}(\psi)|$ is the empirical class distribution in the training data D_{n_ϵ} for the child node n_ϵ. The optimum

$\psi^* \triangleq \arg\max_\psi G(\psi; D_n)$ is found by exhaustive search after proper quantization of thresholds τ_n. Trees are grown up to a predefined maximum depth, or until the number of training examples reaching a node is below a given threshold.

Last but not least, random forests introduce randomization in the training of each tree via feature and data *bagging*. For the t-th tree and at node $n \in \mathcal{V}_t$, only a random subset $\Theta' \subsetneq \Theta$ of candidate features is considered for training [1,7]. Similarly, only a random subset $D_n' \subsetneq D_n$ of training examples sampled with(out) replacement is used [3]. Data bagging is implemented both at an image level (random image subsets) and at a voxel level (random voxel subsets).

It is important to note that we do *not* make use of class rebalancing schemes. Training samples are often weighted according to the relative frequency of their class. This strategy aims to correct classifier bias in favor of the more frequent class, in cases where there is a large class imbalance. Of course, class rebalancing induces the opposite bias against more prevalent classes, which cannot be avoided in a multilabel classification setting. Section 5.2 discusses an alternative strategy to naturally correct for distribution imbalance.

3   Fast Scale-Space Context-Sensitive Features

We revisit scale-space representations to craft fast, expressive, compactly parameterized features, as a simple alternative to the popular integral or Haar-like features [19].

Background: integral features. Integral features are based on intensity averages within anisotropic cuboids offset from the point of interest [5]. Cuboid averages are computed in constant time by probing the value of a precomputed integral map at the cuboid vertices [19]. For instance, $f(\mathbf{x}, \boldsymbol{\theta}) \triangleq \sum_{x' \in \mathcal{C}_2} I_{j_2}(x') - \sum_{x' \in \mathcal{C}_1} I_{j_1}(x')$ computes the difference of responses in cuboids $\mathcal{C}_1$ and $\mathcal{C}_2$ of size $s_1 = (s_1^x, s_1^y, s_1^z)$ and $s_2 = (s_2^x, s_2^y, s_2^z)$, centered at offset locations $x + o_1$ and $x + o_2$, in distinct channels I_{j_1} and I_{j_2}. Here $\boldsymbol{\theta} = (j_1, j_2, o_1, o_2, s_1, s_2)$ is a 14-dimensional feature.

Proposed scale-space representation. During node training, it is crucial for sufficiently strong weak-learners to be computable within the budget allocated to feature sampling and optimization. Therefore, reducing the feature parameterization while maintaining expressiveness is key. For integral features, the sophistication of probing anisotropic cuboids with a continuous range of edge lengths comes at a cost w.r.t. parametric complexity. We restrict ourselves to a small *finite* range of *isotropic* averages. We augment the original set of c input channels with their smoothed counterparts under separable Gaussian filtering at scales σ_1, σ_2 etc. Given s scales, $f(\mathbf{x}, \boldsymbol{\theta}) \triangleq I_{j_2}(x + o_2) - I_{j_1}(x + o_1)$ computes the difference of responses in different channels at different scales and offsets from the voxel of interest ($j \in \{1 \ldots c \times s\}$ flatly indexes channels and scales). Here $\boldsymbol{\theta} = (j_1, j_2, o_1, o_2)$ is an 8-dimensional feature.

A single point is probed for every 8 cuboid vertices probed under integral features, as well as circumventing many boundary checks. For all practical purposes

($s = 2, 3$), `byte[]` storage of scale-space maps limits the memory overhead relative to integral maps (`short[]` storage).

Fast rotation invariant features. We can go beyond *directional* context and account for natural local invariances with fast, multiscale, approximately rotation invariant feature. Let $\phi_1 \cdots \phi_{12}$ stand for the coordinates of an axis-aligned, centered icosahedron of radius r. Denoting by $\boldsymbol{\theta} = (j_1, j_2, r)$ the 3-dimensional feature, $f(\mathbf{x}, \boldsymbol{\theta}) \triangleq \text{Median}_{v=1}^{12} |I_{j_2}(x + \phi_v) - I_{j_1}(x)|$ gives a robust summary of intensity variations around point x and probes 13 points only.

4   Lifting Decision Forests by Minimizing Cross-Validation Error Estimates

4.1   A Cautionary Look at Information Gain Maximization

We follow the notation introduced in Sect. 2, but drop the node index n for convenience. Information gain maximization w.r.t. (feature, threshold) parameters $\psi = (\boldsymbol{\theta}, \tau)$ can be shown to be equivalent to a joint maximum likelihood estimation (MLE) of $\phi \triangleq (\psi, p_L, p_R)$, the node parameters and children' class predictors. We omit the details for the sake of brevity. Essentially, decision trees are usually grown by greedily, recursively splitting leaf nodes by likelihood maximization:

$$\phi^* = \arg\max_{\phi} \mathcal{C}(D; \phi) \triangleq \arg\max_{\phi} \frac{p(D; \phi)}{p^*(D)} . \tag{2}$$

In Eq. (2), the denominator is the data likelihood using the current leaf node predictor, whereas the numerator is the data likelihood when splitting this node with parameters ϕ into left and right children. The denominator is constant w.r.t. ϕ, as optimization of the current node has precedence in the recursive schedule.

MLE runs the risk of overfitting. At a node-level, weak learners with poor generalization may be selected. The deeper the trees, the more likely it is to happen, since the training data is split between an exponentially increasing number of nodes. At a tree-level, the lack of principled method for controlling model capacity negatively impacts generalization. Indeed, the information gain is strictly positive (the likelihood ratio of Eq. (2) is > 1) as long as: (1) training samples remain at the node of interest, and (2) the data distribution is not pure. As a result, trees generally grow to the maximum allowed depth, with little control over generalization. Medical image segmentation tasks often require large trees of weak learners to be grown (tree depth 20–30, millions of nodes). Due to computational constraints, few such trees can be grown (a few dozens at most). For this reason, model averaging across randomized trees is insufficient to balance tree overfitting. As an efficient alternative to MLE that can be directly used to control tree growth and generalization, we propose to maximize the predictive score as obtained from *cross-validation* estimates.

4.2   Maximizing Cross Validation Estimates of Generalization

We derive Cross-Validation Estimates (CVE) of the predictive score as follows. At any given node, the (potentially bagged) training data $D = D^V \coprod D^T$ is randomly divided into two disjoint subsets, a tuning subset D^T and a validation subset D^V. The optimization problem is then defined as:

$$\phi^* = \arg \max_{\phi} \frac{p(D^V; \boldsymbol{\theta})}{p^*(D^V)}, \quad \text{s.t.}$$
$$(\tau_{\boldsymbol{\theta}}, p_\epsilon(\cdot; \boldsymbol{\theta})) = \arg \max_{\tau, p_\epsilon} p_\epsilon(D^T_\epsilon; \phi) \tag{3}$$

where $p(D^V; \boldsymbol{\theta}) \triangleq p(D^V; \boldsymbol{\theta}, \tau_{\boldsymbol{\theta}}, p_\epsilon(\cdot; \boldsymbol{\theta}))$. The key change is that parameters are now constrained to be tuned on D^T, whereas the final feature score is computed on D^V. While a *k-fold* estimate could be used instead in Eq. (3), the *hold-out* procedure has the benefit of efficiency and added randomness.

Key to the proposed approach is that the quantity in Eq. (3) takes values ≤ 1 whenever no candidate split yields superior generalization to the current leaf node model. Based on this, we implement a greedy scheme to control the tree complexity, where branches that do not increase the score are pruned in a single bottom-up pass as post-processing, similarly to [12]. We further use a simple heuristic to drastically reduce training time, growing trees *in stages* up to any desired maximum depth, successively pruning score-decreasing branches and regrowing remaining, non-pruned ones.

5   Auto-Context Forests for Brain Tumour Segmentation

We investigate cascaded DF architectures, made of layers of DFs partially or fully connected via their output posterior maps. This architecture naturally interleaves high-level *semantic* reasoning with *intensity*-based low-level reasoning. We demonstrate this via two ideas: (a) *auto-context*: allowing downstream layers to reason about semantics captured in upstream layers, and (b) *decision pathway clustering*: latent data-space semantics are revealed by clustering decision pathways and cluster-specific DFs are trained.

5.1   Building and Training Auto-Context Forests

The process of cascading DFs is illustrated in Fig. 1. Since DFs rely on generic context-sensitive features that disregard the exact nature of input channels (cf. Sect. 3), we simply proceed by augmenting the set of input channels for subsequent layers with output posterior maps from previous layers.

Layers are trained sequentially, one at a time in a greedy manner (following Sects. 2 and 4.2). Specifically, for the BRATS challenge, class labels follow a *nested* structure: the whole tumour (WT) consists of the edema (ED) and tumour core (TC). The tumour core itself is subdivided into enhancing tumour parts (ET), and other parts of the core that are only indirectly relevant to the

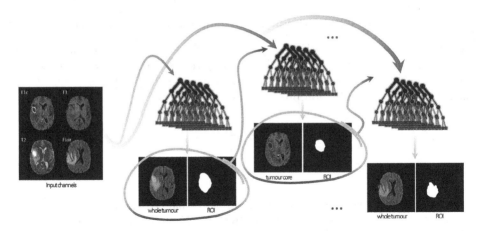

Fig. 1. Auto-Context segmentation Forests. In this schematic example, layer 2 solves a segmentation task distinct from that of layers 1, 3 but the interleaving allows to exploit joint dependencies.

task: the necrotic core (NC) and non-enhancing remaining parts (NE). Usually, these labels would be interpreted as mutually exclusive classes (ED, ET, NC, NE and the background BG) so as to formulate the task as a multilabel classification problem. Instead, our proposed framework directly uses these hierarchical relations. While many variants can reasonably be built, the final architecture that we used for the BRATS challenge consists of layers of binary DFs, alternating between predictions of WT, TC and ET (Sect. 6.2).

5.2 Exposing Latent Semantics in Decision Forests for Guided Bagging

Given Auto-Context Forests, a natural idea is to progressively refine the region of interest (ROI) after each layer, starting from an initial over-approximation of the ROI (*e.g.*, the full image). Downstream DFs are trained on more refined ROIs that exclude irrelevant background clutter, thereby increasing accuracy. Such an approach runs the risk of excluding false negatives, creating a trade-off between coarser ROIs (high recall) and tighter ROIs (high precision). We investigate a complementary strategy to circumvent this limitation. ROI refinement remains as a computational convenience.

The proposed approach exposes and exploits the latent semantics already captured within a given DF as follows. Each data point is identified with the collection of tree paths that it traverses. A metric d_{DP} is defined over such collections of tree paths (*decision pathways*), assigning smaller distance between points following similar paths across many trees, and data clusters are identified by k-means w.r.t. d_{DP}. Then, cluster-specific DFs are trained over the corresponding training data. At test time, data points are assigned to the cluster with closest centroid and the corresponding DF is used for prediction.

Our key insight is that data points that are clustered together will share common underlying semantics, as they jointly satisfy many predicates (see Fig. 2). A wide range of metrics can be designed and for the sake of simplicity, we define (given a collection $\mathcal{T}$ of trees):

$$d_{\mathrm{DP}}^{\mathcal{T}}(\mathbf{x}_i, \mathbf{x}_j) \triangleq \sum_{t=1}^{|\mathcal{T}|} \left(\frac{1}{2}\right)^{\mathrm{depth}_t^{\mathcal{T}}(\mathbf{x}_i, \mathbf{x}_j)} , \qquad (4)$$

where $\mathbf{x}_i, \mathbf{x}_j$ are two points, and $\mathrm{depth}_t^{\mathcal{T}}(\mathbf{x}_i, \mathbf{x}_j)$ is the depth of the deepest common node in both paths for the t-th tree ($+\infty$ if the paths are identical).

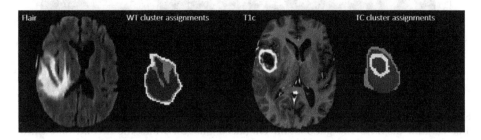

Fig. 2. Voxel cluster assignments for an example subject. Clusters for WT and TC binary forests are learned independently. 4 clusters are used for each and assignments are colour coded in gray levels. On this task clusters naturally appear to relate to "boundary" regions of higher uncertainty and higher certainty regions ("inside" the tumour or the BG).

6 BRATS Challenge: Framework Details

6.1 Training Dataset (BRATS 2015)

The BRATS 2015 dataset was available to participants of the challenge. It contains 274 images together with their ground truth annotations. One of the interesting aspects of the dataset is the nature of ground truth annotations: 30 images (from the BRATS 2013 dataset) were manually annotated, and the remaining were annotated using a consensus of segmentation algorithms [9]. While the ground truth is often of good quality, we note with interest that the consensus of algorithms generally fails at correctly labelling post-resection cavities as in Fig. 3 (bottom row). This is likely due to the fact that there is only *one* such training example in the original BRATS 2013 dataset (Fig. 3, top row).

We paid particular attention to such training examples. For these cases, we favoured a qualitative, visual assessment of correctness over quantitative metrics (DICE overlap or Hausdorff distance) when tuning our pipeline. These cases and similar observations motivate the two following choices: (1) An unsupervised SMM/MRF (see below) is trained on the 30 manually annotated BRATS

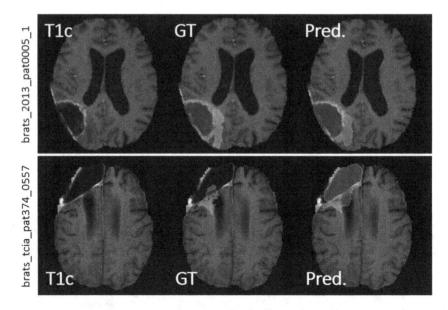

Fig. 3. Example images with resection cavities in the BRATS 2015 training set. The first column displays the gadolinium enhanced images, while the second and third respectively display the ground truth annotations and algorithm predictions. Top row: manual annotation. Bottom row: consensus annotation.

2013 images, to initialize the segmentation pipeline. For the background class, SMM weights are spatially varying, so that the model proves reasonably effective to disambiguate potential post-resection cavities from, say, ventricles, and (2) 70 images from the BRATS 2015 dataset ground truth with high quality annotations are chosen and used for training of the final model. While leading to a slight decrease in quantitative performance of the algorithm, it also qualitatively somewhat improves segmentation results (Fig. 3, last column). The same qualitative observations are made on the BRATS 2016 test set.

6.2   Pipeline, Model and Parameter Settings

Preprocessing. Image masks are defined from the FLAIR modality, masking out 0-intensity voxels. The intensity range is standardized: the distribution of voxel intensities within the mask is normalized to a common median and mean absolute deviation by affine remapping. As a mostly implementation specific step, we further window intensity values to make threshold quantization easier when training DFs: intensities are thresholded and brought within a byte range.

Initialization: SMM/MRF. A Student Mixture Model (SMM) with Markov Random Field (MRF) spatial prior is used to locate the region of interest (ROI) for the whole tumor. The likelihood for each of the five mutually exclusive ground truth classes is modelled by an SMM with spatially varying (BG) or fixed (other classes) proportions [2], as a suitably modified variant of [4]. An MRF prior is assumed over BG, ED and TC. The model is similar in spirit to [10,20]. It is unsupervised: the current implementation does not use white/grey matter and cerebro-spinal fluid labels, but the resulting components for the background SMM are highly correlated to those labels. Variational Bayesian inference is used at training and test time. The MRF defines fully connected cliques over the image, with Gaussian decay of pairwise potentials w.r.t. the distance of voxel centers. For this choice of potentials, the dependencies induced by MRF priors in variational updates can be efficiently computed via Gaussian filtering. Inference over $3D$ volumes is fast at training (seconds or minutes) and test time (seconds).

Auto-context architecture. 9 layers of binary DFs are cascaded, cycling between WT, TC and ET probabilities. All layers use the original, raw image channels. The input of the first layers is augmented with probability maps from the upstream SMM/MRF, the subsequent layers use probability maps output by previous layers. For instance, the second TC layer uses the output of the first TC, ET layers and of the second WT layer. In addition, the prior probability "atlas" maps returned by the spatially-varying background SMM/MRF model are passed to the first three layers. Many variants of this architecture were informally tested without a significant effect on accuracy.

ROI refinement. For computational convenience, subsequent layers are run on ROIs rather than the full image. For instance, the second BG vs. WT binary forest only tests points within the mask provided by the first BG vs. WT forest. Similarly at training time, the second layer is trained on subsets of image voxels within the respective image ROIs output by the first layer. Each layer uses masks obtained as dilated versions of the segmentation masks output by the previous layer (dilated resp. by 15 mm, 10 mm, 5 mm).

Parameter settings. DFs come with a number of parameters, many of which do not seem to strongly affect the pipeline accuracy after informal experiments. Five feature types are used: intensity in a given channel (respectively, at scale s), difference of intensities between the voxel of interest (VOI) at scale s_1 and an offset voxel at scale $s_2 > s_1$ in a given channel, median of the intensity difference (respectively, absolute difference) between the VOI at scale s_1 and the radius-r icosahedron vertices (scale $s_2 > s_1$) in a given channel. Between 100 and 200 candidate features are sampled per node. We use 2 scales: 1 mm and 2 mm for the first layers, 0.5 mm and 1 mm for the second and final layers. The offset along each direction (or the icosahedron radius) is sampled uniformly between 0 mm and 50 mm. The range of feature responses is quantized using 50 thresholds. The maximum tree depth is set at 12, and is seldom reached. The number of decision pathways clusters (Sect. 5.2) is set to 4. They are created using the first layer of WT, TC, ET (separately for each classification task). 50 trees are trained per layer per cluster-specific DF[1]. The subsampling rate for data bagging is adjusted based on the desired computation time. At each node, the training voxels from 25 random images serve as tuning set and similarly 30 (distinct) random images are used for validation (the remaining images are not used to train the node).

6.3   Test Dataset (BRATS 2016)

The pipeline described above is fully automated. To our knowledge, the BRATS 2015 training dataset pre-processing includes rigid registration (as well as resampling to a common image geometry), bias field correction and skull stripping [9]. The BRATS 2016 test dataset contains a number of unprocessed or partially pre-processed images (cf. Fig. 4). To cope with that, the pipeline was modified to include rigid registration and resampling, bias field correction [16] and skull stripping as part of a semi-automatic pre-processing step.

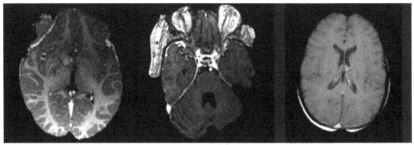

brats_2013_pat0103_0   brats_cbica_patAAM_416   brats_klhd_pat165_2

Fig. 4. BRATS 2016 test data: example of variability not seen in the training set. (Left) Bias field, (Middle) Partial skull stripping, (Right) Rigid misalignment, different geometry.

7   Results

The proposed approach is implemented in a .NET based DF framework which we call Bonsai. All experiments were performed on a 3.6 GHz Intel Xeon processor system with 16 GB RAM running Microsoft Windows 10. Training on the BRATS 2015 dataset takes around 6 to 7 h (including "testing" on the whole dataset). Testing takes about 20 s per image. The model is trained as described previously on 70 images from the BRATS 2015 training set (about 1/4th). Table 1 reports accuracy over the remaining of the BRATS 2015 dataset.

---

[1] As an illustration on WT layers. The 4 (WT) clusters are obtained from (the single DF of) the first WT layer. The second and third WT layers each consist of 4 distinct (50-tree) DFs, each of which is trained on cluster-specific data. At test time, voxels $\mathbf{x}$ pass through the first WT layer and are assigned a cluster $k_{\mathbf{x}} \in \{1 \cdots 4\}$. Then for the second and third layers, they are sent through the DF specific to the $k_{\mathbf{x}}$-th cluster. The same process is followed for TC and ET layers.

Table 1. Hold-out accuracy on the BRATS 2015 dataset for the model entered in the challenge *i.e.*, statistics over the remaining of the BRATS 2015 dataset after training on 70 images.

Dice	WT	TC	ET
Avg ± Std.	84% ± 15%	72% ± 26%	71% ± 29%
Median (IQR)	90% (13%)	82% (28%)	82% (30%)

These numbers are comparable to those reported in the recent state-of-the-art *e.g.* [8]. It is informative to compare the predicted accuracy (on validation data) against the performance on the BRATS 2016 test set. Rough estimates of the median DICE scores are as follows (exact numbers are not available): about 80% for WT, 60% for TC and over 70% for ET. Proper delineation of the tumour core seems to remain the most challenging task, perhaps due to the high variability of appearance across images and glioma types.

8   Conclusion

We described a principled method to train DFs using hold-out estimates of the predictive error, lifting the accuracy and generalization of individual nodes and of the DF altogether. We find that shallow lifted trees formed of a few dozens or hundreds of nodes favorably compare to conventional deep trees formed of millions of nodes. This is of practical interest: it makes training, tuning and experimenting with randomized DFs much more straightforward. We exploit this benefit to experiment within the framework of auto-context forests, on challenging multi-class and multi-organ medical image segmentation tasks. We report our experience using this approach in the MICCAI 2016 BRATS challenge, where it belongs to the top performers.

Acknowledgment. The authors would like to thank the Microsoft–Inria Joint Centre for partially funding this work.

A   BRATS 2015 Dataset: Training IDs

For completeness, the identifiers of images from the BRATS 2015 dataset that were used for training (Sect. 6.1) are listed below.

2013_pat0001_1, 2013_pat0002_1, 2013_pat0003_1, 2013_pat0004_1, 2013_pat0005_1, 2013_pat0006_1, 2013_pat0007_1, 2013_pat0008_1, 2013_pat0009_1, 2013_pat0010_1, 2013_pat0011_1, 2013_pat0012_1, 2013_pat0013_1, 2013_pat0014_1, 2013_pat0015_1, 2013_pat0022_1, 2013_pat0024_1, 2013_pat0025_1, 2013_pat0026_1, 2013_pat0027_1, tcia_pat105_0001, tcia_pat117_0001, tcia_pat124_0003, tcia_pat133_0001, tcia_pat149_0001, tcia_pat153_0181, tcia_pat165_0001, tcia_pat170_0002, tcia_pat260_0129, tcia_pat260_0244, tcia_pat260_0317, tcia_pat265_0001, tcia_pat290_0580, tcia_pat296_0001, tcia_pat300_0001, tcia_pat314_0001, tcia_pat319_0001, tcia_pat370_0001, tcia_pat372_0001, tcia_pat375_0001, tcia_pat377_0001, tcia_pat396_0139, tcia_pat396_0176, tcia_pat401_0001, tcia_pat430_0001, tcia_pat491_0001, 2013_pat0001_1, 2013_pat0004_1, 2013_pat0006_1, 2013_pat0008_1, 2013_pat0011_1, 2013_pat0012_1, 2013_pat0013_1, 2013_pat0014_1, 2013_pat0015_1, tcia_pat101_0001, tcia_pat109_0001, tcia_pat141_0001, tcia_pat241_0001, tcia_pat249_0001, tcia_pat298_0001, tcia_pat307_0001, tcia_pat325_0001, tcia_pat346_0001, tcia_pat354_0001, tcia_pat393_0001, tcia_pat402_0001, tcia_pat408_0001, tcia_pat413_0001, tcia_pat442_0001, tcia_pat449_0001,

References

1. Amit, Y., Geman, D.: Shape quantization and recognition with randomized trees. Neural Comput. **9**(7), 1545–1588 (1997)
2. Archambeau, C., Verleysen, M.: Robust Bayesian clustering. Neural Netw. **20**(1), 129–138 (2007)
3. Breiman, L.: Bagging predictors. Mach. Learn. **24**(2), 123–140 (1996)
4. Cordier, N., Delingette, H., Ayache, N.: A patch-based approach for the segmentation of pathologies: application to glioma labelling. IEEE Trans. Med. Imaging **35**(4), 1066–1076 (2015)
5. Criminisi, A., Robertson, D., Konukoglu, E., Shotton, J., Pathak, S., White, S., Siddiqui, K.: Regression forests for efficient anatomy detection and localization in computed tomography scans. Med. Image Anal. **17**(8), 1293–1303 (2013)
6. Geremia, E., Menze, B.H., Ayache, N.: Spatially adaptive random forests. In: 2013 IEEE 10th International Symposium on Biomedical Imaging, pp. 1344–1347. IEEE (2013)
7. Ho, T.K.: The random subspace method for constructing decision forests. IEEE Trans. Pattern Anal. Mach. Intell. **20**(8), 832–844 (1998)
8. Kamnitsas, K., Ledig, C., Newcombe, V.F.J., Simpson, J.P., Kane, A.D., Menon, D.K., Rueckert, D., Glocker, B.: Efficient multi-scale 3D CNN with fully connected CRF for accurate brain lesion segmentation. Med. Image Anal. **36**, 61–78 (2017). Elsevier
9. Menze, B., Jakab, A., Bauer, S., Kalpathy-Cramer, J., Farahani, K., Kirby, J., Burren, Y., Porz, N., Slotboom, J., Wiest, R., et al.: The multimodal brain tumor image segmentation benchmark (BRATS). IEEE Trans. Med. Imaging **34**(10), 1993–2024 (2015)
10. Menze, B.H., Leemput, K., Lashkari, D., Weber, M.-A., Ayache, N., Golland, P.: A generative model for brain tumor segmentation in multi-modal images. In: Jiang, T., Navab, N., Pluim, J.P.W., Viergever, M.A. (eds.) MICCAI 2010. LNCS, vol. 6362, pp. 151–159. Springer, Heidelberg (2010). doi:10.1007/978-3-642-15745-5_19
11. Pereira, S., Pinto, A., Alves, V., Silva, C.A.: Deep convolutional neural networks for the segmentation of gliomas in multi-sequence MRI. In: Crimi, A., Menze, B., Maier, O., Reyes, M., Handels, H. (eds.) BrainLes 2015. LNCS, vol. 9556, pp. 131–143. Springer, Cham (2016). doi:10.1007/978-3-319-30858-6_12
12. Quinlan, J.R.: Simplifying decision trees. Int. J. Man. Mach. Stud. **27**(3), 221–234 (1987)
13. Shotton, J., Johnson, M., Cipolla, R.: Semantic texton forests for image categorization and segmentation. In: IEEE Conference on Computer Vision and Pattern Recognition (CVPR), pp. 1–8. IEEE (2008)
14. Tu, Z.: Auto-context and its application to high-level vision tasks. In: IEEE Conference on Computer Vision and Pattern Recognition (CVPR), pp. 1–8. IEEE (2008)

15. Tu, Z., Bai, X.: Auto-context and its application to high-level vision tasks and 3D brain image segmentation. IEEE Trans. Pattern Anal. Mach. Intell. **32**(10), 1744–1757 (2010)
16. Tustison, N., Gee, J.: N4ITK: Nicks N3 ITK implementation for MRI bias field correction. Insight J. (2009). http://hdl.handle.net/10380/3053
17. Tustison, N.J., Shrinidhi, K., Wintermark, M., Durst, C.R., Kandel, B.M., Gee, J.C., Grossman, M.C., Avants, B.B.: Optimal symmetric multimodal templates and concatenated random forests for supervised brain tumor segmentation (simplified) with ANTsR. Neuroinformatics **13**(2), 209–225 (2015)
18. Tustison, N., Wintermark, M., Durst, C., Avants, B.: Ants and arboles. Multimodal Brain Tumor Segmentation, p. 47 (2013)
19. Viola, P., Jones, M.: Rapid object detection using a boosted cascade of simple features. In: Proceedings of the 2001 IEEE Computer Society Conference on Computer Vision and Pattern Recognition (CVPR), vol. 1, p. I-511. IEEE (2001)
20. Zhang, Y., Brady, M., Smith, S.: Segmentation of brain MR images through a hidden Markov Random Field model and the Expectation-Maximization algorithm. IEEE Trans. Med. Imaging **20**(1), 45–57 (2001)
21. Zikic, D., et al.: Decision forests for tissue-specific segmentation of high-grade gliomas in multi-channel MR. In: Ayache, N., Delingette, H., Golland, P., Mori, K. (eds.) MICCAI 2012. LNCS, vol. 7512, pp. 369–376. Springer, Heidelberg (2012). doi:10.1007/978-3-642-33454-2_46

Segmentation of Gliomas in Pre-operative and Post-operative Multimodal Magnetic Resonance Imaging Volumes Based on a Hybrid Generative-Discriminative Framework

Ke Zeng$^{(\boxtimes)}$, Spyridon Bakas$^{(\boxtimes)}$, Aristeidis Sotiras, Hamed Akbari, Martin Rozycki, Saima Rathore, Sarthak Pati, and Christos Davatzikos

Section of Biomedical Image Analysis, Perelman School of Medicine, Center for Biomedical Image Computing and Analytics, University of Pennsylvania, Philadelphia, USA
{Ke.Zeng,S.Bakas,Aristeidis.Sotiras,Hamed.Akbari,Martin.Rozycki, Saima.Rathore,Sarthak.Pati,Christos.Davatzikos}@uphs.upenn.edu

Abstract. We present an approach for segmenting both low- and high-grade gliomas in multimodal magnetic resonance imaging volumes. The proposed framework is an extension of our previous work [6,7], with an additional component for segmenting post-operative scans. The proposed approach is based on a hybrid generative-discriminative model. Firstly, a generative model based on a joint segmentation-registration framework is used to segment the brain scans into cancerous and healthy tissues. Secondly, a gradient boosting classification scheme is used to refine tumor segmentation based on information from multiple patients. We evaluated our approach in 218 cases during the training phase of the BRAin Tumor Segmentation (BRATS) 2016 challenge and report promising results. During the testing phase, the proposed approach was ranked among the top performing methods, after being additionally evaluated in 191 unseen cases.

Keywords: Segmentation · Brain tumor · Glioma · Multimodal MRI · Gradient boosting · Expectation maximization · Probabilistic model · BRATS challenge

1 Introduction

Glioma is a common type of brain tumors that originates in the glial cells that surround and support neurons. Gliomas are divided into different types based on the degree of their growth rate and histopathology. Commonly, they are classified into low- and high-grade gliomas (LGGs and HGGs). LGGs are less common than HGGs, constitute approximately 20% of central nervous system glial tumors and almost all of them eventually progress to HGGs [28]. HGGs are rapidly progressing malignancies, divided based on their histopathologic features into anaplastic gliomas and glioblastomas (GBMs) [38].

© Springer International Publishing AG 2016
A. Crimi et al. (Eds.): BrainLes 2016, LNCS 10154, pp. 184–194, 2016.
DOI: 10.1007/978-3-319-55524-9_18

Gliomas are typically diagnosed by multimodal magnetic resonance imaging (MRI), where two main pathological regions may be identified, the tumor core and the peritumoral edematous area. The tumor core typically consists of enhancing (note that LGGs do not always include this part), non-enhancing and necrotic parts. Edema is the response to infiltrating tumor cells, as well as angiogenic and vascular permeability factors released by the spatially adjacent tumor cells [2].

Accurate segmentation of these pathological regions may significantly impact treatment decisions, planning, as well as outcome monitoring. However, this is a highly challenging task due to tumor regions being defined by intensity changes relative to the surrounding healthy tissue, and such intensity information being disseminated across various modalities for each region. Manually delineating tumor boundaries is a highly laborious task that is prone to human error and observer bias [8]. Computer-assisted segmentation, on the other hand, has the potential to reduce expert burden and raters' variability.

The literature on computer-assisted tumor segmentation is abundant. Most methods can be categorized as being either generative or discriminative. Under a generative setting, a probabilistic model is designed for generating the underlying multimodal intensity images. The statistical model often incorporates prior knowledge of appearance and of spatial distribution of healthy brain tissues. Human knowledge for the abnormal tissues is usually encoded through tumor-specific designs (see for example [16,30,32]). Others, however, (e.g. [13,35]) choose to segment tumors as outlier classes not well represented by models for healthy tissues. In a discriminative scenario, a decision function is directly learned from manually annotated training images to characterize the difference between cancerous and normal tissues. A broad spectrum of algorithms have been used for learning the decision function (see for example [1,3,18,27,34,39]). In recent years, convolutional neural networks [1,18,20,21,34] have become an extremely popular choice as the base learner, achieving high rankings in BRATS competitions.

The method proposed in this paper is an extension of our previously published method called GLISTRboost [6,7]. When designing GLISTRboost, we restricted our attention to pre-operative baseline scans, whereas here we introduce an approach for segmenting gliomas in post-operative scans as well. Segmenting residual and recurrent tumors is a task significantly different from segmenting tumors on pre-operative baseline scans. This segmentation task is extremely challenging due to the presence of surgically-imposed cavities and non-neoplastic contrast enhancements on the cavity boundaries. These two tissue classes are not modeled in GLISTRboost. Additionally, GLISTRboost requires the manual initialization of at least one seed point where the tumor initially originated. However, such seed points cannot be identified in many post-operative scans, unless there is an apparent recurrent tumor. Lastly, the mass effect in many post-operative scans has been substantially relaxed due to the removal of the tumor bulk. Therefore, the component of GLISTRboost that models the mass effect is no longer required for segmenting post-operative scans. Due to these important differences, segmenting brain tumors in post-operative scans cannot be tackled by GLISTRboost. To address these differences, we develop here a framework that specifically targets the segmentation of gliomas in post-operative scans. The design follows the generative-discriminative principle of GLISTRboost.

The remainder of this paper is organized as follows: Sect. 2 details the provided data, while Sect. 3 presents the proposed segmentation strategy. The experimental validation setting is described in Sect. 4 along with the obtained results. Finally, Sect. 5 concludes the paper.

2   Materials

186 pre- and 88 post-operative multimodal MRI scans of patients with gliomas (54 LGGs, 220 HGGs) were provided as training images for the BRATS 2016 challenge, from the Virtual Skeleton Database [22]. Specifically, the dataset is a combination of the pre-operative baseline training set (10 LGGs and 20 HGGs) evaluated in the BRATS 2013 challenge [29], 44 LGG and 112 HGG pre-operative baseline scans provided from the National Institutes of Health (NIH) Cancer Imaging Archive (TCIA) and evaluated in the BRATS 2015 challenge, as well as 88 HGG post-operative NIH-TCIA scans evaluated in BRATS 2016. The post-operative scans describe longitudinal observations from 27 patients at multiple time points. The inclusion of these longitudinal scans will allow for the characterization of these tumors, based on expert neuroradiologists and the evaluation of the volumetric segmentations, in 'progressing,' 'stable disease,' or 'shrinking.'

In addition to the training set, 191 multimodal volumetric images were provided as the testing set for BRATS 2016 challenge, comprising 92 pre-operative baseline and 99 post-operative scans. The partition of the testing set into pre- and post-operative was done based on visual confirmation of a surgically imposed cavity.

The data of each patient consists of native and contrast-enhanced (CE) T1-weighted, as well as T2-weighted and T2 Fluid-attenuated inversion recovery (FLAIR) MRI volumes. Finally, ground truth (GT) segmentations for the training set were also provided. Specifically, the data from BRATS 2013 were manually annotated, whereas data from NIH-TCIA were automatically annotated by fusing the approved by experts results of the segmentation algorithms that ranked high in the BRATS 2012 and 2013 challenges [29]. The GT segmentations comprise the enhancing part of the tumor (ET), the tumor core (TC), which is defined as the union of necrotic, non-enhancing and enhancing parts of the tumor, and the whole tumor (WT), which is the union of the TC and the peritumoral edematous region.

In this study, we only considered 32 out of the 88 provided post-operative HGG cases in the experiments, as labeling errors were found in the automatically generated GT for the other 56 samples. The most common mislabeling in those cases is surgically imposed cavities being segmented as part of the tumor core.

3 Methods

In this section, we describe the extended GLISTRboost segmentation framework that addresses tumor segmentation in both pre-operative baseline and post-operative multimodal volumes.

Firstly, all the provided MRI volumes are skull-stripped, co-registered and filtered to reduce intensity noise in regions of uniform intensity profile [37]. The intensity histograms of all modalities of all patients are then matched to the corresponding modality of a single reference patient [31]. Pre-operative baseline and post-operative volumes are handled differently after the common pre-processing pipeline.

A pre-operative baseline scan is segmented by applying GLISTRboost [6,7], our previously published method that ranked 1st in the BRATS 2015 challenge. GLISTRboost is a hybrid generative-discriminative segmentation framework, in which a generative approach is used to compute probabilistic segmentations of the brain scans into cancerous, as well as healthy tissue. This generative approach is based on GLISTR [14–16,23,25], a joint segmentation-registration scheme that incorporates a glioma growth model to deal with the tumor mass effect [19]. A gradient boosting classification (discriminative) scheme is then used to refine the probabilistic segmentations based on information learned from multiple patients [10,11]. Lastly, a probabilistic Bayesian strategy, inspired by [4,5], is employed to refine further and finalize the tumor segmentation based on within-patient brain-specific intensity statistics. Interested readers are referred to [7] for detailed information on GLISTRboost.

Although GLISTRboost performs well on segmenting pre-operative baseline scans, it is not applicable to the task of segmenting post-operative volumes. Specifically, GLISTR is not designed to handle the two extra tissue classes present in post-operative scans, namely surgically-imposed cavities and non-neoplastic contrast enhancement on cavity boundaries. Moreover, it requires manual initialization of at least one seed point to approximate the center of the tumor, and such points cannot be identified in many post-operative scans unless there is an apparent recurrent tumor. Lastly, the mass effect, modeled by a computationally demanding tumor growth model in GLISTR, is expected to be substantially relaxed in most post-operative scans, where the tumor bulk is resected.

The generative part of GLISTRboost is adjusted accordingly to address these differences. Specifically, two additional classes, namely non-enhancing cavity and enhancing cavity, are introduced to the Gaussian mixture model within the joint segmentation-registration scheme to address the presence of surgically-imposed cavities and non-neoplastic enhancement on their boundaries. We have also removed the requirement for at least one manually placed tumor seed point and introduced a new option for specifying approximately the center and radius of the cavity. Lastly, the glioma growth model is taken out of the joint segmentation-registration scheme due to the absence of severe mass effect. We note that the time required for the joint segmentation-registration scheme to converge is substantially reduced after removing the computationally intensive growth model [19]. These modifications were also previously considered as a subcomponent of a registration framework that aligns pre-operative to post-recurrence brain scans of glioma patients [24, 26].

We continue using the gradient boosting machine to learn a classifier for the discriminative step. The predictor variables proposed in GLISTRboost, augmented with two additional features, are used to learn the classifier. The original feature set considered in GLISTRboost comprises five components; image intensity, image derivative, geodesic information [12], texture features, and the GLISTR posterior probability maps. The intensity component includes the raw intensity value of each voxel, as well as inter-modality differences. The image derivative component consists of image gradient magnitude and the Laplacian of Gaussian. The geodesic information at a given voxel v_i was computed as its geodesic distance to the tumor center v_s manually seeded for running GLISTR. Specifically, the geodesic distance between v_i and v_s was defined as $\min_\gamma \int P(\gamma(s))ds$, where γ can be any path connecting v_i to v_s. We set the weight P at each voxel to be proportional to its gradient magnitude, and the optimization was solved using the fast marching method [9, 36]. Furthermore, the texture features describe the first and second order texture statistics computed from a gray-level co-occurrence matrix [17]. Two additional features have been included specifically for segmenting post-operative volumes, namely the geodesic distance of every voxel to the center of the cavity and the posterior probability of a voxel in the image being cavity (as computed by the generative step).

Finally, it should be noted that separate models have been trained for pre-operative baseline and post-operative scans.

4   Experiments and Results

To assess the segmentation performance of our method on the provided training data, we evaluated the overlap, both qualitatively and quantitively through the Dice coefficient, between the tumor labels computed by the proposed method and the GT in three regions, *i.e.*, WT, TC, and ET, as suggested in [29]. Figure 1a showcases examples of the provided multimodal pre-operative baseline scans, along with their corresponding GT and their segmentation labels as computed by our method, for four patients (two HGGs and two LGGs). We visually note the highest overlap in the edematous region while observing some disagreement in the enhancing and non-enhancing parts of the tumor between the suggested segmentations and the GT. Figure 1b illustrates representative post-operative examples of two patients with resection cavities and two with recurrent tumors. We note in the resection cases that the cavity itself and its enhancing boundary have almost identical intensity characteristics with the non-enhancing and enhancing parts of the tumor, respectively. As a result, they were partially misclassified as cancerous regions they resemble by the proposed method.

To further evaluate the performance of the proposed method, we quantitatively validated the per-voxel overlap between the GT and the proposed segmentation using the Dice coefficient. Figure 2 summarizes the distributions of the

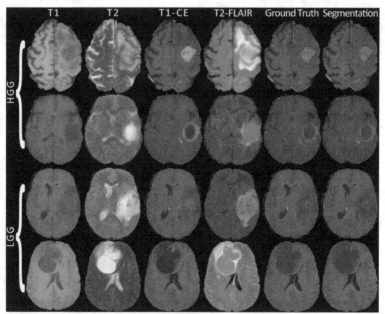

a. Pre-operative baseline multimodal scans.

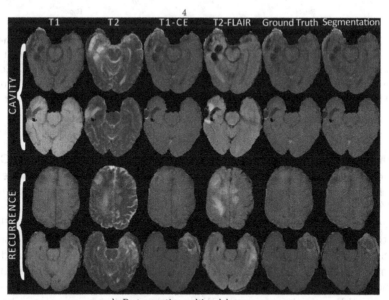

b. Post-operative multimodal scans.

Fig. 1. Representative example segmentation results for four pre-operative baseline and four post-operative multimodal scans. Green, red and blue masks denote the edema, the enhancing tumor and the union of the necrotic and non-enhancing parts of the tumor, respectively. (Color figure online)

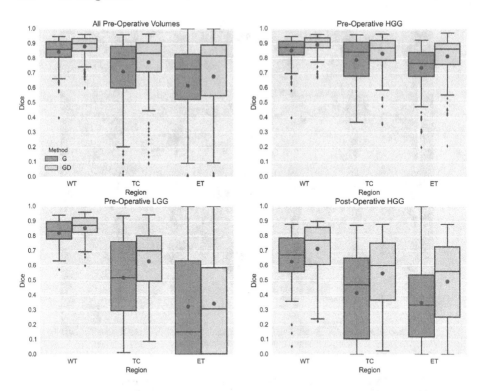

Fig. 2. Distributions of the Dice coefficient across patients for each step of the proposed method, each tissue label and different groupings of data. The different steps are described by the boxes colored in green and yellow for the generative only step (G) and the complete generative-discriminative method (GD), respectively. The dot and the line inside each box denote the mean and median values, respectively. (Color figure online)

cross-validated Dice coefficient scores for each region of interest (WT, TC, and ET) and across patients of the training set while using only the generative step, as well as the complete method. The results are presented for four different groupings of the data, comprising all pre-operative baseline scans, the pre-operative baseline HGGs, the pre-operative baseline LGGs and the post-operative HGGs. We note a definite improvement after application of the discriminative step in both the mean and median Dice coefficient values for all tissue labels and data groupings. Furthermore, it is observed that the segmentation results for the ET label vary significantly between LGGs and HGGs, with the former showing lower and less consistent results. We hypothesize that segmenting enhancing tumor is more challenging in LGGs because they are characterized by a distinct pathophysiological phenotype that often manifests as small ill-defined areas of enhancement or absence of it altogether. Nevertheless, the segmentation of the WT label in the LGGs is comparable to that of the HGGs.

One may also notice that the segmentation quality for post-operative HGG volumes is inferior to and less consistent than that for pre-operative baseline HGG volumes. Such phenomenon is in line with the visual inspections in Fig. 1, again highlighting the challenging nature of segmenting post-operative scans. It is also worth noting that we have excluded 56 out of the 88 post-operative scans for validation purposes due to labeling errors in their GT. Therefore, we believe that the difference in the number of training scans available (32 vs. 132) also affects the segmentation accuracy, and we expect to obtain improved performance by increasing the number of post-operative training samples.

A software implementation of the proposed method is available in www.cbica.upenn.edu/sbia/software/glistrboost through the Imaging Processing Portal (IPP) of Center for Biomedical Image Computing and Analytics (ipp.cbica.upenn.edu). The Cancer and Phenomics Toolkit (CapTk) [33] (www.cbica.upenn.edu/sbia/software/CAPTk) is used for the manual initialization of the proposed method. It showcases some of the highlight applications from CBICA along with advanced visualization and interactive capabilities to make it a complete radiological tool. CapTk is available in www.nitrc.org/projects/captk.

5   Conclusion

We presented a semi-automated approach based on a generative-discriminative framework towards providing a reliable and highly accurate segmentation of gliomas in both pre- and post-operative multimodal MRI volumes. The first step in the proposed approach is to compute a probabilistic segmentation for the given patient by a generative joint segmentation-registration scheme. This probabilistic segmentation is subsequently refined by a discriminative approach, taking into account population-wide tumor label appearance statistics that are learned by employing the gradient boosting machine.

The proposed method was validated on the BRATS 2016 training dataset, which is a mixture of pre-operative baseline HGG and LGG scans, as well as post-operative HGG scans. For all scan types and all regions of interests (WT, TC, and ET), the coupled generative-discriminative framework significantly improves the segmentation generated by the generative approach alone, achieving higher Dice coefficients with a clear margin in all cases.

The generative-discriminative method segmented whole tumor and tumor core with consistently high accuracy for both pre-operative baseline HGGs and LGGs. However, the difference between the performances on HGGs and LGGs is more pronounced in the enhancing tumor region, with the segmentation accuracy on LGGs being lower and less consistent. Such difference in performance suggests that segmenting enhancing tumor is much more challenging in LGGs than in HGGs, possibly because the former is characterized by a distinct pathophysiological phenotype that often manifests as small ill-defined areas of enhancement or absence of enhancement altogether while the HGGs often feature clearly defined enhancing regions. One may also note that the segmentation accuracy of the post-operative HGGs was inferior to that for the pre-operative baseline HGGs in all three areas of interests, due to their more challenging nature and fewer available training samples. Overall, the proposed method produced high-quality segmentations for whole tumor, tumor core and enhancing tumor on the full dataset.

References

1. Agn, M., Puonti, O., Rosenschöld, P.M., Law, I., Leemput, K.: Brain tumor segmentation using a generative model with an RBM prior on tumor shape. In: Crimi, A., Menze, B., Maier, O., Reyes, M., Handels, H. (eds.) BrainLes 2015. LNCS, vol. 9556, pp. 168–180. Springer, Cham (2016). doi:10.1007/978-3-319-30858-6_15
2. Akbari, H., Macyszyn, L., Da, X., Wolf, R.L., Bilello, M., Verma, R., O'Rourke, D.M., Davatzikos, C.: Pattern analysis of dynamic susceptibility contrast-enhanced MR imaging demonstrates peritumoral tissue heterogeneity. Radiology **273**(2), 502–510 (2014)
3. Ayachi, R., Ben Amor, N.: Brain tumor segmentation using support vector machines. In: Sossai, C., Chemello, G. (eds.) ECSQARU 2009. LNCS (LNAI), vol. 5590, pp. 736–747. Springer, Heidelberg (2009). doi:10.1007/978-3-642-02906-6_63
4. Bakas, S., Chatzimichail, K., Hunter, G., Labbe, B., Sidhu, P.S., Makris, D.: Fast semi-automatic segmentation of focal liver lesions in contrast-enhanced ultrasound, based on a probabilistic model. In: Computer Methods in Biomechanics and Biomedical Engineering: Imaging & Visualization, pp. 1–10 (2015)
5. Bakas, S., Labbe, B., Hunter, G.J.A., Sidhu, P., Chatzimichail, K., Makris, D.: Fast segmentation of focal liver lesions in contrast-enhanced ultrasound data. In: Proceedings of the 18th Annual Conference on Medical Image Understanding and Analysis (MIUA), pp. 73–78 (2014)
6. Bakas, S., Zeng, K., Sotiras, A., Rathore, S., Akbari, H., Gaonkar, B.,Rozycki, M., Pati, S., Davazikos, C.: Segmentation of gliomas in multimodal magnetic resonance imaging volumes based on a hybrid generative-discriminative framework. In: Proceedings of the Multimodal Brain Tumor Image Segmentation Challenge (BRATS) 2015, pp. 5–12 (2015)
7. Bakas, S., Zeng, K., Sotiras, A., Rathore, S., Akbari, H., Gaonkar, B., Rozycki, M., Pati, S., Davazikos, C.: GLISTRboost: combining multimodal MRI segmentation, registration, and biophysical tumor growth modeling with gradient boosting machines for glioma segmentation. In: Crimi, A., Menze, B., Maier, O., Reyes, M., Handels, H. (eds.) BrainLes 2015. LNCS, vol. 9556, pp. 144–155. Springer, Cham (2016). doi:10.1007/978-3-319-30858-6_13
8. Deeley, M.A., Chen, A., Datteri, R., Noble, J.H., Cmelak, A.J., Donnelly, E.F., Malcolm, A.W., Moretti, L., Jaboin, J., Niermann, K., Yang, E.S., Yu, D.S., Yei, F., Koyama, T., Ding, G.X., Dawant, B.M.: Comparison of manual and automatic segmentation methods for brain structures in the presence of space-occupying lesions: a multi-expert study. Phys. Med. Biol. **56**(14), 4557–4577 (2011)
9. Deschamps, T., Cohen, L.D.: Fast extraction of minimal paths in 3D images and applications to virtual endoscopy. Med. Image Anal. **5**(4), 281–299 (2001)
10. Friedman, J.H.: Greedy function approximation: a gradient boosting machine. Ann. Stat. **29**(5), 1189–1232 (2001)
11. Friedman, J.H.: Stochastic gradient boosting. Comput. Stat. Data Anal. **38**(4), 367–378 (2002)

12. Gaonkar, B., Macyszyn, L., Bilello, M., Sadaghiani, M.S., Akbari, H., Attiah, M.A., Ali, Z.S., Da, X., Zhan, Y., O'Rourke, D., Grady, S.M., Davatzikos, C.: Automated tumor volumetry using computer-aided image segmentation. Acad. Radiol. **22**(5), 653–661 (2015)

13. Gering, D.T., Grimson, W.E.L., Kikinis, R.: Recognizing deviations from normalcy for brain tumor segmentation. In: Dohi, T., Kikinis, R. (eds.) MICCAI 2002. LNCS, vol. 2488, pp. 388–395. Springer, Heidelberg (2002). doi:10.1007/3-540-45786-0_48

14. Gooya, A., Biros, G., Davatzikos, C.: Deformable registration of glioma images using EM algorithm and diffusion reaction modeling. IEEE Trans. Med. Imaging **30**(2), 375–390 (2011)

15. Gooya, A., Pohl, K.M., Bilello, M., Biros, G., Davatzikos, C.: Joint segmentation and deformable registration of brain scans guided by a tumor growth model. Med. Image Comput. Comput.-Assist. Interventions **14**(2), 532–540 (2011)

16. Gooya, A., Pohl, K.M., Bilello, M., Cirillo, L., Biros, G., Melhem, E.R., Davatzikos, C.: GLISTR: glioma image segmentation and registration. IEEE Trans. Med. Imaging **31**(10), 1941–1954 (2012)

17. Haralick, R.M., Shanmugam, K., Dinstein, I.H.: Textural features for image classification. IEEE Trans. Syst. Man Cybern. **6**, 610–621 (1973)

18. Havaei, M., Davy, A., Warde-Farley, D., Biard, A., Courville, A., Bengio, Y., Pal, C., Jodoin, P.M., Larochelle, H.: Brain tumor segmentation with deep neural networks. Med. Image Anal. **35**, 18–31 (2017). http://www.sciencedirect.com/science/article/pii/S1361841516300330

19. Hogea, C., Davatzikos, C., Biros, G.: An image-driven parameter estimation problem for a reaction-diffusion glioma growth model with mass effects. J. Math. Biol. **56**(6), 793–825 (2008)

20. Kamnitsas, K., Ferrante, E., Parisot, S., Ledig, C., Nori, A., Criminisi, A., Rueckert, D., Glocker, B.: Deepmedic on brain tumor segmentation

21. Kamnitsas, K., Ledig, C., Newcombe, V.F., Simpson, J.P., Kane, A.D., Menon, D.K., Rueckert, D., Glocker, B.: Efficient multi-scale 3D CNN with fully connected CRF for accurate brain lesion segmentation. Med. Image Anal. **36**, 61–78 (2017). http://www.sciencedirect.com/science/article/pii/S1361841516301839

22. Kistler, M., Bonaretti, S., Pfahrer, M., Niklaus, R., Büchler, P.: The virtual skeleton database: an open access repository for biomedical research and collaboration. J. Med. Internet Res. **15**(11), e245 (2013)

23. Kwon, D., Akbari, H., Da, X., Gaonkar, B., Davatzikos, C.: Multimodal brain tumor image segmentation using GLISTR. In: MICCAI Brain Tumor Segmentation (BraTS) Challenge Manuscripts, pp. 18–19 (2014)

24. Kwon, D., Niethammer, M., Akbari, H., Bilello, M., Davatzikos, C., Pohl, K.M.: Portr: pre-operative and post-recurrence brain tumor registration. IEEE Trans. Med. Imaging **33**(3), 651–667 (2014)

25. Kwon, D., Shinohara, R.T., Akbari, H., Davatzikos, C.: Combining generative models for multifocal glioma segmentation and registration. Med. Image Comput. Comput.-Assist. Interventions **17**(1), 763–770 (2014)

26. Kwon, D., Zeng, K., Bilello, M., Davatzikos, C.: Estimating patient specific templates for pre-operative and follow-up brain tumor registration. Med. Image Comput. Comput.-Assist. Interventions **2**, 222–229 (2015)

27. Lee, C.-H., Wang, S., Murtha, A., Brown, M.R.G., Greiner, R.: Segmenting brain tumors using pseudo–conditional random fields. In: Metaxas, D., Axel, L., Fichtinger, G., Székely, G. (eds.) MICCAI 2008. LNCS, vol. 5241, pp. 359–366. Springer, Heidelberg (2008). doi:10.1007/978-3-540-85988-8_43

28. Louis, D.N.: Molecular pathology of malignant gliomas. Ann. Rev. Pathol. Mech. Dis. **1**, 97–117 (2006)

29. Menze, B.H., et al.: The Multimodal Brain Tumor Image Segmentation Benchmark (BRATS). IEEE Trans. Med. Imaging **34**(10), 1993–2024 (2015). doi:10.1109/TMI. 2014.2377694

30. Moon, N., Bullitt, E., van Leemput, K., Gerig, G.: Model-based brain and tumor segmentation. In: Object Recognition Supported by User Interaction for Service Robots. vol. 1, pp. 528–531 (2002)

31. Nyul, L.G., Udupa, J.K., Zhang, X.: New variants of a method of mri scale standardization. IEEE Trans. Med. Imaging **19**(2), 143–150 (2000)

32. Parisot, S., Duffau, H., Chemouny, S., Paragios, N.: Joint tumor segmentation and dense deformable registration of brain MR images. In: Ayache, N., Delingette, H., Golland, P., Mori, K. (eds.) MICCAI 2012. LNCS, vol. 7511, pp. 651–658. Springer, Heidelberg (2012). doi:10.1007/978-3-642-33418-4_80

33. Pati, S., Rathore, S., Kalarot, R., Sridharan, P., Bergman, M., Shinohara, T., Yushkevich, P., Fan, Y., Verma, R., Kontos, D., Davatzikos, C.: Cancer and Phenomics Toolkit (CAPTk): a software suite for computational oncology and radiomics. In: Radiological Society of North America 2016 Scientific Assembly and Annual Meeting, November 27 - December 2, 2016, Chicago IL (2016). http://archive.rsna.org/2016/16014589.html

34. Pereira, S., Pinto, A., Alves, V., Silva, C.A.: Brain tumor segmentation using convolutional neural networks in MRI images. IEEE Trans. Med. Imaging **35**(5), 1240–1251 (2016)

35. Prastawa, M., Bullitt, E., Ho, S., Gerig, G.: A brain tumor segmentation framework based on outlier detection. Med. Image Anal. **8**(3), 275–283 (2004). http://dx.doi.org/10.1016/j.media.2004.06.007

36. Sethian, J.A.: A fast marching level set method for monotonically advancing fronts. Proc. Nat. Acad. Sci. U.S.A. **93**(4), 1591–1595 (1996)

37. Smith, S.M., Brady, J.M.: SUSAN - a new approach to low level image processing. Int. J. Comput. Vis. **23**(1), 45–78 (1997)

38. Wen, P.Y., Kesari, S.: Malignant gliomas in adults. New England J. Med. **359**(5), 492–507 (2008)

39. Zikic, D., Glocker, B., Konukoglu, E., Criminisi, A., Demiralp, C., Shotton, J., Thomas, O.M., Das, T., Jena, R., Price, S.J.: Decision forests for tissue-specific segmentation of high-grade gliomas in multi-channel MR. In: Ayache, N., Delingette, H., Golland, P., Mori, K. (eds.) MICCAI 2012. LNCS, vol. 7512, pp. 369–376. Springer, Heidelberg (2012). doi:10.1007/978-3-642-33454-2_46

Interactive Semi-automated Method Using Non-negative Matrix Factorization and Level Set Segmentation for the BRATS Challenge

Dimah Dera[1], Fabio Raman[2], Nidhal Bouaynaya[1],
and Hassan M. Fathallah-Shaykh[2,3,4,5(✉)]

[1] Department of Electrical and Computer Engineering,
Rowan University, Glassboro, NJ, USA
[2] Department of Biomedical Engineering,
University of Alabama at Birmingham, Birmingham, AL, USA
hfshaykh@uabmc.edu
[3] Department of Neurology, University of Alabama at Birmingham,
Birmingham, AL, USA
[4] Department of Electrical Engineering,
University of Alabama at Birmingham, Birmingham, AL, USA
[5] Department of Mathematics, University of Alabama at Birmingham,
Birmingham, AL, USA

Abstract. The 2016 BRATS includes imaging data on 191 patients diagnosed with low and high grade gliomas. We present a novel method for multimodal brain segmentation, which consists of (1) an automated, accurate and robust method for image segmentation, combined with (2) semi-automated and interactive multimodal labeling. The image segmentation applies Non-negative Matrix Factorization (NMF), a decomposition technique that reduces the dimensionality of the image by extracting its distinct regions. When combined with the level-set method (LSM), NMF-LSM has proven to be an efficient method for image segmentation. Segmentation of the BRATS images by NMF-LSM is computed by the Cheaha supercomputer at the University of Alabama at Birmingham. The segments of each image are ranked by maximal intensity. The interactive labeling software, which identifies the four targets of the challenge, is semi-automated by cross-referencing the normal segments of the brain across modalities.

1 Introduction

Image analysis and segmentation is challenging because of the unpredictable appearance and shape of brain tumors from multi-modal imaging data. Among different segmentation approaches in the literature, it is hard to compare existing methods because of the variability of the quality of the images, validation datasets, the type of lesion, and the state of the disease (pre- or post-treatment).

© Springer International Publishing AG 2016
A. Crimi et al. (Eds.): BrainLes 2016, LNCS 10154, pp. 195–205, 2016.
DOI: 10.1007/978-3-319-55524-9_19

The Multimodel Brian Tumor Image Segmentation Benchmark (BRATS) challenge, [6], is organized to gauge the state-of-the-art in brain tumor segmentation and compare between different methods.

Non-negative matrix factorization (NMF) has shown promise as a robust clustering and data reduction technique in DNA microarrays clustering and classification [1] and learning facial features [5]. NMF is distinguished from the other methods, such as principal components analysis and vector quantization, by its use of non-negativity constraints. These constraints lead to a parts-based representation because they allow only additive, not subtractive, combinations. The first use of NMF for image segmentation was pioneered by our group in [3].

The level set method (LSM) is one of the most powerful and advanced methods to extract object boundaries in computer vision [2,7]. The basic idea of LSM is to evolve a curve in the image domain around the object or the region of interest until it locks onto the boundaries of the object. The level set approach represents the contour as the zero level of a higher dimensional function, referred to as the "level set function" (LSF). The segmentation is achieved by minimizing a functional that tends to attract the contour towards the objects features. The advantages of NMF-LSM is that it: (i) is robust to noise, initial condition, and intensity inhomogeneity because it relies on the distribution of the pixels rather than the intensity values and does not introduce spurious or nuisance model parameters, which have to be simultaneously estimated with the level sets, (ii) uses NMF to discover and identify the homogeneous image regions, (iii) introduces a novel spatial functional term that describes the local distribution of the regions within the image, and (iv) is scalable, i.e., able to detect a distinct region as small as desired.

In this paper, we briefly explain NMF as a region discovery and clustering used to detect the homogeneous regions in the image [4]. The framework for segmenting the data of 191 patients (flair, t1, t1c, and t2 MRI images) in a limited time frame is achieved in two steps. The first step is applying the NMF-LSM segmentation method on each image using 264 processors at the UAB Super Computer; all the images were segmented in less than 12 h. The second step is the labeling, where the segments are labeled using a multimodal, user-friendly, and interactive software as (1) for necrosis, (2) for edema, (3) for tumor core, (4) for enhancing tumor, and (0) for everything else.

The paper is organized as follows: Sect. 2 describes briefly how the clustering and region discovery performed using NMF. Section 3 demonstrates the variational level set model. Section 4 elucidates the high performance computing (HPC) implementation. Section 5 describes the interactive semi-automated and multimodal method for labeling the targets/regions of interest. We proceed to the challenges in Sect. 6 and a summary of this paper is provided in Sect. 7.

2   NMF-based Clustering

The NMF-LSM method is fully automated, pixel-wise accurate, less sensitive to the initial selection of the contour(s) or initial conditions compared to state-of-the-art LSM approaches, robust to noise and model parameters, and able to detect as small distinct regions as desired (for a detailed description, please see [4]). These advantages stem from the fact that NMF-LSM method relies on histogram information instead of intensity values and does not introduce nuisance model parameters. We have applied the NMF-LSM method to analyze the MRIs of two patients with grade 2 and 3 non-enhancing oligodendroglioma and compared its measurements to the diagnoses rendered by board-certified neuroradiologists; the results demonstrate that NMF-LSM can detect earlier progression times and may be used to monitor and measure response to treatment [4].

The basic schemes of the NMF-based clustering are summarized in Fig. 1, where the image is divided into equally sized blocks and the histogram of each block is computed to build the data matrix V. Then, NMF generates matrices W and H that include key information on the number and histograms of the regions in the image and on their local distribution. These key information is used to build an accurate and pixel-wise variational level set segmentation model.

3   Energy Minimization and Segmentation

Segmentation is achieved by minimizing the energy functional $\mathcal{F}$ in Eq. 1 with respect ot the level set function (LSF) ϕ [4]. The minimization is achieved by solving the gradient flow equation: $\frac{\partial \phi}{\partial t} = -\frac{\partial \mathcal{F}}{\partial \phi}$.

$$\mathcal{F}(\phi, b) = \alpha \sum_{i=1}^{k} \left[\int_{\Omega} e_i(\boldsymbol{x}, b) M_i(\phi) d\boldsymbol{x} \right] + \alpha \sum_{i=1}^{k} \sum_{j=1}^{m} \left(\int_{\Omega} \mathcal{I}_{S_j}(\boldsymbol{x}) M_i(\phi) d\boldsymbol{x} - \frac{h_{ij}a}{\sum_{i=1}^{k} h_{ij}} \right)^2$$
$$+ \frac{\beta}{2} \int_{\Omega} (|\nabla \phi| - 1)^2 d\boldsymbol{x} + \gamma \int_{\Omega} g |\nabla H(\phi)| d\boldsymbol{x}. \tag{1}$$

By calculus of variations, we compute the derivative $\frac{\partial \mathcal{F}}{\partial \phi}$ as follows:

$$\frac{\partial \phi}{\partial t} = -\alpha \sum_{i=1}^{k} \sum_{j=1}^{m} \left[I_{S_j} \frac{\partial M_i(\phi)}{\partial \phi} \left(I_{S_j} M_i(\phi) - \frac{h_{ij}a}{\sum_{i=1}^{k} h_{ij}} \right) \right] + \beta (\nabla^2 \phi - div(\frac{\nabla \phi}{|\nabla \phi|})) + \gamma \delta(\phi) \, div(\frac{\nabla \phi}{|\nabla \phi|}). \tag{2}$$

In the implementation, the membership function $M_i(\phi)$ is approximated by $H_\epsilon(\boldsymbol{x}) = 0.5 \sin(\arctan(\frac{x}{\epsilon})) + 0.5$, and its derivative, the dirac delta function, is estimated by $\delta_\epsilon(\boldsymbol{x}) = 0.5 \cos(\arctan(\frac{x}{\epsilon})) \frac{\epsilon}{\epsilon^2 + x^2}$.

$\mathcal{I}_{S_j}(\boldsymbol{x})$ is the indicator function of block S_j, and is defined as follows:

$$\mathcal{I}_{S_j}(\boldsymbol{x}) = \begin{cases} 1, & \text{if } \boldsymbol{x} \in S_j \\ 0, & \text{otherwise}. \end{cases} \tag{3}$$

The entries of the H matrix are h_{ij}, and α, β, and γ, are weighting constants. The function $e_i(\boldsymbol{x}, b)$ is defined as follows:

$$e_i(\boldsymbol{x}, b) = \log(\sqrt{2\pi}\sigma_i) + \frac{(I(x) - \mu_i b(x))^2}{2\sigma_i^2}, \tag{4}$$

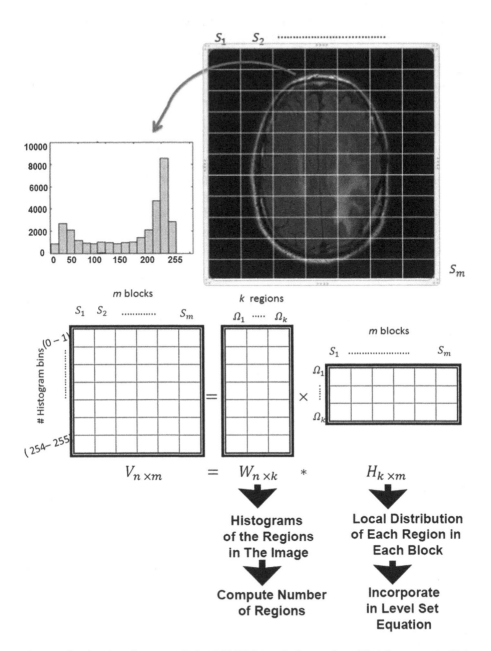

Fig. 1. The basic schemes of the NMF-based clustering. The data matrix V is built from the histograms of the blocks of the image. NMF of V generates W and H; the former, including the histograms of the regions in the image, is applied to compute the number of regions. H, which includes information on the local distribution of the regions in each of the blocks, is used to modify the level set equation.

where μ_i and σ_i are the mean and standard deviation of region i computed from the matrix W in the NMF factorization. For more details about the model, please refer to [4].

4 Super Computer Implementation

The dataset for each of 191 patients consists of four MRIs: FLAIR, T2, T1, and T1c at each brain section for every patient. In order to reduce computational times, the MRIs were pre-processed to select the images that include tumor, necrosis or edema. We wrote a software that displays all four modalities for each patient and allows the user to quickly identify the range of the 2D images to be sent for segmentation. The UAB super computer (high performance computing cluster) Cheaha has 3120 CPU cores that provide over 120 TFLOP/s of combined computational performance, and 20 TB of memory. All 191 patients were segmented by 265 processors in about 12 h. A single PC processed a single MRI in about 3 h. Four PCs can also process a patient's four MRIs in about 3 h.

5 Interactive, Multimodal, Semi-automated, Labelling Software

We have devised an interactive and semiautomated software for labelling the target regions; we were driven by the heterogeneity of the quality of the datasets and by our desire to exclude brain abnormalities (like hemorrhage) that are not related to the four target regions. For example, the poor quality of the flair or t1 sequences of some of the subjects limited their usability; in these cases, we relied on other modalities. Furthermore, some MRIs showed subdural hematomas, which are unrelated to the tumor, producing high signal on t1 and t1c images. Our objective is to sketch and illustrate the basic concepts of the interactive labelling method. We do not plan on covering every single subject, but rather the general tools that we have developed. The overall quantitative analysis of this method is presented by the organizers of the challenge. We have chosen the following examples to illustrate the methodology and to point out inconsistencies in the tumor core.

5.1 Over-Segmentation, Ranking of Segments, and Combining Segments

The datasets in the BRATS 2016 challenge are highly heterogenous in quality and form, which made the segmentation task challenging. To ensure that the tumor structures are detected and separated from the normal structures of brain (gray and white matter), we over-segment by instructing the NMF-LSM method to generate 8 segments for each image. The number of segments is a parameter in the NMF-LSM software. The 8 segments are generated by one NMF-LSM process. These segments are ranked based on their maximum intensity values.

It is fairly easy to combine segments to obtain the specified regions/targets, *i.e.* edema, enhancement, tumor core, and necrosis.

Figure 2(I) shows the flair image and its 8 segments ranked in order of their maximal intensity values from (max = 26, rank = 1) to (max = 255, rank = 8). By combining the segments in Figs. 2(I-i), (I-j), and (I-k), we obtain the edema region shown in Fig. 2(I-b). Figure 2(I-c) shows the final result.

Figure 2(II) shows the t1c image and its 8 segments ranked based on their maximal intensity values. By combining the segments whose ranks are 3 and 4 (Figs. 2(II-f) and (II-g), we obtain the necrosis region with the gray and white matter as shown in Fig. 2(II-b). We will subtract the normal brain structures in steps that follow. Combining the segments whose ranks are ≥ 5 gives us the region of contrast enhancement shown in Fig. 2(II-c).

Figure 2(III-a) shows the t1 image with its 8 segments ranked based on their maximum intensity values. By combining the segments whose ranks are 3 and 4, we obtain the tumor core region and the gray matter as shown in Fig. 2(III-b). We will subtract the gray matter in order to obtain the tumor core region as shown in the final result in Fig. 2(I-c).

5.2 Identification and Using Brain Structures to Semi-automate Labelling

We recognized from the case of Fig. 2 that we need to: (1) define the location of the normal structure of the brain, *i.e.* gray and white matter, in the image, and (2) the ranks of the segments that include the target regions. This goal will help us subtract/remove the normal structures of the brain and isolate the target regions.

Coordinates of White and Gray Matter. The segmentation of the t2 sequence yields the coordinates of the normal white and gray matter. By examining Fig. 2(IV), we notice that the normal white matter is identified by the segment whose rank and maximal intensity are 2 and 70 respectively. Furthermore, the gray matter is delineated by the segment whose rank and maximal intensity are 3 and 95, respectively. This is not surprising given the distribution of the intensities of white and gray matter in t2 sequences. These normal gray and white matter can be subtracted from the segments that include necrosis, tumor core, and enhancing tumor.

Automating the Discovery of the Ranks of Interest. Recall that NMF-LSM method processes each 2D slice separately to generate its segments, which are ranked by their maximal intensities. Furthermore, the interactive software processes each 2D slice separately. Having the coordinates of the normal white matter and gray matter from the segmentation of t2, yields the ranks of the segments of t1c, t1, and flair that correspond to these structures. For example, we can identify the rank of the segment of the t1c image that corresponds to white matter; this can be easily computed by finding the segment having the largest intersection with the white matter. We denote the rank of this segment

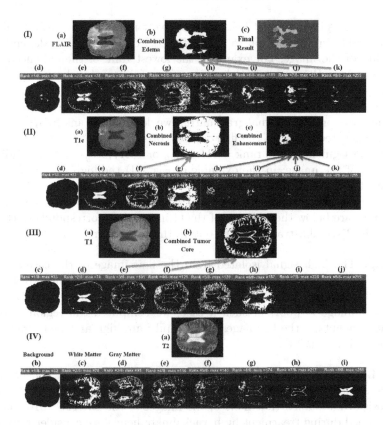

Fig. 2. Illustrative High Grade Case 1. The flair image (I-a) and its 8 segments ((I-d) to (I-k)) obtained by NMF-LSM. The images are ranked by their maximal intensities (shown). (I-b) shows the combination of segments (I-i) to (I-k), which gives us the region including the edema, tumor, and a part of the necrosis. (I-c) shows the final segmentation result including the four regions, edema (yellow), tumor core (orange), enhancement (red), and necrosis (blue). The t1c image (II-a) and its 8 segments ((II-d) - (II-k) are obtained by NMF-LSM. The images are ranked by their maximal intensities (shown). (III-b) displays the combination of the segments whose ranks are 3 and 4 (Figs. (II-f) and (II-g)), which gives us the regions of necrosis combined with the gray and white matter, which will be subtracted later. (II-c) shows the combination of the segments whose ranks are 5–8 (Figs. (III-h) - (III-k)), which gives us the region of contrast enhancement. The t1 image (III-a) and its 8 segments ((III-c) - (III-j)) are obtained by NMF-LSM. The images are ranked by their maximal intensities (shown). (II-b) shows the combination of segments whose ranks are 3 and 4 (Figs. (III-e) and (III-f)), giving us the region of the tumor core. The t2 image (IV-a) and its 8 segments ((IV-b) - (IV-i)) obtained by NMF-LSM. The images are ranked by their maximal intensities (shown). (IV-b) shows the segment corresponding to the background, whose rank and maximal intensity are 1 and 32, respectively. (IV-c) shows the segment whose rank and maximal intensity are 2 and 70, respectively; this segment corresponds to the normal white matter. (IV-d) shows the segment whose rank and maximal intensity are 3 and 95, respectively; this segment corresponds to the normal gray matter. The gray (IV-d) and white (IV-c) matter from the t2 image are applied to discover the ranks of the segments corresponding to the FLAIR signal and enhancement, respectively. (Color figure online)

by $Rt1c_{wm}$. This is important because the lowest rank of the contrast enhancement in the t1c image is equal to either $Rt1c_{wm}$ or $Rt1c_{wm} + 1$, depending on the quality of the image. For example, the lowest rank of the enhancement in Fig. 2(II) is $5 = Rt1c_{wm} + 1$. Below, we give an example where the contrast enhancement is detected at a rank $= Rt1c_{wm}$.

Similarly, we can define the highest rank of the segment of the flair image that has an intersection with normal gray matter; we denote this rank by $Rflair$. Typically, the elevated signal in the flair image, corresponding to the edema, starts either in the segment whose rank $= Rflair_{gm}$ or $= Rflair_{gm} + 1$, depending on the quality of the image; in the example of Fig. 2(I) the high signal in the flair image starts at the segment whose rank $= Rflair + 1$.

The tumor core is defined from the t1 image. It is included in the segments whose ranks are below the segment of the t1 image that corresponds to the gray matter; Fig. 2(III) illustrates how to obtain the tumor core.

Masking. The high signal isolated from the flair image of the case shown in Figs. 2(I) can serve as a mask that filters the parts of the t1 and t1c that are positioned outside its outer borders. This approach is not applicable if the quality of the flair image is poor; in such a case, we computed the region of edema from the segments of the t2 images whose ranks are high and we extracted the cerebrospinal fluid (CSF).

Cystic Lesions in Low Grade Tumors. Because pathological necrosis has profound clinical implications, we did not label cystic lesions in low grade tumors as necrosis. We assumed that none of the images of the BRATS 2016 challenge were obtained during treatment by bevacizumab; hence, we consider a tumor as low grade if it lacks contrast enhancement.

6   Challenges

6.1   Tumor Core in High Grade Tumors

The ranks of the segments containing the high signal in the flair image of Fig. 3(II) are from $Rflair = 4$ to 8. The contrast enhancement is detected in the segments of the t1c image whose ranks are $Rt1c_{wm} = 4$ to 8. For the tumor core, applying the same rule as in case 1 above, yields the sum of the segments whose ranks are 3–5 (Figs. 3(IV-e)-(IV-g)), which essentially covers most of the region of the edema. Hence, we select the segments whose ranks are 3 and 4 (Figs. 3(IV-e)-(IV-f)); the final result is shown in Fig. 3(I-b). Notice that extracting the tumor core from the segments of the t2 image, whose ranks and 4 and 5 (Figs. 3(I-f)-(I-g)) would have given us a different result.

6.2   Tumor Core in Low Grade Tumors

The next case illustrates the challenge of computing the tumor core from low grade gliomas. The coordinates of the normal white matter are computed from

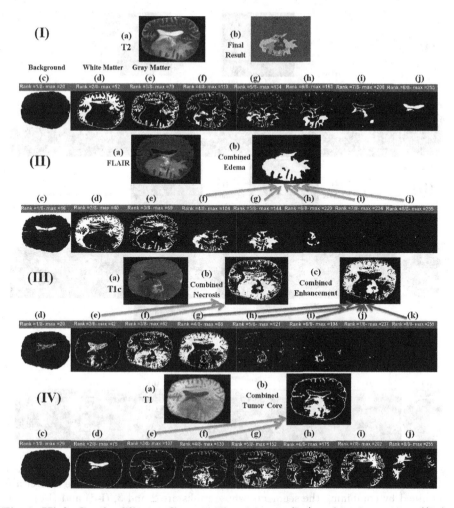

Fig. 3. High Grade Glioma Case 2. The t2 image (I-a) and its 8 segments ((I-c) - (I-j)) are produced by NMF-LSM. The images are ranked by their maximal intensities (shown). The coordinates of the normal white matter and gray matter are determined by the segments whose ranks are 2 (I-d) and 3 (I-e), respectively. (I-b) shows the final segmentation result including the four regions, edema (yellow), tumor core (orange), enhancement (red), and necrosis (blue). The flair image (II) and its 8 segments are ranked by their maximal intensities (shown). (II-b) shows the combination of the segments whose ranks are ≥ 4, (II-f) to (II-j), which gives us the region including the edema. The t1c image is shown in (III); its 8 segments (are also ranked by their maximal intensities (shown); necrosis is includes in segments 2 and 3 while the enhancement is included in the combination of the segments whose ranks are ≥ 4. The t1 image is shown in (IV); its 8 segments are also ranked by their maximal intensities (shown). (IV-b) shows the combination of segments whose ranks are 3 and 4, giving us the region of the tumor core. The gray (I-d) and white (I-e) matter from the t2 image are applied to discover the ranks of the segments corresponding to the FLAIR signal and enhancement, respectively. (Color figure online)

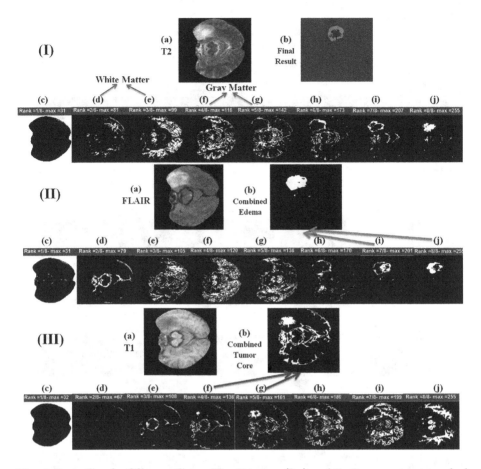

Fig. 4. Low Grade Glioma Case. The t2 image (I-a) and its 8 segments are ranked by their maximal intensities (shown). The coordinates of the normal white matter are determined by combining the segments whose ranks are 2 and 3, (I-d) and (I-e). The segments whose ranks are 4 and 5 yield the coordinates of the normal gray matter, (I-f) and (I-g). (I-b) shows the final segmentation result including the four regions, edema (yellow), tumor core (orange), enhancement (red), and necrosis (blue). The flair image is shown in (II); its 8 segments are ranked by their maximal intensities (shown). (II-b) shows the combination of segments whose ranks are ≥ 7, (II-h) to (I-J), which gives us the region including the edema. The t1 image is shown in (III); its 8 segments are ranked by their maximal intensities (shown). (III-b) shows the combination of segments whose ranks are 4 and 5 (III-f) and (III-g), giving us the region of the tumor core. (Color figure online)

combining the segments of t2 whose ranks are 2 and 3; the gray matter is configured from the segments of t2 images whose ranks = 4 and 5 (see Fig. 4(I)). The region for edema is computed from the flair image as detailed above by combining the segments whose ranks are 7 and 8. The region of the tumor core was extracted from the segments of t1 whose ranks are 4 and 5; the final result is shown in (Fig. 4(I-b)). Notice that the tumor core, extracted from t1, corresponds to region 8 of the t2 image, whose maximal intensity = 255 (Fig. 4(I-j)), which is paradoxical because the segments that include high signal in the t2 of the high grade glioma case shown in Fig. 3(I-h)-(I-j) do not correspond to the tumor core.

7   Conclusion

We have applied our novel NMF-LSM segmentation approach to segment the BRATS 2016 data sets [4]. We describe an interactive and semi-automated scheme for extracting the four targets/regions from the multimodal segments. The latter are ranked by their maximal intensities; the normal structures of the brain (white and gray matter) are discovered and are applied to semi-automate the identification of the segments that include the targets/regions of interest. Here, we have used the approach of over-segmentation followed by combining segments using the interactive software (see Figs. 2, 3 and 4). The interactive method lends itself to the development of logical and medically relevant criteria/standards for image analysis. Computations of the tumor core have generated paradoxical results; we suggest either abandoning it or redefining its meaning.

References

1. Bayar, B., Bouaynaya, N., Shterenberg, R.: Probabilistic non-negative matrix factorization: theory and application to microarray data analysis. J. Bioinform. Comput. Biol. **12**, 25 (2014)
2. Cohen, L.D., Cohen, I.: Finite-element methods for active contour models and balloons for 2-D and 3-D images. IEEE Trans. Pattern Anal. Mach. Intell. **15**(11), 1131–1147 (1993)
3. Dera, D., Bouaynaya, N., Fathallah-Shaykh, H.M.: Level set segmentation using non-negative matrix factorization of brain MRI images. In: IEEE International Conference on Bioinformatics and Biomedicine (BIBM), Washington, D.C., pp. 382–387 (2015)
4. Dera, D., Bouaynaya, N., Fathallah-Shaykh, H.M.: Automated robust image segmentation: level set method using non-negative matrix factorization with application to brain mri. Bull. Math. Biol. **78**, 1–27 (2016)
5. Lee, D.D., Seung, H.S.: Learning the parts of objects by non-negative matrix factorization. Nature **401**, 788–793 (1999)
6. Menze, B., et al.: The multimodal brain tumor image segmentation benchmark (brats). IEEE Trans. Med. Imaging **34**, 1993–2024 (2015)
7. Tsai, A., Yezzi, A.S., Willsky, A.: Curve evolution implementation of the mumford-shah functional for image segmentation, denoising, interpolation and magnification. IEEE Trans. Image Process. **10**, 1169–1186 (2001)

Brain Tumor Segmentation by Variability Characterization of Tumor Boundaries

Edgar A. Rios Piedra[1,2,3(✉)], Benjamin M. Ellingson[2,3],
Ricky K. Taira[1,2,3], Suzie El-Saden[1,2,3], Alex A.T. Bui[1,2,3],
and William Hsu[1,2,3]

[1] Medical Imaging Informatics Group, Department of Radiological Sciences,
University of California, Los Angeles, USA
edgar.riosp@engineering.ucla.edu
[2] Department of Radiological Sciences, David Geffen School of Medicine,
University of California, Los Angeles, USA
[3] Department of Bioengineering, University of California, Los Angeles, USA

Abstract. Automated medical image analysis can play an important role in diagnoses and treatment assessment, but integration and interpretation across heterogeneous data sources remain significant challenges. In particular, automated estimation of tumor extent in glioblastoma patients has been challenging given the diversity of tumor shapes and appearance characteristics due to differences in magnetic resonance (MR) imaging acquisition parameters, scanner variations and heterogeneity in tumor biology. With this work, we present an approach for automated tumor segmentation using multimodal MR images. The algorithm considers the variability arising from the intrinsic tumor heterogeneity and segmentation error to derive the tumor boundary and produce an estimate of segmentation error. Using the MICCAI 2015 dataset, a Dice coefficient of 0.74 was obtained for whole tumor, 0.55 for tumor core, and 0.54 for active tumor, achieving above average performance in comparison to other approaches evaluated on the BRATS benchmark.

Keywords: Glioblastoma · Brain tumor · Segmentation variability · Automatic segmentation

1 Introduction

Quantitative measurement and assessment of medical images can play an important part in diagnosis of a disease, treatment planning, and clinical monitoring. As imaging technology and standards have been rapidly changing and increasing in complexity within the field of neuro-oncology, it has become extremely burdensome for clinicians to manually review imaging studies. In addition to increased labor and expense, manual measurements can have a high degree of measurement variability [1] due to the inconsistency and diversity of MRI acquisition parameters (e.g. echo time, repetition

Funded by the National Institutes of Health (NIH) under the award number R01CA1575533.

A. Crimi et al. (Eds.): BrainLes 2016, LNCS 10154, pp. 206–216, 2016.
DOI: 10.1007/978-3-319-55524-9_20

time, etc.) and strategies (2D vs. 3D) along with hardware variations (e.g. field strength, gradient performance, etc.) that change the appearance characteristics of the tumor [2]. The increased variability in measurement from multiple imaging sources, combined with the need for faster interpretation, may potentially result in errors with treatment decisions or conclusions about of potential therapeutic benefits.

Simplistic two-dimensional measurements used to characterize therapeutic changes in the Response Assessment in Neuro Oncology (RANO) criteria [3] have been used for several years. Despite the need for an automated characterization, an accurate classification of brain tumors remains challenging for automated approaches as it has also proven difficult for expert neuroradiologists as well [4].

In this paper, we hypothesize the inherent variability in tumor volume measurements can be leveraged to provide a more accurate assessment of tumor burden and produce an estimate of tumor segmentation variability. While multiple automated segmentation techniques are being actively developed [3], a method that accounts for the variability in tumor burden estimation has not been entirely investigated [5]. We explored a different perspective towards the identification of tumor boundaries and developed a knowledge-based approach that considers a series of brain tissue probability distribution maps as prior information to inform the location and boundaries of brain tumors. This algorithm uses superpixel-based morphological features and the prior statistical maps to generate a preliminary tumor region. The areas of highest variation inside this preliminary region are iteratively measured to create a Tumor Variability Map (TVM), which represents the image heterogeneity along the tumor boundary (measure of uncertainty).

2   Methods

We developed a processing pipeline to automate the segmentation from the raw MRI images to create tumor variability maps that indicate tumor extent. This pipeline is illustrated on Fig. 1 and PseudoCode 1.

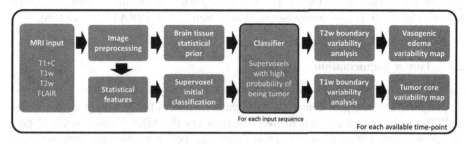

Fig. 1. Overall segmentation process from input multimodal MRI, feature extraction, preliminary tumor ROI calculation by supervoxel classification, and a tumor histogram variability analysis to generate segmentation error estimates for the overall tumor boundary and different tumor components. The process is repeated for all time-points available for an input subject. The output variability maps are a graphical representation that reflect the likely location of a heterogeneous tumor boundary.

Pseudo Code 1: Brain Tumor segmentation through estimation of variability

---

for each follow up: $d = \{d_1, \ldots d_{t-1}, d_t\}$
    // **Data preprocessing**
    Read directory and load MRI Sequences $\rightarrow$ FLAIR, T1, T1+C, T2
    Register and skull strip all volumes;
    Normalize and denoise all volumes;
    Calculate tissue probability masks for white and gray matter $\rightarrow$ WM, GM
    Obtain Subtraction map T1+C - T1 $\rightarrow$ DeltaMap
    // **Preliminary ROI identification**
    for sequences: m = {FLAIR, T2, DeltaMap}
        for orientations x = {axial, coronal, sagittal}
            Obtain brain tissue distributions(WM,GM)
            Cluster volume using SLIC (input volume(m,x), k=10) $\rightarrow$ Volume superpixels
            Extract image features(m,x) $\rightarrow$ Histogram, Symmetry, Inhomogeneity
            Find tumor preliminary ROI by using extracted image features $\rightarrow$ 3DtumorROI
        end
    end
    // **Tumor segmentation**
    for tumor regions: z = {Edema, Enhancing, Necrosis}
        Get tissue distribution inside ROI (3DtumorROI, WM, GM)
        Evaluate rate of change on tumor region z $\rightarrow$ top regions of intensity variation (t(i))
        Apply thresholds at intensity t(i) inside ROI(z) $\rightarrow$ Tumor subregion variability map
    end
    Obtain binary tumor masks by obtaining mask consensus on variability maps
    Locate unclassifed regions inside tumor area $\rightarrow$ Non-enhancing tumor
    Warp back all volumes to original scan space
end

The system is divided into a series of preprocessing strategies followed by the proposed tumor segmentation algorithm. This approach finds an approximate tumor ROI by using the knowledge-based approach proposed in this paper. Afterwards, the intensity variation observed on the approximate tumor ROI is analyzed to find the possible tumor boundaries for the TVM. This approach was evaluated using the 2015 Multimodal Brain Tumor Image Segmentation Benchmark (BRATS) dataset [6].

2.1   Tumor Segmentation

As first step, the algorithm selects all MR modalities of interest including pre-contrast T1-weighted images, post-contrast T1-weighted images (T1+C), T2-weighted images, and T2-weighted fluid attenuated inversion recovery (FLAIR). Then, a series of pre-processing steps are performed as preliminary step before running the proposed segmentation approach, including intra-subject image registration [7], skull stripping [8], intra-subject intensity normalization (z-scores), and image denoising (bias-field correction and soft Gaussian smoothing) [8]. Note that the data for the BRATS benchmark has already been preprocessed.

Afterwards, a series of tissue probability masks are generated to provide context/ knowledge about the approximate distribution of normal cerebral tissues including gray matter, white matter and cerebrospinal fluid (CSF), using this information for tumor identification [10]. The tissue distribution information models image intensities as a mixture of k Gaussians, modelled by a mean (μ_k), standard deviation (σ_k) and a mixing proportion. Following this, Bayes rule is employed to produce the posterior probability of each tissue class. Using this model, the probability of observing an element with intensity y_i on the kth Gaussian is given by:

$$P(y_i|k = \mu_k, \sigma_k) = \frac{1}{\sqrt{2\pi\sigma_k^2}}\exp\left(-\frac{(y_i - \mu_k)^2}{2\sigma_k^2}\right) \qquad (1)$$

Finally, the probability of obtaining the pixel y on a Gaussian is maximized with respect to μ, σ and γ by the minimization of the cost function [10]:

$$\varepsilon = -\log P(y|\mu, \sigma, \gamma) = -\sum_{i=1}^{I}\log\left(\sum_{k=1}^{K}\frac{\gamma_k}{\sqrt{2\pi\sigma_k^2}}\exp\left(-\frac{(y_i - \mu_k)^2}{2\sigma_k^2}\right)\right) \qquad (2)$$

where K is the total number of Gaussian distributions (one for each tissue), and I is the total number of image elements. The update of the mixture proportion (γ_k) is performed by the expectation maximization (EM) algorithm and generates pixel-wise probability maps for cerebral gray matter, white matter and cerebrospinal fluid. These maps (obtained using SPM [9]) let us devise the likely tumor distribution so subsequent analysis and statistics can be performed only on the image patches that are the most likely to correspond to the tumor.

After this step is completed, using the information provided by the tissue distribution probability maps as well as imaging features from each MR volume an initial tumor ROI is obtained. This process involves the partition of the images into superpixels by using the SLIC algorithm [11], a popular method that implements an adaptation of the k-means clustering approach that provides and efficient and fast segmentation of an input image while combining color and spatial proximity to generate the superpixels. By default, in a simple implementation of the SLIC algorithm, only one parameter has to be set (the number of superpixels to be extracted) before being able to use it. In this work, we modified the approach to automatically select the number of clusters based on the histogram distribution of the input imaging volume (3D), setting an initial histogram partition parameter k at 10, roughly based on the type of normal and tumor tissues present on the input images [12].

Afterwards, the preliminary tumor ROI is obtained by selecting the superpixels that represent the regions with the lowest probability of being normal brain tissue according to the information provided by the described distribution probability maps for normal cerebral tissues (including gray matter, white matter and cerebrospinal fluid) [13]. This process is iterated under different orientations (axial, coronal, sagittal) to increase the accuracy of the initial ROI, hypothesizing that different tumor shapes may be easier for the algorithm to identify if visualized under different perspectives (e.g., a u-shaped tumor might be visualized as two different small structures on the axial view but as a

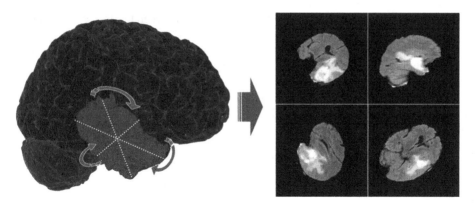

Fig. 2. To have multiple estimates of the tumor boundaries, multiple rotations are found along the tumor major axes so at the end of this process these measurements can be aggregated into the measurement variability map. In this work, the segmentation occurs on the three main tumor axes and ten random rotations on each axis.

continuous and more defined mass on the coronal view, as shown in Fig. 2). Finally, the preliminary tumor ROI is then obtained by taking the union of all regions generated across different perspectives, resulting in a single volumetric ROI.

2.2   Multimodal Tumor Boundary Selection

The next step involves identifying a set of tumor boundaries for the total tumor mass as well as for the tumor sub-regions (i.e., edema, necrosis, enhancing and non-enhancing tumor) using the preliminary tumor ROI defined in the previous step. This approach intends to represent the tumor heterogeneous boundary by doing multiple measurements and then combine them into a TVM to quantify uncertainty associated with segmentation boundaries.

The specific tumor boundaries are obtained as follow: A single definition for T2 abnormality was used to define a "T2 abnormal ROI" using the preliminary ROIs found on the FLAIR and T2 contrast images. Regions of edema are extracted by ranking the intensity rate of change on the preliminary tumor ROI histogram, defining as boundaries the locations where the highest total variation across the histogram corresponding to the tumor region are found. The tumor variability map is produced by aggregating the different binary ROIs obtained at each of these identified values on the tumor histogram.

The same process is followed to locate the enhancing and necrotic regions but using the post-contrast T1 sequence or a subtraction map (defined as T1+c - T1 volumes) [13]. Similarly, the TVM for these regions is then obtained by aggregating these different approximations of the tumor boundary (Fig. 3). A binary representation of the tumor mask is obtained by using the following approach on the TVM:

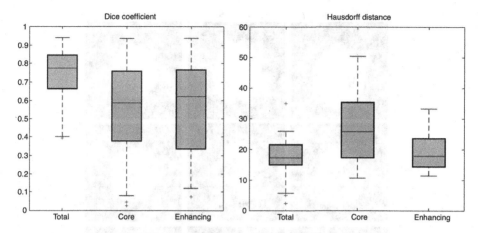

Fig. 3. Box-plots showing the proposed method's performance for the BRATS 2015 dataset. It plots the Dice similarity coefficient on the left (higher is better) and Hausdorff distance on the right (lower is better) when comparing a binarized tumor mask generated by the proposed approach and a segmentation gold standard. Label "Total" refers to all tumor components (edema, enhancing, necrosis and non-enhancing tumor), "Core" refers to the tumor core (excluding regions of vasogenic edema), and 'Enhancing' refers to active tumor cells with microvascular proliferations.

$$I = \begin{cases} P_{i,j} \geq \frac{n}{2} \therefore I_{i,j} = 1 \\ P_{i,j} < \frac{n}{2} \therefore I_{i,j} = 0 \end{cases} \tag{3}$$

where I is the output binary image, $P_{i,j}$ is the intensity at pixel location i,j of the TVM P and n is the number of discrete probability levels defined in the variability map. The output is a set of masks that represent the tumor extent and the different sub-regions with the possibility to calculate variability metrics (e.g., agreement ratio, standard deviation, statistical change measurement, and others).

3 Results

This proposed approach was tested on all 220 cases in the BRATS 2015 dataset and evaluated on three components: whole tumor, tumor core (enhancing and necrotic components) and active tumor (enhancing component). The Dice coefficient for total tumor mass of 0.74 (median: 0.77, 1st quartile: 0.66, 3rd quartile: 0.84), 0.54 for the tumor core (median: 0.57, 1st quartile: 0.37, 3rd quartile: 0.75) and 0.54 for the active tumor (median: 0.60, 1st quartile: 0.29, 3rd quartile: 0.76). Figure 3 shows the Dice coefficient as well as the Hausdorff distance metric for this dataset.

On Fig. 4 some examples of input images and the output tumor variability maps for edema, enhancing and necrotic regions of the tumor as well as the representation of these tumor compartments overlaid on the image as binary masks. This binary representation of the TVMs (as previously described) is done with the purpose of similarity

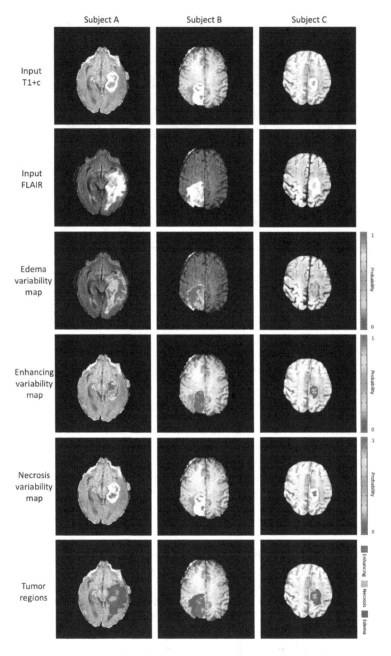

Fig. 4. Tumor segmentation results for three different subjects. First and second rows represent the input post-contrast T1-weighted and FLAIR scans respectively for each subject (column), rows three to five show the result of the variability analysis to find different boundary estimations on each tumor (edema, enhancing and necrosis respectively) (non-enhancing tumor is not shown in this example). The color bar represents the pixel-wise probability for each tumor tissue. Finally, the bottom row displays a color coded binary mask that represents the total abnormality (all components) and subclasses (enhancing shown in red, vasogenic edema in blue and necrosis in green). (Color figure online)

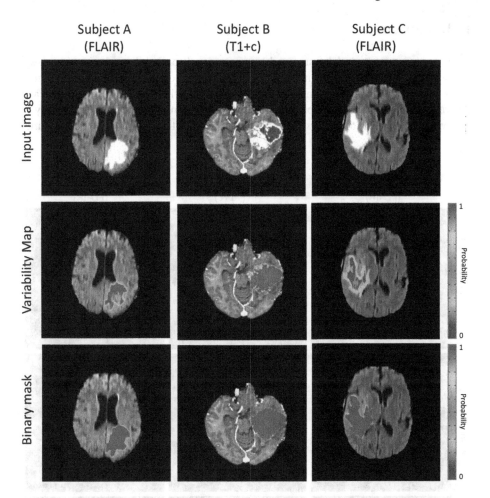

Fig. 5. Examples of brain tumor segmentation results for total tumor mass on three different cases. The first row shows one of the four imaging sequences that are used to perform the tumor segmentation (FLAIR is used on this example for the examples on the left and right and T1+c is used for the example on the center). The tumor variability map is displayed for total tumor on the second row, highlighting on red the regions where the algorithm is most certain that there is an abnormality in that pixel region and showing other color intensities for decreased belief in tumor abnormality according to the color bar located on the right. Finally, the third row shows the binarization of the variability map, according to a majority agreement of the different estimates (that is using a threshold of 0.5), this enables comparison with binary gold standards to evaluate accuracy and also allows for other more standard metrics and use the results in other processing pipelines. (Color figure online)

computations against binary gold standards as well as an easy integration with other processing pipelines (e.g. evaluation of clinical variables, genetic algorithms, etc.) or statistical approaches that require a binary input (Fig. 5).

4 Discussion

We proposed a multimodal framework for automated, probabilistic brain tumor segmentation by using variability in estimates of the tumor boundary. By exploiting tumor heterogeneity from different imaging sources, this algorithm is able to automatically generate tumor probability maps or alternatively add a measurement of uncertainty to binary tumor segmentations. As the proposed approach iteratively measures the tumor

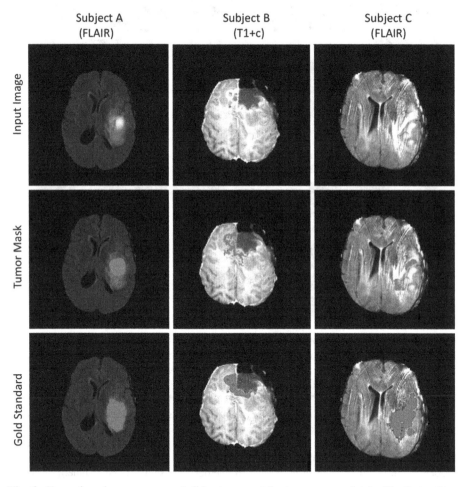

Fig. 6. Examples where our approach did not segment the tumor appropriately. The first column shows an example where the tumor is under segmented, we believe this is because a miscalculation on the prior information that is obtained as a preprocessing step and only the hyper intense edema was selected as part of the tumor, leaving the darker parts unselected. The second column shows a resection cavity on which the full area of enhancement is not captured and the third column shows how image artifacts can also cause problems while trying to segment the tumor.

boundaries, it is able to better detect and capture the heterogeneity found on brain tumors (e.g., being able to capture the shape of tumors with eccentric outlines). By explicitly quantifying the error associated with any given segmentation, we believe that this added information is critical to understand and judge the actual tumor extent by a radiologist or neuro-oncologist when interpreting the follow-up imaging data in the clinical setting.

When evaluating the results with other approaches proposed in previous years, our results are comparable to or surpass the mean performance of other algorithms [6] (Reza, Meier, Cordier, Bauer, Festa, Geremia, Buendia, Taylor, Shin). As a method to improve our results, we are also developing a classifier based on Convolutional Neural Networks (CNN) [14] to help in the definition of the preliminary tumor ROI and also to help reduce the number of false positives during the tumor boundary selection. Combining the result of our knowledge-based approach and the result of the CNN (trained to classify whether an individual voxel is part of a brain tumors using an independent dataset) might contribute towards better results on the different tumor contours (some examples where the proposed approach did not segment the tumor accurately are shown in Fig. 6).

The inclusion of variability calculations into segmentation methodologies can lead to better results and ultimately provide more meaningful data to clinicians as the knowledge of a measurement variation is fundamental to make more objective decisions. Future work includes the evaluation of variability on tumor biomarkers (such as

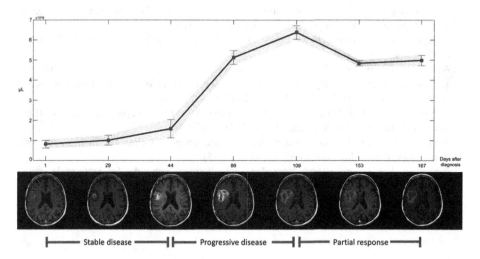

Fig. 7. Example of tumor progression over time. Showing volume measurement for each time-point with its respective error estimate. As time passes it becomes critical to evaluate if the action taken at a given point in time (e.g., chemotherapy, radiotherapy) had a significant effect on the tumor characteristics observed on the following MRI scans. The proposed segmentation method with analysis of tumor boundary variability enables clinicians to have different estimates of tumor characteristics (e.g., tumor volume, grow rate) and statistically define if there has been significant change over time or not (e.g., analysis of variance), essential for subsequent treatment planning.

tumor volume, thickness of enhancing margin, necrosis proportion, etc.) and impact on medical decision making to provide automated evaluations of tumor progression over time (as shown in Fig. 7) to be able to better evaluate treatment effectiveness and increase the radiologist's efficiency at evaluating imaging studies.

References

1. Omuro, A., DeAngelis, L.M.: Glioblastoma and other malignant gliomas: a clinical review. JAMA **310**(17), 1842–1850 (2013)
2. Inda, M., Bonavia, R., Seoane, J.: Glioblastoma multiforme: a look inside its heterogeneous nature. Cancers **6**(1), 226–239 (2014)
3. Wen, P.Y., et al.: Updated response assessment criteria for high-grade gliomas: response assessment in neuro-oncology working group. JCO **28**(11), 1963–1972 (2010)
4. Bauer, S., et al.: A survey of MRI-based medical image analysis for brain tumor studies. Phys. Med. Biol. **58**(13), R97 (2013)
5. Huo, J., et al.: Ensemble segmentation for GBM brain tumors on MR images using confidence-based averaging. Med. Phys. **40**(9), 093502 (2013)
6. Menze, B.H., et al.: The multimodal brain tumor image segmentation benchmark (BRATS). IEEE Trans. Med. Imaging **34**(10), 1993–2024 (2015)
7. Jenkinson, M., Bannister, P.R., Brady, J.M., Smith, S.M.: Improved optimization for the robust and accurate linear registration and motion correction of brain images. NeuroImage **17**(2), 825–841 (2002)
8. The AFNI program (Analysis of Functional NeuroImages). National Institute of Health, USA. https://afni.nimh.nih.gov/afni/. Accessed Sept 2016
9. Vaseghi, S.V.: Advanced Digital Signal Processing and Noise Reduction. Wiley, Hoboken (2008)
10. Ashburner, J., Friston, K.J.: Unified segmentation. Neuroimage **26**(3), 839–851 (2005)
11. Ji, S., et al.: A new multistage medical segmentation method based on superpixel and fuzzy clustering. Comput. Math. Methods Med. **2014**, 01–15 (2014)
12. Achanta, R., et al.: SLIC superpixels compared to state-of-the-art superpixel methods. IEEE Trans. Pattern Anal. Mach. Intell. **34**(11), 2274–2282 (2012)
13. Nechifor, R.E., et al.: Novel magnetic resonance imaging techniques in brain tumors. Top. Magn. Reson. Imaging **24**(3), 137–146 (2015)
14. Simonyan, K., Zisserman, A.: Very deep convolutional networks for large-scale image recognition. arXiv preprint arXiv:1409.1556 (2014)

Ischemic Stroke Lesion Image Segmentation

Predicting Stroke Lesion and Clinical Outcome with Random Forests

Oskar Maier[1,2(✉)] and Heinz Handels[1]

[1] Institute of Medical Informatics, Universität zu Lübeck, Lübeck, Germany
maier@imi.uni-luebeck.de
[2] Graduate School for Computing in Medicine and Life Sciences,
Universität zu Lübeck, Lübeck, Germany

Abstract. The treatment of ischemic stroke requires fast decisions for which the potentially fatal risks of an intervention have to be weighted against the presumed benefits. Ideally, the treating physician could predict the outcome under different circumstances beforehand and thus make an informed treatment decision. To this end, this article presents two new methods: one for lesion outcome and one for clinical outcome prediction from multispectral magnetic resonance sequences. After extracting tailored image features, a random forest classifier respectively regressor is trained. Both approaches were submitted to the Ischemic Stroke Lesion Segmentation (ISLES) 2017 challenge and obtained a first and third place. The outcome underlines the robustness of our designed features and stresses the approach's resilience against overfitting when faced with small training datasets.

Keywords: Ischemic stroke · Lesion segmentation · Lesion outcome · Clinical outcome · mRS · Magnetic resonance imaging · Brain MR · Random forest · RDF · ISLES 2016

1 Introduction

Stroke is the second most frequent cause of death worldwide and one of the major contributors to disability in the elderly. An ischemic stroke is caused by an obstruction in the cerebral blood supply and the subsequent underperfusion of the affected brain tissue, which ultimately results in infarction. The available treatment options are thrombolysis, the breakdown of blood clots by pharmacological means, and thrombectomy, their surgical removal by means of a catheter. Unfortunately, both are only affective if applied in a relatively small time window of a few hours after stroke onset and are moreover associated with a number of potentially fatal complications, such as rupture of the vessel wall.

Desirable would be a mechanism, with which the treating physician could estimate the intervention's success beforehand, and thus weight the potential gain against the involved risks for an informed treatment decision. To this end, a method is sough that allows to compare the outcome under treatment against

© Springer International Publishing AG 2016
A. Crimi et al. (Eds.): BrainLes 2016, LNCS 10154, pp. 219–230, 2016.
DOI: 10.1007/978-3-319-55524-9_21

the untreated outcome. Since the involved processes are highly complex and poorly understood, no manual solution is feasible. This raises the question of whether a computer assisted algorithm can reliably predict the outcome under varying conditions.

The Ischemic Stroke Lesion Segmentation (ISLES) 2016 challenge, held in conjunction with the Conference on Medical Image Computing and Computer Assisted Intervention (MICCAI) 2016 in Athens, aims to answer this question. Researchers are called upon to submit their solutions, which are applied to a representative, freely available dataset and subsequently compared in a fair and direct manner. All participants are supplied with acute magnetic resonance (MR) imaging data, including diffusion and perfusion scans, and a number of associated clinical parameters, namely the time-since-stroke (TSS), time-to-treatment (TTT) and standardized Thrombolysis in Cerebral Infarction (TICI) scale, which rates the reperfusion success. The challenge is divided into two tasks, which both employ the same input data (see Fig. 1 for a graphical representation)[1].

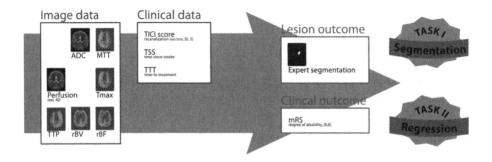

Fig. 1. Schema of the ISLES 2016 tasks.

Task I is the prediction of the lesion outcome. For the gold standard, three month follow-up MR scans, which denote the final lesion outcome, were acquired, segmented by two clinical experts, and co-registered to the acute images. These final lesion outcome binary masks constitute the endpoints of the first task. Any algorithm successfully solving this task, e.g., by reaching inter-rater accuracy, could be used to assess an intervention's gain in brain tissue based solely on the acute MR images acquired at the time of patient admission.

While the quantity of salvaged brain tissue is a favorable measure on which to base a treatment decision, the real benefit for the patient's life quality is denoted by the qualitative clinical outcome, two factors which do not necessarily correlate. Hence, for **Task II**, the participants are called upon to predict the clinical outcome as measured by the widely used 90 days Modified Rankin Scale (mRS) disability assessment.

Most existing approaches from the clinical domain which are concerned with tissue fate after stroke are based on simple thresholding and are thus unable

---

[1] For more details on the ISLES 2016 challenge, see http://www.isles-challenge.org.

to model the effects of an intervention [5]. An exception is the work of Kemmling et al. (2015) [7], where the authors approach lesion outcome prediction based on CT perfusion data using a general linear model (GLM). While reporting respectable results, their proposal is missing a suitable quantitative evaluation and the authors fail to make their data publicly available. Furthermore, a GLM might be too simple a model for the problem's complexity. To our best knowledge, the second task of estimating the mRS scores directly from the acute data has never been attempted. An approach to derive the mRS score from the follow-up lesion masks by considering overlap with predefined brain regions is reported in Forkert et al. (2015) [4].

This article describes our participation in the ISLES 2016 challenge. By treating the lesion outcome prediction as a segmentation task, we approach Task I with our previously published brain lesion segmentation framework [12,13], which is based on a random forest (RF) classifier. The method already participated successfully [14] in the previous year's edition of the challenge [11]. For Task II, we extend our application by appending a random regression forest (RRF), which makes use of the lesion outcome mask computed for Task I to extract a number of tailored regression features to ultimately predict the mRS score for each testing case.

2   Method

In this section, we describe the data and introduce our methods developed for the two ISLES 2016 tasks.

2.1   Data

The data consists of 30 training and 19 testing cases from two medical centers. Each case represents an acute stroke case before treatment and consists of a set of MR sequences acquired during the stroke lesion's acute phase as well as a number of additional clinical parameters (see Fig. 1). Diffusion properties are represented by the apparent diffusion coefficient (ADC) map, which is assumed to reveal approximately the area of already infarcted brain tissue. To assess the perfusion properties, the raw 4D perfusion weighted imaging (PWI) data, as acquired through dynamic contrast-enhanced perfusion imaging, as well as the derived perfusion maps mean transit time (MTT), time-to-peak (TTP), time-to-maximum (Tmax), relative blood volume (rBV), and relative blood flow (rBF), are provided. These are assumed to enable the assessment of the underperfused brain region. All images are provided co-registered and skull-stripped. The clinical parameters denote the time already passed at the point of image acquisition, the time that will still pass till the treatment is performed, and the success of the treatment in terms of reperfusion.

The gold standard is only released for the training data, while the evaluation for testing dataset was performed by the challenge organizers. As gold standard for Task I, two sets of expert segmentation delineated in the three month follow-up scans are provided. For Task II, the 90 day mRS scores serve as endpoints.

2.2 Random Forest Framework

Any prediction task makes the silent assumption that all information required to anticipate the lesion's further evolution is already available from the present acute data situation. Under this premise, the lesion outcome prediction task can be treated as a segmentation problem. We therefore adapt our existing brain lesion segmentation framework, which already proved its competitive performance in MS [10], glioma [14], and acute as well as sub-acute stroke [13] segmentation, to the new problem.

Lesion Outcome Prediction Through Classification. The segmentation framework's basic steps are depicted in Fig. 2 and follow the classical machine learning schema of separate training and application phases. The RF method [1,2], as implemented in the sklearn Python package [15], is employed for voxel-wise classification of the multispectral image data. Since the images are already skull-stripped and co-registered, the image features can be extracted directly without any need for further preprocessing. Bias-field correction or intensity range standardization are not required for ADC and perfusion maps (see [14]).

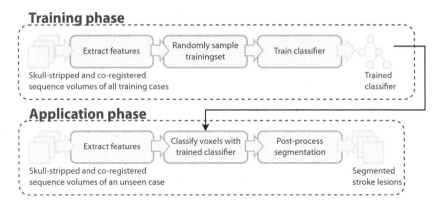

Fig. 2. Framework for lesion outcome prediction.

Image features. Brain lesions differ strongly in shape, location, homogeneity, and intensities. Even for a single pathology, the lesion appearance can vary greatly [11]. We employ in this work a set of features chosen to model a human observers discriminative criteria and specifically developed for the purpose of brain lesion segmentation.

First feature is the voxel's unprocessed intensity value. Next, the Gaussian weighted local average in an area of 3, 5 and 7 mm around each voxel is extracted to obtain regional information. Then, the medial longitudinal fissure is roughly estimated and the intensity difference between corresponding voxels of the two brain hemispheres obtained. To assess the voxels' rough location in the brain's anatomy, the 2D centerdistance is computed once for each of the three dimensions. Finally, the local histogram feature provides information about the local intensity distribution in a small area around each voxel. All of these features are described in detail in Maier et al. (2015) [13] and a free implementation is available as part of the MedPy library [9].

All features are extracted voxel-wise from the ADC as well as the five perfusion maps. The 4D raw PWI data is not used in this work, neither are the clinical parameters. The implications of this choice and the circumstances that led to this decision are discussed in Sect. 4.

Classifier training. We employ the previously introduced stratified random sampling scheme to reduce the amount of training samples without reducing the represented variance [13]. The resulting 2.5 million samples are passed to the classifier for training. A total of 200 trees is trained to avoid overfitting due to the small number of training cases. No growth restriction is imposed. Node splits are performed with $\sqrt{F}$ of the F available features and the Gini criterion is used for node split optimization.

Classifier application & postprocessing. At application time, the same feature extraction steps are performed, just as depicted in Fig. 2. The trained classifier then produces a posteriori class probability map. This is thresholded at a value of 0.3 to counter an observed undersegmentation tendency. The only postprocessing step applied is the closing of structural 3D holes in the resulting binary segmentation mask, as stroke lesions are known to be solid objects.

Clinical Outcome Prediction Through Regression. To predict the clinical outcome of an ischemic stroke case, we employ RRFs, which are thoroughly described in Criminisi and Shotton (2013) [2] and implemented in the sklearn Python package [15]. As input, these regressors take a number of hand-crafted features representing the processed case, and return a real number as output that can be interpreted as the sought mRS score. The framework's schema is depicted in Fig. 3.

Regression features. Just as RFs, the RRFs require a number of features which constitute the information they have available to base their regression process on. These feature must be chosen to be representative and allow the prediction of the clinical outcome.

For achieve an accurate mRS prediction, we decided to extract information about 1. the state of the lesion itself, 2. the state of a band around the lesion whose fate is unclear and 3. the state of the remainder of the brain. These three regions of interest (ROI) are not defined, but we have access to the lesion outcome mask returned by the lesion outcome prediction method, from which we can estimate the desired regions. To this end, the probability map resulting from the first task is thresholded at a value of 0.1. Secondly, this inner region mask is extended with a binary dilation of size 5 mm, resulting in a banded region

Training phase

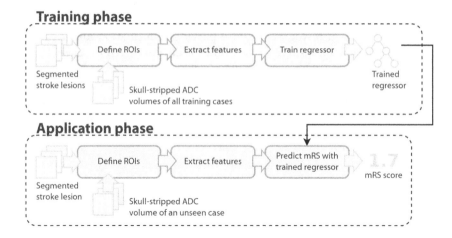

Application phase

Fig. 3. Framework for clinical outcome prediction.

denoting roughly the desired band around the lesion. Finally, the remaining brain forms the third region. Figure 4 denotes this process. By comparing image attributes between these three regions and by considering their shape characteristics, we aim to predict the clinical outcome.

From the ADC image, we extract the same features as previously for the lesion outcome task. These are voxel-wise image features and cannot be employed directly. Instead, we consider statistics of these features' values in the three regions, namely 10 percentile values, the standard deviation, the variance and a histogram of 10 bins. These image based features amount to a total of 1650.

Furthermore, we extract shape characteristics from the three regions, as the lesion outcome is considered to have an influence on the clinical outcome. These

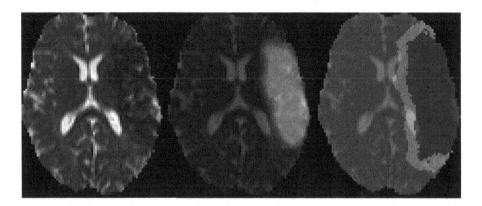

Fig. 4. The three ROIs at the example of training case 06: Left original ADC image, middle the probability map of the lesion outcome task, and right the three derived regions.

are region area, perimeter, roundness, and equivdiameter, which amount to a total of 12 additional features.

Regressor training. First, the lesion outcome prediction method is applied to each of the training cases to obtain the lesion probability maps. Based on these, the three ROIs are computed and the above described regression features extracted. Then, the RRF is trained on all training cases with the mRS score as training endpoint.

Since the amount of training data is very limited with only 30 cases, a large number of 200 trees is trained to avoid overfitting. No growth-restriction is imposed. The mean squared error is employed as node optimization term.

Regressor application. The application of the regressor to a formerly unseen training case follows the same steps as the training (see Fig. 3). The output of the forest is the final estimated mRS score.

3   Evaluation and Results

3.1   Evaluation Metrics

For Task I, the employed evaluation metrics are the Dice's coefficient (DC), which denotes the volume overlap, the average symmetric surface distance (ASSD), denoting the volume surface distance, and the Hausdorff distance (HD), revealing outliers. For a detailed definition of these metrics, please refer to the challenge's web page. It contains furthermore a description of the employed rankings scheme, which combines these three measure into a relative rank used for the leaderboard. For Task II, the average absolute error compared to the known mRS score is computed. The reported rank is the average rank over all cases.

3.2   Results Task I

After submitting the predicted lesion outcome as binary masks, the evaluation was performed by the challenge organizers against the hidden gold standard segmentations to allow for a fair and direct comparison of the participating methods. The final results as published at the day of the challenge's workshop are shown in Table 1 and Fig. 5 shows an exemplary visual result. Our method obtained the third place according to the leaderboard.

3.3   Results Task II

After submitting the predicted mRS scores, the evaluation was performed by the challenge organizers against the hidden gold standard to allow for a fair and direct comparison of the participating method. The final results as published at the day of the challenge's workshop are shown in Table 2. Our method obtained the first place according to the leaderboard.

Table 1. ISLES Task I testing dataset average results with standard deviation. Our method is highlighted. [1]: the rank was computed as described in [11], taking all three evaluation metrics into account. [2]: the average ASSD and HD values were computed only for the cases for which the segmentation results had an at least partial overlap with the gold standard segmentation. [3]: these three submission are variants of the same method and were considered as one in the leaderboard.

Rank[1]	Team	cases[2]	ASSD (mm)	DC [0,1]	HD (mm)
3.34	KR-SUL[3]	18/19	6.38 ± 4.18	0.31 ± 0.24	34.09 ± 21.08
3.42	KR-SUK[3]	18/19	6.23 ± 3.55	0.31 ± 0.24	32.84 ± 15.68
3.68	KR-SUC[3]	18/19	6.46 ± 4.38	0.30 ± 0.25	37.70 ± 21.61
4.38	CH-UBE	19/19	7.10 ± 4.19	0.26 ± 0.19	44.30 ± 24.64
4.60	**DE-UZL**	18/19	7.57 ± 4.17	0.30 ± 0.23	36.88 ± 16.84
4.98	UK-CVI	18/19	7.56 ± 4.34	0.29 ± 0.23	35.91 ± 17.04
6.03	HK-CUH	19/19	10.56 ± 5.92	0.27 ± 0.22	59.44 ± 38.27
6.22	PK-PNS	19/19	9.12 ± 5.46	0.26 ± 0.22	78.04 ± 18.11
7.97	US-SFT	18/19	13.96 ± 6.14	0.19 ± 0.20	76.28 ± 22.61
	inter-rater	19/19	3.00 ± 2.48	0.58 ± 0.20	24.87 ± 15.48

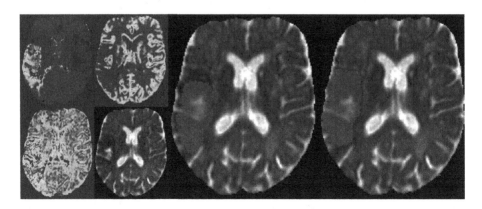

Fig. 5. Example result on training case 12: On the left are shown the MR sequences Tmax, rBF, ADC, and MTT, from top-left clockwise; in the middle the segmentation result overlaid on the ADC map; and on the right the gold standard segmentation overlaid on the ADC map.

4   Discussion and Conclusion

We presented a method based on RFs for lesion as well as clinical outcome prediction for acute ischemic stroke. The placement obtained in both tasks shows the developed algorithm to rank among the best existing solutions with a first and third place.

Table 2. ISLES Task II testing dataset average results with standard deviation. Our method is highlighted. [1]: the rank was computed as an average rank over the ranks obtained for each testing case.

Rank[1]	Team	cases[2]	average absolute error
1.5	**DE-UZL**	19/19	1.05±0.62
1.6	KR-SUL	19/19	1.10 ± 0.70
1.8	KR-SUK	19/19	1.26 ± 0.81
2.3	KR-SUC	19/19	1.37 ± 1.00
2.5	PK-PNS	19/19	1.26 ± 0.87

Lesion outcome prediction through classification. The proposed method, which was previously employed in various brain lesion segmentation tasks, proved to be equally suited for brain lesion outcome prediction. Compared to the other participating approaches, only a convolutional neural network (CNN) and a second RF solution reached higher scores. The statistical evaluation presented at the day of the challenge's workshop revealed no significant difference between our and the second placed method. Despite the small training set, all participating methods used algorithms from machine learning. The stroke evolution process might be simply to complex to be modeled explicitly.

Two observations stand out. First, the results from the ISLES 2015 challenge [11] showed that the worst outcome can be predicted with high accuracy from acute data. Other studies reported similar results for the best possible outcome as estimated by the already infarcted ADC lesion [16]. Hence, the task should be feasible. This view is challenged by the low evaluation scores obtained by all teams, which are far from the inter-observer performance. Second, in Sect. 2.2, we stated that the task is making the silent assumption that all information required for the prediction is provided by the acute data. After the evaluation, this can neither be confirmed nor rejected. Owing to the high complexity of stroke lesion evolution, which depends on many interdependent factors often yet poorly understood, it is unknown what exactly would be required to make a reliable prediction. Both of these failures to draw a speaking conclusion from the obtained results can be attributed to the small training set size. The prediction task encompasses small and large strokes, interventions with different levels of success, interventions at different timepoint of the stroke evolution, and a range of patients with varying constitutions. To suitably represent the variance of the problem, a few hundred sample cases would likely be required.

Perfusion maps are essentially representations of the parameters of a curve, which represents the pass of a contrast agent bolus through a tissue voxel. To this end, various parametric models have been proposed, all of which make at least some simplifications. Hence, it could be assumed that the raw 4D PWI data contains more information than the derived perfusion maps. During a number of preliminary experiments, we did not found the 4D PWI to improve the prediction results. In fact, its addition decreased the accuracy slightly. This result is consistent with the observation reported by Forkert et al. (2014) [3]. Thus, either the forest is unable to model the time curve of a passing bolus implicitly or the approximations made during the computation of the perfusion maps are successfully revealing the real underlying model.

All three of the supplied clinical parameters are considered major contributors to the final stroke lesion outcome. Surprisingly, the addition of TSS, TTT and TICI did not have any effect on the prediction accuracy and were subsequently left out. We can only assume that the small training set size impeded the efficient use of the clinical parameters. Unfortunately, this does leaver with which the physicians were assumed to vary the lesion outcome for the purpose of comparing successful against failed interventions at different moments in stroke evolution.

Clinical outcome prediction through regression. The obtained first place could be considered to prove the suitability of our approach for predicting the clinical outcome in ischemic stroke. However, the results of this task should be interpreted with care. Clinical outcome prediction is a very complex task, where the final results are the sum of many interdependent factors. First, there are the patients general state of health, gender, age, and predisposition to ischemic attacks among others. Then there are the lesion and brain characteristics, such as lesion age, location, size, shape, supporting perfusion through peripheral arteries [8], and the yet poorly understood molecular processes involved in ischemic cell death [6]. Final, there is the intervention itself, how it is conducted, its success and timing. As already observed for Task I, with only 30 training and 19 testing cases, the challenge's dataset is too small to draw a general conclusion. All participating methods are based on machine learning algorithm, which require sufficient training data.

During our experiments, we found that adding the clinical parameters to the regression training set did not change the results in any significant way. Considering the temporal development of stroke lesions, the TSS, TTT and TICI parameters were expected to have a major influence on the clinical outcome. That this assumption could not be confirmed is likely to be an effect of the problem's underrepresentation through the small dataset, rather than a new observation challenging the benefit of established stroke treatments.

Our method is based on the definition of three ROIs, which are rather arbitrarily chosen and do neither reflect any anatomical, nor any lesion properties. That we still obtained the first place is another confirmation of the rather ill posed problem. Still, we consider our approach a promising base from which to derive a good clinical outcome prediction algorithm when more training and testing data becomes available.

Conclusion. We presented a lesion outcome prediction and a clinical outcome prediction solution. Despite the difficulty of the task and the small training dataset, high ranks were obtained. This shows our method to be competitive and to successfully avoid overfitting. The second characteristic proved especially important for the second task of mRS score estimation with only 30 training cases and was awarded with a first place.

For the future, we plan to obtain a larger dataset for both tasks that sufficiently covers the problem's complexity. For the regression task, we aim to study the molecular processed involved in stroke evolution and derive some tailored image features. Finally, we would like to take the in the first task predicted lesion's exact location into account when predicting the mRS, which was shown to have a beneficial effect on the accuracy [4].

References

1. Breiman, L.: Random forests. Mach. Learn. **45**(1), 5–32 (2001)
2. Criminisi, A., Shotton, J.: Decision Forests for Computer Vision and Medical Image Analysis, 1st edn. Springer, London (2013)
3. Forkert, N.D., Siemonsen, S., Dalski, M., et al.: Is there more valuable information in PWI datasets for a voxel-wise acute ischemic stroke tissue outcome prediction than what is represented by typical perfusion maps? In: Molthen, R.C., Weaver, J.B. (eds.) SPIE Medical Imaging, vol. 9038, p. 903810. International Society for Optics and Photonics (2014)
4. Forkert, N.D., Verleger, T., Cheng, B., et al.: Multiclass support vector machine-based lesion mapping predicts functional outcome in ischemic stroke patients. PLOS ONE **10**(6), e0129569 (2015)
5. Galinovic, I.: Evaluation of automated and manual perfusion MRI post-processing: the search for accurate tissue fate prediction in acute ischemic stroke. Ph.D. thesis, Medizinische Fakultät Charité-Universitätsmedizin Berlin (2013)
6. Gonzalez, R.G., Hirsch, J.A., Koroshetz, W.J., Lev, M.H., Schaefer, P.W. (eds.): Acute Ischemic Stroke - Imaging and Intervention, 2 edn. Springer, Berlin (2006)
7. Kemmling, A., Flottmann, F., Forkert, N.D., et al.: Multivariate dynamic prediction of ischemic infarction and tissue salvage as a function of time and degree of recanalization. J. Cereb. Blood Flow Metab. **35**(9), 1397–1405 (2015)
8. Maas, M.B., Lev, M.H., Ay, H., et al.: Collateral vessels on CT angiography predict outcome in acute ischemic stroke. Stroke **40**(9), 3001–3005 (2009)
9. Maier, O.: MedPy - Medical image processing in Python (2016)
10. Maier, O., Handels, H.: MS-lesion segmentation in MRI with random forests. In: Pham, D. (ed.) Longitudinal Multiple Sclerosis Lesion Segmentation Challenge, ISBI (2015)
11. Maier, O., Menze, B.H., von der Gablentz, J., et al.: ISLES 2015 - a public evaluation benchmark for ischemic stroke lesion segmentation from multispectral MRI. Med. Image Anal. **35**, 250–269 (2017)
12. Maier, O., Schröder, C., Forkert, N.D., Martinetz, T., Handels, H.: Classifiers for ischemic stroke lesion segmentation: a comparison study. PLOS ONE **10**(12), e0145118 (2015)
13. Maier, O., Wilms, M., von der Gablentz, J., et al.: Extra Tree forests for sub-acute ischemic stroke lesion segmentation in MR sequences. J. Neurosci. Methods **240**, 89–100 (2015)

14. Maier, O., Wilms, M., Handels, H.: Image features for brain lesion segmentation using random forests. In: Crimi, A., Menze, B., Maier, O., Reyes, M., Handels, H. (eds.) BrainLes 2015. LNCS, vol. 9556, pp. 119–130. Springer, Cham (2016). doi:10.1007/978-3-319-30858-6_11
15. Pedregosa, F., Varoquaux, G., Gramfort, A., et al.: Scikit-learn: machine learning in python. J. Mach. Learn. Res. **12**, 2825–2830 (2011)
16. Straka, M., Albers, G.W., Bammer, R.: Real-time diffusion-perfusion mismatch analysis in acute stroke. J. Magn. Reson. Imaging **32**(5), 1024–37 (2010)

Ensemble of Deep Convolutional Neural Networks for Prognosis of Ischemic Stroke

Youngwon Choi[1], Yongchan Kwon[1], Hanbyul Lee[1], Beom Joon Kim[2], Myunghee Cho Paik[1], and Joong-Ho Won[1(✉)]

[1] Department of Statistics, Seoul National University, Seoul 08826, Korea
wonj@stats.snu.ac.kr
[2] Department of Neurology and Cerebrovascular Center,
Seoul National University Bundang Hospital, Seongnam 13620, Korea

Abstract. We propose an ensemble of deep neural networks for the two tasks of automated prognosis of post-treatment ischemic stroke, as imposed by the ISLES 2016 Challenge. For lesion outcome prediction, we employ an ensemble of three-dimensional multiscale residual U-Net and a fully convolutional network, trained using image patches. In order to handle class imbalance, we devise a multi-step training strategy. For clinical outcome prediction, we combine a convolutional neural network (CNN) and a logistic regression model. To overcome the small sample size and the need for whole brain image, we use the CNN trained using patches as a feature extractor and trained a shallow network based on the extracted features. Our ensemble approach demonstrated an appealing performance on both problems, and is ranked among the top entries in the Challenge.

Keywords: Fully convolutional networks · U-Net · 3D convolutional kernels · Patchwise learning · Multi-phase training · Class imbalance · Ensemble

1 Introduction

The success of an ischemic stroke treatment is highly dependent on the time delay between its onset and the recanalization of occluded cerebral arteries. Timely and precise decision-making, which should be made on the scene within a several minutes, is therefore of paramount importance for patients' outcomes [19]. In this regard, an automated method that reliably and precisely delineates the extent of ischemic lesions would be an invaluable resource for the successful treatment. Our study thus focuses on automatic prognosis of ischemic stroke after treatment. As a participant of the ISLES 2016 Challenge [1], we devoted our efforts to build a reliable machine learning model that serves for this purpose.

The Challenge was two-fold: (1) predicting the lesion outcome, as measured by regions in the magnetic resonance imaging (MRI) scan, (2) predicting the

---

Y. Choi, Y. Kwon and H. Lee—Contributed equally.

© Springer International Publishing AG 2016
A. Crimi et al. (Eds.): BrainLes 2016, LNCS 10154, pp. 231–243, 2016.
DOI: 10.1007/978-3-319-55524-9_22

clinical outcome, as measured by the modified Rankin Scale (mRS), both measured in more than 90 days after treatment. Clinical informations such as Time-Since-Stroke (TSS), Time-To-Treatment (TTT), and thrombolysis in cerebral infarction (TICI) were available as predictors, together with preprocessed MRI images in 7 types: Apparent Diffusion Coefficient (ADC), Perfusion Weighted Image (PWI), relative cerebral Blood Flow (rBF), relative cerebral Blood Volume (rBV), Mean Transit Time (MTT), Time To Peak (TTP), and Time To Maximum (Tmax). There were thirty (30) training cases given, for which the ground truth for the lesions and the mRS for clinical outcome were available. The task is to predict these outcomes for 19 test cases. The evaluation measures for lesion prediction were Dice's coefficient (DC), the average symmetric surface distance (ASSD) and the Hausdorff distance (HD). On the other hand, the evaluation measure for clinical outcome prediction was the average of absolute errors between the true and predicted mRSes.

Recently, Convolutional Neural Networks (CNN) have achieved great success in medical image analysis [17]. These approaches do not depend on hand-crafted features, and make it possible to extract features from raw images automatically. Especially, the Fully Convolutional Network (FCN) [16] and the U-net [3,18] are mainly used in image segmentation problems. The FCN extends the CNN model that operates on images with a fixed size, to handle those of arbitrary sizes. The U-Net has an unique U-shaped topology consisting of a contracting path that can capture the context, and an expanding path that can localize interesting features.

Our tasks were challenging in the sense that the sample size is very small compared to common CNN applications, and that there is a large variation in lesion sizes and clinical score among cases. To alleviate these difficulties, we adopted an ensemble method, which helps reducing prediction variance.

2   The Lesion Outcome Prediction

We considered an ensemble of two different CNN models and applied a patchwise approach in order to increase the effective sample size. Two models, one based on the three-dimensional (3D) multiscale residual U-net and the other the FCN, are different in the interpretation of the problem. For the residual U-net, we interpreted the lesion outcome prediction as a voxel-wise segmentation problem. Negative DC was used as the loss function for segmentation. For the FCN, we regarded the problem as a patch-wise classification problem and used the cross entropy as the loss function. This difference causes distinct drawbacks of two models. For instance, the prediction from the FCN could be noisy, while the U-net might cause artifacts. We expected these drawbacks to be improved by the ensemble of models.

A significant amount of heterogeneity was observed in the dimension of the images because they were collected from disparate machines and institutions. We used 6 out of 7 available types of images; namely ADC, rBF, rBV, MTT, TTP, and Tmax, which are all three-dimensional. We ignored the four dimensional

PWI, because it is hard to handle the time axis. We resized all images to the same dimension: (width × height × depth) = (256 × 256 × 32).

Usually the stroke lesion is small compared to the whole brain. This causes a severe imbalance in the training dataset. With uniformly sampled patches, prediction will tend to be overwhelmed by healthy parts at initial time. To resolve this problem, we considered multi-phase learning [7], a novel technique dividing training procedure into several steps. In each training phase, the network architecture remained the same but was trained with the different input data. In one of the phases, we used patches oversampled near the lesions.

2.1 3D Multiscale Residual U-Net

Preprocessing. To segment 3D images, both two-dimensional (2D) or 3D patches can be used [7,8,13,15]. We trained our model with both kinds of patches and found a better performance with 3D patches. This is interesting because there is a deficiency in the depth resolution. We sampled patches in two different scales in order to capture both short- and long-range spatial correlation. For a given center voxel, a "local" patch was extracted from its $32 \times 32 \times 8$ neighborhood; a "global" patch was obtained from the $64 \times 64 \times 16$ neighborhood, and then 8-to-1 downsampled to maintain the same number of inputs. We call this technique multiscale input following [13]. This multiscale approach was partially motivated practically by the lack of GPU memory. For our purpose it showed better performance than increasing the patch size. This multiscale approach instead of increasing the patch size improved the performance much better and was practically more feasible. The maximum size of patches was restricted because of the lack of GPU memory. For data augmentation, we only used sagittal axis reflection; other methods such as translation and rotation did not improve performance much.

Main Architecture. The U-net has shown an impressive performance in many biomedical image segmentation applications [3,18]. Our proposed architecture was to supplement U-net by residual shortcut paths making deeper networks [9,11]. Thus the proposed model incorporates two different blocks: the convolutional block and the residual block. A convolutional block consisted of a 3D convolutional layer followed by an exponential linear unit activation [4] and a batch normalization layer [12]. A residual block consisted of two paths, one for an identity operator and the other for a residual operator [20]. The output of the residual block is computed as the sum of the values in the two paths. The proposed method processes 3D multiscale input images through two pathways. The proposed network used 42 layers with approximately 100,000 parameters. The network architecture and main blocks are shown in Fig. 1.

Sample Imbalance. We implemented multi-phase learning with two phases to address the imbalance in the training dataset. In the first step, we trained the model by using patches oversampled near the lesions. In the second stage, we tuned the trained network by using patches sampled uniformly from the training set.

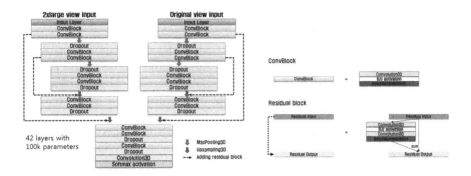

Fig. 1. (Left) Illustration of the main architecture, 3D multiscale residual U-net (Right) Two main blocks, a convolutional block and a residual block.

Prediction. Prediction for the test cases was conducted by a sliding window method. We preprocessed input images into patches, and computed aggregated scores ranging between 0 and 1 by feeding them to the trained network. A voxel was classified as 1 (part of a lesion) if the score was greater than 0.5, 0 otherwise.

Implementation Details. All the weights in the network were initialized by drawing from the zero-mean normal distribution with variance inversely proportional to number of input neurons [10]. The Adam optimizer [14] was used with learning rate of 0.0001. For regularization, dropout, batch normalization, and early stopping rule with 5-epoch patience were applied. We anticipated L1 and L2 regularizations on the layers to improve prediction accuracy, but it turned out not effective. We used negative DC as the target function; the cross entropy, a more common choice in binary segmentation problem, often resulted failures in training. Nonetheless, computing the Dice score for each patch tended to produce extreme scores when the lesion inside the patch was small. To resolve this, we constructed a single 3D patch by concatenating all the inputs in the batch and computed DC for it. This stabilized the training procedure, mitigating the extremities. It required 5 h to fully train the network, while it took and only 10 s per case to predict on a workstation equipped with thirty two Intel(R) Xeon(R) CPU E5-2630 v3 @ 2.40 GHz processors and four NVIDIA GeForce GTX TITAN X GPUs which have 3072 CUDA cores, 1 GHz and 12 GB memory. All the implementations were based on python and Keras [2].

2.2   Fully Convolutional Networks

In the proposed FCN model, the goal was to predict whether the patch contained a lesion, rather than voxel-wise segmentation. We set a binary label for each patch and used the binary cross entropy as the loss function. This converted the segmentation problem to a binary classification problem, thus we could reduce the number of parameters. Furthermore, clinical variables could be easily incorporated into the problem. We utilized the FCN architecture in [16] that uses shift-and-stitch rather than a decoding arm: at the training time, our network is a regular CNN; after the training, we transformed the fully connected layers into convolutional layers of size $(1 \times 1 \times 1)$. The FCN model had two local pathways, pretrained with two kinds of datasets for which a patch is labeled differently. To obtain a voxel-wise prediction, we interlaced predicted volumes from shifted inputs [16].

Preprocessing. Before extracting patches from the data, we scaled the image to make intensity levels to lie between 0 and 1. Extremely high levels were substituted by 1. Due to the difference in the interpretation of the problem, the optimal patch sizes were smaller than the residual U-net model; see Sect. 2.3 for details. The prediction from the models with small-size patches tend to be noisy, while those from using large-size patches tend to lose accuracy.

Main Architecture. The FCN model had two pathways, and each pathway was obtained from a single CNN pretrained with different dataset. We first labeled a patch as 1 if there was a lesion within the patch. We trained a single CNN to construct a local pathway using the dataset labeled in this way. We call this labeling strategy as full view method. For the other local pathway, we labeled a patch as 1 if there was a lesion at the center voxel, and trained the other single network. We call this labeling strategy as small view method. Both networks consisted of 3D convolutional, 3D max-pooling, and fully connected layers. Clinical information was fed into the penultimate layer. To construct the full model, we removed the last fully connected layers from both pathways and added three fully connected layers to the last convolutional layers in order to combine the features from the local pathways. The maxout regularization [6] were applied to the fully connected layers. The maxout pool sizes were 2. To train the full model, we freezed the weights of convolutional layers from single model, and only trained the fully connected layers. After training the full model, we converted all the fully connected layers of the model to the 3D convolutional layers with kernels of size $(1 \times 1 \times 1)$ to handle images of arbitrary sizes. The architectures of the local pathways and the full FCN model are illustrated in Fig. 2.

Sample Imbalance. We implemented the multi-phase learning [7] with three phases to address the sample imbalance. In the first phase, we constructed a training set with an even class distribution. In this step, the goal was to place the initial weight for the next phase near the optimum. In the second phase, we collected the false positive samples from the model trained in the first phase, augmented them by sagittal axis reflection [13]. Then we constructed a training set by resampling the positive (1), negative (0), and the false positive samples (0) equally likely. In the last phase, a fine-tuning was conducted using patches uniformly sampled from the original training set.

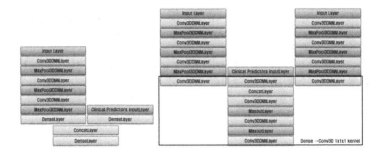

Fig. 2. (Left) Single model. The clinical information applied before the last layer. (Right) Multiview model. The full view regarding a patch as 1 if there was a lesion, and the small view regarding a patch as 1 if there was a lesion in central voxel. After training, the fully connected layers of full models were converted to $(1 \times 1 \times 1)$ size 3D convolutional kernels.

Prediction. The resulting network consisted only of convolutional and pooling layers, and a voxel-wise prediction was possible for an image of an arbitrary size. In order to achieve a voxel-wise segmentation at the original resolution, we used the shift-and-stitch method [16], which stitches outputs from many shifted versions of the input. That is, if the output was downsampled by a factor of f, we shifted the input by x voxels to the right, y voxels down and z voxels to the back, for every (x, y, z) such that $0 \leq x, y, z < f$. By processing each of these f^3 inputs and interlacing the outputs, we could produce a volume of prediction. Each value on the volume represented the voxel-wise probability of the input volume to be a lesion. While this prediction required f^3 forward passes, because we used the maximum patch size of $(9 \times 9 \times 3)$, prediction took only a few seconds for each MRI image.

Implementation Details. The rectified linear unit (ReLU) was employed for the activation function in the convolutional layers and fully-connected layers. In the last fully-connected layer, the softmax function was used to yield prediction. Dropout layers and early stopping rules with 5-epoch patience were applied for regularization. The Adadelta optimizer [21] were used for each training phase. We trained one model with one Intel(R) Xeon(R) CPU E5-2680 v2 @ 2.80 GHz processor and one NVIDIA GeForce 980 GPU which has 2048 CUDA cores, 1 GHz and 4 GB memory. It required an hour for the whole training, and few seconds for testing. All the implementations were based on python and Lasagne [5].

2.3   Ensemble

To obtain a better predictive performance, we used an ensemble method with multiple algorithms derived from the two models described in Sects. 2.1 and 2.2.

There were a total of 12 models in the ensemble. For the FCN, we used a total of eight models, which used one of the four patch sizes of $(3 \times 3 \times 3)$, $(5 \times 5 \times 3)$,

$(7 \times 7 \times 3)$, and $(9 \times 9 \times 3)$, and produced one of the two predictions using the shift-and-stitch method or the FCN's low resolution output. The details of the single CNN models for the local pathway were summarized in Table 1, and the hyperparameters of fully connected layers in the full models were summarized in Table 2. For the U-net, we considered four variants of the main architecture in Sect. 2.1, with different widths of the patches, number of patches per case, and number of filters in the first convolutional layer. For details, see Table 3.

A majority vote is common for ensemble, but we performed a slightly modified voting scheme by taking a weighted average of the models. The formula was as follows:

$$mean = \frac{0.8 \cdot \sum_{i=1}^{2} FCN_i + \sum_{i=3}^{8} FCN_i + weight \cdot \sum_{j=1}^{4} Unet_j}{1.6 + 6 + weight \cdot 4}$$

$$\begin{cases} \text{segment } 1 & \text{if } mean > threshold \\ \text{segment } 0 & \text{if } mean \leq threshold \end{cases}$$

where FCN_i and $Unet_j$ were the variables with a value of 0 or 1, and $mean$ had a value between 0 and 1. In particular, for the two FCN models using patches of size $(3 \times 3 \times 3)$, the prediction outputs were too noisy, so we started with a weight of 0.8.

Table 1. Hyperparameters for the CNN models of the local pathway.

Patch size	$3 \times 3 \times 3$		$5 \times 5 \times 3$		$7 \times 7 \times 3$		$9 \times 9 \times 3$	
	Filter	Features	Filter	Features	Filter	Features	Filter	Features
Conv 1	$3 \times 3 \times 3$	64	$3 \times 3 \times 3$	64	$3 \times 3 \times 3$	64	$3 \times 3 \times 3$	64
Max-pool 1	$2 \times 2 \times 2$	64	$2 \times 2 \times 2$	64	$2 \times 2 \times 1$	64	$2 \times 2 \times 1$	64
Conv 2	$1 \times 1 \times 1$	64	$1 \times 1 \times 1$	64	$1 \times 1 \times 1$	64	$1 \times 1 \times 3$	64
Max-pool 2	-	-	$2 \times 1 \times 1$	64	$1 \times 1 \times 2$	64	$2 \times 2 \times 2$	64
Conv 3	$1 \times 1 \times 1$	64	$1 \times 1 \times 1$	64	$1 \times 1 \times 1$	64	$1 \times 1 \times 1$	64
Max-pool 3	-	-	-	-	$2 \times 2 \times 1$	64	$2 \times 2 \times 1$	64
	Number of units		Number of units		Number of units		Number of units	
FC 1	80		100		100		80	
FC-info	3		3		3		3	
FC 2	2		2		2		2	

We considered the weights of 2 for the U-net to effectively make the number of U-nets equal to that of FCN models used, and 1.5 as the case of a compromise between the arithmetic average and the "doubling". The threshold for the final prediction was chosen to minimize ASSD and HD and to maximize DC.

As a result, we obtained two ensemble models: one with (1.5, 0.67) for the weight and the threshold, and the other with (2, 0.71).

Table 2. Hyperparameters for the full models.

	Number of units			
Patch size	$3 \times 3 \times 3$	$5 \times 5 \times 3$	$7 \times 7 \times 3$	$9 \times 9 \times 3$
Dense 1	16	32	32	32
Dense 2	16	32	32	32
Dense 3	2	2	2	2

Table 3. The width of patches, the number of patches per case, and the number of filters in the first convolutional layer used for the four instances of the main architecture used in final submission model.

	Width	# of patches	# of filters
Model 1	32	300	16
Model 2	32	300	12
Model 3	24	500	24
Model 4	24	300	24

2.4   Evaluation

The top panel of Fig. 3 shows that an artifact in a U-net output in one training case (GT 10) was removed. The bottom panel indicates that the noisy output from the FCN in another case (GT 16) was cleaned up after applying the ensemble method. This indicates the effectiveness of the ensemble approach.

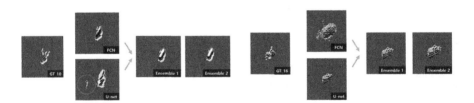

Fig. 3. (Left) A case that an artifact in a U-net output was removed. (Right) A case that the noisy output from the FCN was cleaned up after ensemble. Ensemble 1 is the model with coefficients (1.5, 0.67), and ensemble 2 with (2, 0.71).

The test outputs from both ensemble models and the U-net-alone model were submitted to the challenge, and all of them were ranked among the top entries (Table 4).

3   The Clinical Outcome Prediction

We interpreted the prediction of mRS as a multiclass classification problem, and used two models utilizing the MRI images and the clinical predictors. To

Table 4. Rank and evaluation results on the segmentation problem. The figures other than the place were calculated by using the test set.

	Rank score	ASSD	Dice	HD	place
U-net	3.42	6.23	0.31	32.84	1st
Ensemble 1	3.68	6.46	0.30	37.70	2nd
Ensemble 2	3.34	6.38	0.31	34.09	3rd

reflect the features from MRI images, we built a CNN model, which classifies the patient's mRS, by using the brain images and the clinical information such as TSS, TTT, and TICI. We also employed a logistic regression model to emphasize the effect of the clinical information. We obtained predicted mRSes from both the CNN and logistic regression models, and chose randomly between the two scores.

3.1 Convolutional Neural Network Model

A full CNN model for mRS prediction required the whole brain as input. This was intractable because of the lack of samples in the dataset. We thus used a CNN as a feature extractor, and a shallow neural network to predict the class based on the extracted features.

Main Architecture. The feature extraction part is a CNN with patch size of $(3 \times 3 \times 3)$ as illustrated in part A of Fig. 4. The CNN model consisted of 3D convolutional layers, 3D max pooling layers, and fully connected layers. The clinical predictors were employed right before the fully connected layers. The details of the CNN model are summarized in Table 5. The number of parameters in this CNN model was kept small compared to the FCN models for the lesion prediction, partly due to the size of the model for classification (Part B in Fig. 4). After training the CNN model, we converted all fully-connected layers in the model to convolutional layers with $(1 \times 1 \times 1)$-sized kernels. The resulting dimension of the output of the CNN part was $(128 \times 128 \times 15)$. The classification part is a shallow fully-connected network with a single hidden layer, which operates on the $(128 \times 128 \times 15)$ "feature volume." Since the number of weights of this part was much larger than the sample size, maxout regularization [6] with a large pooling size (16) was essential. As there were only 5 classes in the training dataset, the number of units in the last layer was set to 5.

Sample Imbalance. The convolutional layers in part A of Fig. 4 had a large number of parameters, comparing to the 30 cases in the training set. Thus we trained this part in a patch-wise fashion to overcome the lack of data. Because the goal of part A is to learn a feature map for the following classification, we trained the CNN to predict the lesion and transferred the learned feature to predict the clinical outcome. Thus there is the same sample imbalance problem as in Sects. 2.1 and 2.2. We applied three-phase training. The training details were the same as for the FCN model in the Sect. 2.2. For part B, because the large number of parameters caused memory problems and overfitting, we froze all the weights from the convolutional layers and trained part B only with the batch size of 1.

Implementation Details. The implementation environment and details are almost the same as Sect. 2.2. It required half an hour for the whole training and a few seconds for testing.

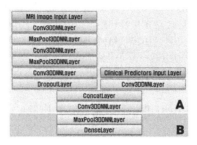

Fig. 4. CNN architecture for the clinical outcome prediction.

Table 5. Hyperparameters for the CNN models in the part A of Fig. 4.

	Filter	Features
Conv 1	$3 \times 3 \times 3$	16
Max-pool 1	$2 \times 2 \times 2$	16
Conv 2	$1 \times 1 \times 1$	8
	Number of units	
FC 1	30	
FC 2	2	

3.2 Logistic Regression Model

We sought to improve the prediction by using ensembles of the CNN's with a simple classification model taking only clinical informations into account. We fit logistic regression model with TICI, TSS, TTT, and the sum of TSS and TTT as predictors to classify mRS. All of the explanatory variables were standardized, except for TICI, which was a categorical variable. The model formula was as follows:

$$logit(p_{i,class}) = \beta_0 + \beta_1 TSS + \beta_2 TTT + \beta_3(TSS + TTT) + \beta_4 I(TICI = 0)$$
$$+ \beta_5 I(TICI = 1) + \beta_6 I(TICI = 2a) + \beta_7 I(TICI = 2b) + \beta_8 I(TICI = 3).$$

Multiclass classification algorithm was a one-vs-rest scheme. Thus we built in total five models to predict mRS.

3.3   Evaluation

The predicted results were evaluated by the average absolute errors between true and predicted mRS. In Table 6, we present the evaluation results from CNN, logistic regression and ensemble of both. The ensemble of two models showed a good performance in the Challenge, holding the second place.

Table 6. Rank and evaluation results on the classification problem. The figures other than the place were calculated by using the test set.

	Rank	Avg abs error	Place
Ensemble	1.6	1.10	2nd
Logistic regression	1.8	1.26	3rd
FCN	2.3	1.37	4th

4   Conclusion

We proposed an ensemble of deep-learning-based models for automatic prognosis of ischemic stroke after treatment. For the lesion outcome prediction, we applied an ensemble of residual U-net and FCN model. The residual U-net produced successful segmentation results based on the Dice coefficient, while it is subject to segmentation artifacts. The FCN was capable of incorporating clinical information as predictors, but the voxel-wise predictions tended to be noisy. Both models possessed complementary strengths and weaknesses. We demonstrated that ensembling them can increase both prediction accuracy and robustness. For the clinical outcome prediction, we combined the image-based features from a CNN with a logistic regression model that explicitly conveys the effect of clinical predictors. In this way, we were able to predict mRS scores in spite of limited sample size. Our ensemble approach showed an appealing performance on both problems, which is confirmed by that all of our models ranked among the top entries in the ISLES 2016 Challange. For a future direction, we may employ multiple GPUs to allow larger models and overcome the memory limit. In this direction, extensive data augmentation may turn out crucial for prediction accuracy.

Acknowledgments. This research was supported by the National Research Foundation of Korea (NRF) grant funded by the Korean government (MSIP, No. 2016012002). Joong-Ho Won's research was partially supported by the National Research Foundation of Korea (NRF) grant funded by the Korean government (MSIP, Nos. 2013R1A1A1057949 and 2014R1A4A1007895).

References

1. ISLES 2016 challenge. http://www.isles-challenge.org/
2. Chollet, F.: Keras (2015). https://github.com/fchollet/keras
3. Çiçek, Ö., Abdulkadir, A., Lienkamp, S.S., Brox, T., Ronneberger, O.: 3D u-net: learning dense volumetric segmentation from sparse annotation. CoRR abs/1606.06650 (2016). http://arxiv.org/abs/1606.06650
4. Clevert, D., Unterthiner, T., Hochreiter, S.: Fast and accurate deep network learning by exponential linear units (ELUs). CoRR abs/1511.07289 (2015). http://arxiv.org/abs/1511.07289
5. Dieleman, S., Schlter, J., Raffel, C., Olson, E., Snderby, S.K., Nouri, D., Maturana, D., Thoma, M., Battenberg, E., Kelly, J., Fauw, J.D., Heilman, M., de Almeida, D.M., McFee, B., Weideman, H., Takcs, G., de Rivaz, P., Crall, J., Sanders, G., Rasul, K., Liu, C., French, G., Degrave, J.: Lasagne: first release. http://dx.doi.org/10.5281/zenodo.27878
6. Goodfellow, I.J., Warde-Farley, D., Mirza, M., Courville, A.C., Bengio, Y.: Maxout networks. ICML **3**(28), 1319–1327 (2013)
7. Havaei, M., Davy, A., Warde-Farley, D., Biard, A., Courville, A., Bengio, Y., Pal, C., Jodoin, P.-M., Larochelle, H.: Brain tumor segmentation with deep neural networks. Med. Image Anal. **35**, 18–31 (2017). Elsevier
8. Havaei, M., Guizard, N., Larochelle, H., Jodoin, P.: Deep learning trends for focal brain pathology segmentation in MRI. CoRR abs/1607.05258 (2016). http://arxiv.org/abs/1607.05258
9. He, K., Zhang, X., Ren, S., Sun, J.: Deep residual learning for image recognition. In: Proceedings of the IEEE Conference on Computer Vision and Pattern Recognition, pp. 770–778 (2016)
10. He, K., Zhang, X., Ren, S., Sun, J.: Delving deep into rectifiers: surpassing human-level performance on imagenet classification. In: Proceedings of the IEEE International Conference on Computer Vision (2015)
11. He, K., Zhang, X., Ren, S., Sun, J.: Identity mappings in deep residual networks. In: Leibe, B., Matas, J., Sebe, N., Welling, M. (eds.) ECCV 2016. LNCS, vol. 9908, pp. 630–645. Springer, Cham (2016). doi:10.1007/978-3-319-46493-0_38
12. Ioffe, S., Szegedy, C.: Batch normalization: accelerating deep network training by reducing internal covariate shift. CoRR abs/1502.03167 (2015). http://arxiv.org/abs/1502.03167
13. Kamnitsas, K., Ledig, C., Newcombe, V.F.J., Simpson, J.P., Kane, A.D., Menon, D.K., Rueckert, D., Glocker, B.: Efficient multi-scale 3D CNN with fully connected CRF for accurate brain lesion segmentation. CoRR abs/1603.05959 (2016). http://arxiv.org/abs/1603.05959
14. Kingma, D.P., Ba, J.: Adam: a method for stochastic optimization. CoRR abs/1412.6980 (2014). http://arxiv.org/abs/1412.6980
15. Lai, M.: Deep learning for medical image segmentation. CoRR abs/1505.02000 (2015). http://arxiv.org/abs/1505.02000
16. Long, J., Shelhamer, E., Darrell, T.: Fully convolutional networks for semantic segmentation. In: Proceedings of the IEEE Conference on Computer Vision and Pattern Recognition, pp. 3431–3440 (2015)
17. Menze, B.H., Jakab, A., Bauer, S., Kalpathy-Cramer, J., Farahani, K., Kirby, J., Burren, Y., Porz, N., Slotboom, J., Wiest, R., et al.: The multimodal brain tumor image segmentation benchmark (brats). IEEE Trans. Med. Imaging **34**(10), 1993–2024 (2015)

18. Ronneberger, O., Fischer, P., Brox, T.: U-net: convolutional networks for biomedical image segmentation. CoRR abs/1505.04597 (2015). http://arxiv.org/abs/1505.04597

19. Saver, J.L., Goyal, M., van der Lugt, A., Menon, B.K., Majoie, C.B., Dippel, D.W., Campbell, B.C., Nogueira, R.G., Demchuk, A.M., Tomasello, A., et al.: Time to treatment with endovascular thrombectomy and outcomes from ischemic stroke: a meta-analysis. Jama **316**(12), 1279–1288 (2016)

20. Shah, A., Kadam, E., Shah, H., Shinde, S.: Deep residual networks with exponential linear unit. In: Proceedings of the Third International Symposium on Computer Vision and the Internet. ACM (2016)

21. Zeiler, M.D.: Adadelta: an adaptive learning rate method. arXiv preprint arXiv:1212.5701 (2012)

Prediction of Ischemic Stroke Lesion and Clinical Outcome in Multi-modal MRI Images Using Random Forests

Qaiser Mahmood$^{(\boxtimes)}$ and A. Basit

Pakistan Institute of Nuclear Science and Technology, Islamabad, Pakistan
qaiserpieas@hotmail.com, abdulbasit1975@gmail.com

Abstract. Herein, we present an automated segmentation method for ischemic stroke lesion segmentation in multi-modal MRI images. The method is based on an ensemble learning technique called random forest (RF), which generates several classifiers and combines their results in order to make decisions. In RF, we employ several meaningful features such as intensities, entropy, gradient etc. to classify the voxels in multi-modal MRI images. The segmentation method is validated on both training and testing data, obtained from MICCAI ISLES-2016 challenge dataset. The evaluation of the method is done by performing two tasks: ischemic stroke lesion outcome prediction (Task I) and clinical outcome prediction (Task II). For Task I, the performance of the method is evaluated relative to the manual segmentation, done by the clinical experts. For Task II, the performance of the method is evaluated relative to the 90 days mRS score, provided as ground truths by ISLES-2016 challenge organizers. The experimental results show the robustness of the segmentation method, and that it achieves reasonable accuracy for the prediction of both ischemic stroke lesion and clinical outcome in multi-modal MRI images.

Keywords: Segmentation · Automatic · MRI · Ischemic stroke lesion · Random forests · ISLES-2016

1 Introduction

Every year, more than 10 million people worldwide have a stroke and a third of these don't survive [1]. Stroke is the second leading cause of death and disability (for examples; paralysis, speech or vision loss) in industrial countries. It is a neurological disorder that is caused by either a clot blocking an artery or a burst blood vessel causing bleeding inside the cranium [2]. The former stroke type is called ischemic stroke and the later type is called hemorrhage stroke. Ischemic stroke is the most common type of stroke, accounting for about 80% of all strokes [3].

Computerized tomography (CT) is presently the gold standard for stroke diagnosis, with magnetic resonance imaging (MRI) often being used when CT does not provide a definitive answer [4]. MRI has a major advantage over CT

© Springer International Publishing AG 2016
A. Crimi et al. (Eds.): BrainLes 2016, LNCS 10154, pp. 244–255, 2016.
DOI: 10.1007/978-3-319-55524-9_23

in that it does not employ ionizing radiation. It generates a 3D image of the human head by exploiting the nuclear magnetic resonance properties of the water contained in the tissues. Because of its high spatial resolution and good contrast for soft tissues, MRI is perfectly suited for detecting the ischemic stroke lesion [5]. Due to this characteristic, it can be helpful for neurosurgeons and physicians in diagnosing the stroke as well as in monitoring the efficacy of clinical treatments for stroke.

Automated and accurate ischemic stroke segmentation in MRI images is a challenging task because of stroke lesion location, shape, size and appearance vary greatly across patients. As a result expert manual segmentation is still a gold standard for quantitative analysis of lesion in stroke patients. However, it is challenging, tedious, labor-intensive, time-consuming task as well as requires expert supervision and impractical for large-scale group study. Moreover, manual segmentation leads to $28\% \pm 12\%$ intra-and $20\% \pm 15\%$ inter-observer variabilities [6].

Development of an accurate and fully automated technique for ischemic stroke lesion segmentation is highly desirable because the lesion volume is an essential end-point for medical trials. In past years, several automated segmentation methods [7–11] have been proposed in literature for different type of stroke lesion segmentation. A review on non-chronic ischemic stroke lesion segmentation techniques has been presented in [8]. A method for chronic stroke lesions segmentation has been proposed in [10], which is based on an outlier search method and the fuzzy clustering. The method is employed on single modal (T1-weighted) MRI datasets for segmenting the chronic lesions. A Bayesian multi-spectral hidden Markov model has been presented in [11] for chronic stroke lesions segmentation. In [7], an extra tree forest has been proposed for chronic stroke lesions segmentation.

However, the performance of above mentioned methods are difficult to directly compare with each other. The reason is that these methods are evaluated on different MRI datasets with using different quantitative measures for stroke detection by their respective authors [12].

In order to make a fair and direct comparison of automated methods for acute ischemic stroke detection, Ischemic Stroke Lesion Segmentation (ISLES) challenge was organized at Medical Image Computing and Computer Assisted Intervention (MICCAI) conference 2016. The ISLES-2016 challenge consists of following two tasks.

Task I: Lesion outcome prediction

Task II: Clinical outcome prediction

We participated in ISLES-2016 challenge and presented an automated method for acute ischemic stroke lesion segmentation using multi-modal MRI images. The method is based on a machine learning technique called random forests (RF). The key contribution in the method is employing a set of meaningful features for segmenting the stroke lesion and the choice of step for post-processing of segmented lesion data.

2 Method

Our segmentation method takes the multi-modal MRI brain images as input. The schematic procedure of method is shown in Fig. 1. The following set of meaningful features (n = 67) is extracted for each voxel in multi-modal MRI images.

1. MRI scans intensities: These features comprise the intensity in the MRI scans (ADC, Perfusion (4D scan), MTT, Tmax, rBF, rBV and TTP) provided by the data sets. The total number of these features was 7.
2. MRI scans smooth intensities: A Gaussian filter with size $5 \times 5 \times 5$ was employed to each MRI scan in order to extract the smooth intensities. The total number of these features was 7.
3. MRI scans median intensities: A median filter with size $5 \times 5 \times 5$ was applied to each MRI scan to obtain the median intensities. The total number of these features was 7.
4. The gradient and magnitude of the gradient: A gradient in the x, y and z direction and their magnitude was computed in order to get the information about the lines and edges in each MRI scan. The total number of these features was 28.
5. Hessian features: These features are extracted by computing the second order derivatives of MRI scan intensity. These features describe information about the local structure. The total number of these features was 4. For these features, we chose only ADC MRI scan because it has good details about the brain structures compared to other MRI scans.
6. Local standard deviation: The standard deviation for each voxel in the MRI scans was computed using the neighborhoods size $5 \times 5 \times 5$. The total number of these features was 7.
7. Local entropy: The entropy for each voxel in the MRI scans was computed using the neighborhoods size $9 \times 9 \times 9$. The total number of these features was 7.

These features are then applied to train the RF [13,14] classifier and classifying the acute ischemic stroke lesion.

The labeled data sets, obtained from the ground truths, are used to train the RF classifier. In RF, multiple decision trees are constructed. This construction is based on a random choice of a subset of features. In each tree, every node is a decision node that comprises a feature and its corresponding threshold except the leaves. Every leaf node has a probabilistic class distribution (histogram of class labels for the voxels that have reached that node).

In RF, the classification (testing) is performed by traversing voxels over the trees, initiating from the root of each tree to a leaf node. The voxels are split at a given node based on the learned feature and a threshold value at that node. In the end, the mean probabilistic decision of the class distribution from all trees yields the final probabilistic class distribution (voxel label in this scenario).

"Number of trees" and "depth of each tree" are two critical parameters of RF. In this work, we set "number of trees" = 90 and "depth of each tree" = 50. The Gini impurity was applied as a splitting criterion and $\sqrt{67}$ features were used at each node for splitting.

For training, a total of 80,000 data samples (10,000 samples per training data) were used to train the RF classifier. These samples were acquired randomly by down sampling the majority class (non ischemic stroke) data in each training data set in order to make their frequencies closer to the minority class (acute ischemic stroke) data.

Lastly, the post-processing is done using the closing (dilation followed by an erosion) operation by employing the 2D $5 \times 5 \times 5$ square structuring elements in order to remove the isolated outlier voxels that treated as stroke lesion.

3   Acute MRI Data

For evaluation of our method, 30 training and 19 testing MRI data are used, provided from the ISLES-2016 challenge organizers. Both training and testing MRI data comprises 7 acute MRI scans: ADC, MTT, perfusion raw 4D data, rBF, rBV, Tmax and TTP.

ADC map is generated from the DWI images whereas rBF, rBV, Tmax and TTP maps are computed from the perfusion data.

For training data, the ground truths (labeled data) are also provided from the ISLES-2016 challenge organizers.

4   Evaluation Measures

The evaluation of the method is done using the online evaluation system, provided by the MICCAI ISLES-2016 challenge organizers. The evaluation is done by performing two tasks: ischemic stroke lesion outcome prediction (Task I) and clinical outcome prediction (Task II). For Task I, the evaluation is done in terms of average symmetric surface distance (ASSD), Dice and the Hausdorff distance. The ASSD denotes the average surface distance the ground truth and automated segmentation. Dice measures the degree of overlap between the ground truth and automated segmentation. Hausdorff distance denotes the maximum distance between the ground truth and automated segmentation surface points.

For Task II, the evaluation is performed in terms of (modified ranking scale) mRS score. For prediction of mRS score, the regression forest is applied. The regression forest is trained by employing the local image features and the stroke lesion characteristics, obtained from the Task I. For regression forest training, the mean squared error function was applied as splitting criterion.

5   Results and Discussion

The training data include 30 acute ischemic stroke lesion cases whilst the testing data comprise 19 acute ischemic stroke lesion cases. The evaluation of the method is first done on training data and then is performed on the testing data.

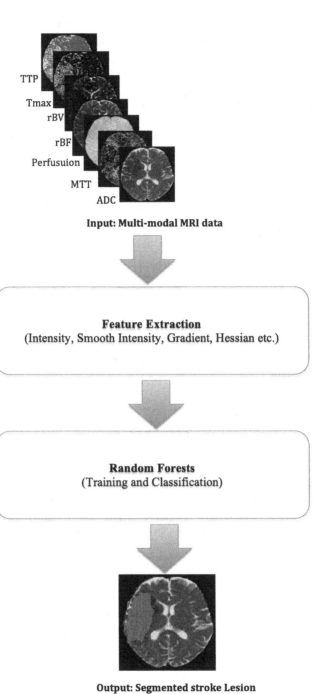

Fig. 1. Schematic procedure of the segmentation method.

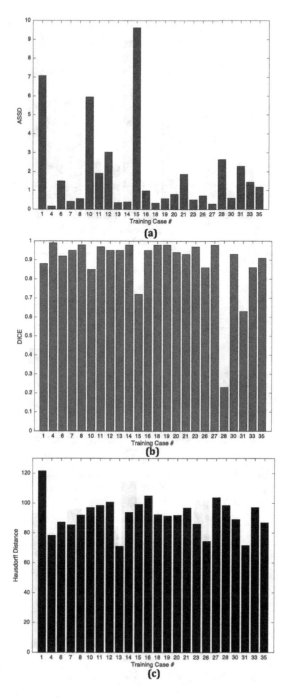

Fig. 2. Quantitative results of our method for Task I for 24 training cases: (a) ASSD (b) Dice and (c) Hausdorff distance.

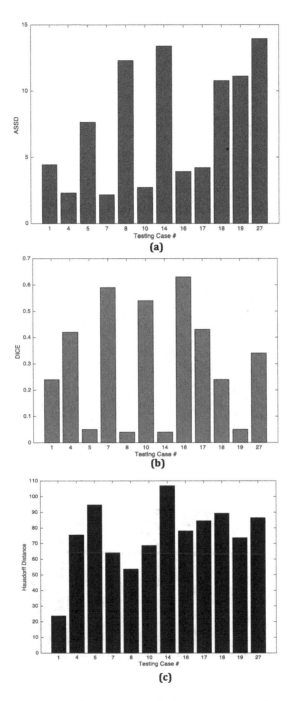

Fig. 3. Quantitative results of our method for Task I for ground truths GT1 from12 test cases: (a) ASSD (b) Dice and (c) Hausdorff distance.

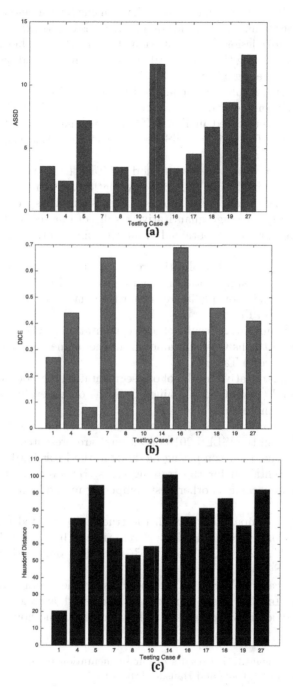

Fig. 4. Quantitative results of our method for Task I for ground truths GT2 from12
test cases: (a) ASSD (b) Dice and (c) Hausdorff distance.

For training data, the evaluation is achieved using leave-one-out cross validation. The classifier, trained from the training data, is applied to the testing data to segment the stroke lesion. The evaluation of our method for both training and testing data is done using the online evaluation system provided by the MICCAI ISLES-2016 challenge organizers.

The quantitative results of our method for Task I for the 24 training cases (obtained from the online evaluation system in terms of ASSD, Dice, and Hausdorff distance) are presented in Fig. 2. They show that our method has poor segmentation (lower Dice, higher ASSD and Hausdorff distance) for the training case "28".

The quantitative results of our method for Task I for the 12 test cases for GT1 and GT2 (obtained from the online evaluation system in terms of ASSD, Dice, and Hausdorff distance) are shown in Figs. 3 and 4 respectively.

Table 1 shows the average quantitative results of our segmentation method over the 24 training cases, obtained from the online evaluation system for Task I.

An example of the good qualitative result of our segmentation method for axial slice "8" of the training case "11" is presented in Fig. 5.

An example of the poor qualitative result for axial slice "19" of the training case "28" is shown in Fig. 6.

The average quantitative results of our segmentation method over the 12 test cases using ground truths GT1 (obtained from the online evaluation system for Task I) are presented in Table 2.

The average quantitative results of our segmentation method over the 12 test cases using ground truths GT2 (obtained from the online evaluation system for Task I) are shown in Table 3.

The average quantitative results of our segmentation method over the all test cases (obtained from the ISLES-2016 organizers) are presented in Table 4.

Compared to the other competing methods in the ISLES-2016 challenge, we have better segmentation for the training cases. However, for the test cases, our method is comparable to other best competing methods in the ISLES-2016 challenge.

For Task II, a comparison between the true and predicted mRS scores for training cases is presented in Table 5. Herein, it can be observed that for the training cases "1", "2", "10", "19", "15" and "28", our method has a false prediction of mRS scores.

For the test cases, Task II is evaluated using the average absolute error of mRS scores. In this study, our method achieved average absolute error $= 1.26 \pm 0.87$, which is comparable to other competing methods in the ISLES-2016 challenge.

Table 1. Average quantitative results of our segmentation method over 24 training cases in terms of ASSD, Dice, and Hausdorff distance.

ASSD (mm)	Dice	Hausdorff distance (mm)
1.88 ± 2.34	0.89 ± 0.26	80.16 ± 11.09

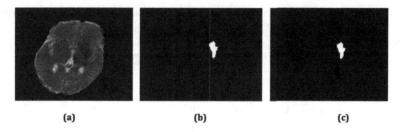

Fig. 5. Qualitative result of our segmentation method for axial slice "8" of the training case "11": (a) ASD (b) ground truth (c) segmented stroke lesion.

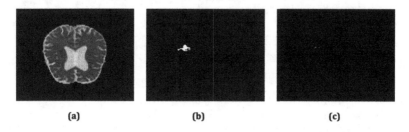

Fig. 6. Qualitative result of our segmentation method for axial slice "19" of the training case "28": (a) ASD (b) ground truth (c) segmented stroke lesion.

Table 2. Average quantitative results of our segmentation method for GT1 over 12 test cases in terms of ASSD, Dice and Hausdorff distance.

ASSD (mm)	Dice	Hausdorff distance (mm)
7.41 ± 4.42	0.30 ± 0.21	74.90 ± 20.60

Table 3. Average quantitative results of our segmentation method for GT2 over 12 test cases in terms of ASSD, Dice and Hausdorff distance.

ASSD (mm)	Dice	Hausdorff distance (mm)
5.68 ± 3.49	0.36 ± 0.20	72.88 ± 21.17

Table 4. Average quantitative results of our segmentation method over all the test cases in terms of ASSD, Dice and Hausdorff distance.

ASSD (mm)	Dice	Hausdorff distance (mm)
9.12 ± 5.46	0.26 ± 0.22	78.04 ± 18.11

Table 5. Task II: Comparison between the true and predicted mRS scores for training cases.

Case	True mRS score	Predicted mRS score
1	1	2
2	1	2
4	4	4
5	2	2
6	1	1
7	2	2
8	1	1
9	1	1
10	1	2
11	1	1
12	1	1
13	2	2
14	2	2
15	0	1
16	1	1
18	4	4
19	0	0
20	1	2
21	1	1
22	3	3
23	1	1
24	2	2
26	2	2
27	3	3
28	1	2
30	3	3
31	3	3
33	3	3
35	2	2

6   Conclusions

Herein, we present an automated method, based on the RF for performing two tasks: ischemic stroke lesion outcome prediction (Task I) and clinical outcome prediction (Task II). We employ a set of meaningful features to train the RF and classify the ischemic stroke lesion. The experimental results show the efficacy of the segmentation method and that it can achieve reasonable accuracy for both stroke lesion outcome prediction and clinical outcome prediction compared to other competing methods in the ISLES-2016 challenge. In the future, we will investigate a more robust set of features in order to improve the accuracy of our segmentation method. The total execution time of our segmentation method is approximately 15 min for segmenting the stroke lesion for each data set using the MATLAB R2015b on a MacBook Pro with an Intel processor (i5, 2.5 GHz) and 4 GB RAM.

References

1. The Atlas of Heart Disease and Stroke. http://www.who.int/cardiovascular_diseases/resources/atlas/en/
2. Fassbender, K., Balucani, C., Walter, S., Levine, S.R., Haass, A., Grotta, J.: Streamlining of prehospital stroke management: the golden hour. Lancet Neurol. **12**, 585–596 (2013)
3. Feigin, V.L., Lawes, C.M., Bennett, D.A., Barker-Collo, S.L., Parag, V.: Worldwide Stroke incidence and early case fatality reported in 56 population-based studies: a systematic review. Lancet Neurol. **8**, 355–369 (2009)
4. Qaiser, M., Shaochuan, L., Andreas, F., Stefan, C., Artur, C., Andrew, M., Mikael, P.: A comparative study of automated segmentation methods for use in a microwave tomography system for imaging intracerebral hemorrhage in stroke patients. J. Electromagn. Anal. Appl. (JEMAA) **7**, 152–167 (2015)
5. Ball, J.B., Pensak, M.L.: Fundamentals of magnetic resonance imaging. Am. J. Otol. **8**, 81–85 (1987)
6. Moumen, T., E., Hashim, M., M.: Tumor segmentation in brain MRI using a fuzzy approach with class center priors. EURASIP J. Image Video Process., online (2014)
7. Oskar, M., Matthias, W., von der Janina, G., Ulrike, M.K., Thomas, F.M., Heinz, H.: Extra Tree forests for sub-acute ischemic stroke lesion segmentation in MR sequences. J. Neurosci. Methods **240**, 89–100 (2014)
8. Rekik, I., Allassonniere, S., Carpenter, T.K., Wardlaw, J.M.: Medical image analysis methods In MR/CT-imaged acute-subacute ischemic stroke lesion: segmentation, prediction and insights into dynamic evolution simulation models. Critical Appraisal. NeuroImage Clinical **1**, 164–178 (2012)
9. Mitra, J., Bourgeat, P., Fripp, J., Ghose, S., et al.: Lesion segmentation from multimodal MRI using random forests following ischemic stroke. NeuroImage **98**, 324–335 (2014)
10. Seghier, M.L., Ramlackhansingh, A., Crinion, J., Leff, A.P., Price, C.J.: Lesion identification using unified segmentation-normalisation models and fuzzy clustering. NeuroImage **41**, 1253–1266 (2008)
11. Forbes, F., Doyle, S., Garcia-Lorenzo, D., Barillot, C., Dojat, M.: Adaptive weighted fusion of multiple MR sequences for brain lesion segmentation. In: IEEE International Symposium on Biomedical Imaging: From Nano to Macro (ISBI), pp. 69–72 (2010)
12. Oskar, M., Björn, M., Matthias, L., Stefan, W., et al.: ISLES 2015 - a public evaluation benchmark for ischemic stroke lesion segmentation from multispectral MRI. Med. Image Anal. **35**, 250–269 (2017)
13. Breiman, L.: Random forests. Mach. Learn. **45**, 5–32 (2001)
14. Criminisi, A., Shotton, J.: Decision forests for Computer Vision and Medical Image Analysis. Advances in Computer Vision and Pattern Recognition. Springer, London (2013)

Mild Traumatic Brain Injury Outcome Prediction

Combining Deep Learning Networks with Permutation Tests to Predict Traumatic Brain Injury Outcome

Y. Cai[1(✉)] and S. Ji[1,2]

[1] Department of Biomedical Engineering,
Worcester Polytechnic Institute, Worcester, MA 01605, USA
{ycai2,sji}@wpi.edu
[2] Thayer School of Engineering, Dartmouth College, Hanover, NH 03755, USA

Abstract. Reliable prediction of traumatic brain injury (TBI) outcome using neuroimaging is clinically important, yet, computationally challenging. To tackle this problem, we developed an injury prediction or classification pipeline based on diffusion tensor imaging (DTI) by combining a novel deep learning approach with statistical permutation tests. We first applied a multi-modal deep learning network to individually train a classification model for each DTI measure. Individual results were then combined to allow iterative refinement of the classification via Tract-Based Spatial Statistics (TBSS) permutation tests, where voxel sum of skeletonized significance values served as a classification performance feedback. Our technique combined a high-performance machine learning algorithm with a conventional statistical tool, which provided a flexible and intuitive approach to predict TBI outcome.

Keywords: Brain image analysis · Brain injury · Deep learning · Permutation test

1 Introduction

An accurate and robust diagnosis of traumatic brain injury (TBI), including mild TBI (mTBI), is important to mitigate this prevailing neurological disease. Unfortunately, objective assessment of the likelihood and severity of mTBI remains lacking, as they are often undetectable using conventional anatomical images such as T1-weighted MRI. Automatic prediction using state-of-the-art pattern recognition and machine learning techniques is a popular research topic at present [1, 2]. However, relying solely on existing machine learning methods appears insufficient to provide a direct assessment of mTBI outcome, due to non-Gaussian spatial-intensity distribution and uncertain cross-subject variation in neuroimages [3, 4]. The performance of the learning algorithms is also typically limited due to the often small training datasets available in mTBI research. On the other hand, conventional statistical tools such as permutation test have been shown to be capable of analyzing neuroimaging changes in cognitive studies, e.g., for identifying minor differences between two or among multiple data groups [5, 6]. The permutation test can also be used to analyze an existing classification (control vs.

© Springer International Publishing AG 2016
A. Crimi et al. (Eds.): BrainLes 2016, LNCS 10154, pp. 259–270, 2016.
DOI: 10.1007/978-3-319-55524-9_24

patient), which is suitable for small datasets. However, the method does not directly provide data classification, by itself.

In this study, we developed an iterative learning approach to predict mTBI outcome. This approach treated mTBI prediction as classification of the neuroimaging data into healthy or concussed groups, and for the latter, further into levels of injury severity. Instead of training a classifier directly from data to label through a learning algorithm, we first trained a sub-optimal classifier using a subset of labeled data. The classifier was further adjusted via group-wise permutation statistics. The adjustment could be performed either by tuning the classifier parameters or by feeding the sub-optimal classifier with newly articulated labeled data. The latter strategy ensured the classification to follow the statistics of the data distribution and also provided a prediction of unlabeled data. The strengthened sub-optimal classifier then proceeded to another round of classification to further generate labeled data for group-wise statistical evaluation. This iterative learning approach was capable of generating sufficient training samples from a relatively small dataset to train the machine learning system. It also helped prediction of weakly or incorrectly labeled data, which was possible in mTBI data collection.

In particular, we chose a multi-modal deep learning network as the basis for our machine learning system and iteratively used results from Tract-Based Spatial Statistic (TBSS) analysis as a refinement feedback to enhance network training. This combination of deep learning training and TBSS-based feedback enabled an objective mTBI outcome prediction using brain diffusion tensor image (DTI) data alone.

2   Related Previous Work

Developing a reliable mTBI imaging biomarker is desirable for predicting brain injury. Diffusion Tensor Imaging (DTI) is a promising MR imaging modality that provides a platform for image-based mTBI outcome prediction.

Image Modality for mTBI detection. Numerous DTI studies have shown significant changes in FA and MD (fractional anisotropy and mean diffusivity, respectively) measures for mTBI patients [7]. This suggests that FA and MD are effective DTI measures for predicting mTBI outcomes. Further, studies have shown that mTBI patients often present changes in FA in various locations in the white matter as well as discontinuity in fibers, either in acute [8] or chronic [9] stages. For patients with moderate/severe TBI, often decrease in FA and increase in AD and RD (axial diffusivity and radial diffusivity, respectively) are found. Generally, it is believed that increased FA may represent axonal swelling or cytotoxic edema, while decreased FA may indicate axonal degradation and discontinuity [10]. Unfortunately, changes in FA/MD have often been identified on a group-wise basis (e.g., control vs. patient), and contradicting findings regarding their increase or decrease [11] precluded a consensus.

Analysis Methods. Often, a region-of-interest (ROI) or voxel-wise analysis is employed to analyze DTI parameter changes in specific white matter structures [12]. In a ROI-based approach, inter- or intra-class correlation [12] or ANOVA statistical analysis [9] is performed to compare the characteristics across different ROIs and/or from different

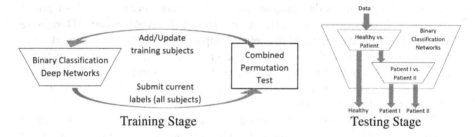

Fig. 1. Overview of the training (left) and cross-validation or testing (right) pipeline.

subject groups. The ROI-based method becomes a voxel-wise approach when DTI volumes under scrutiny are properly registered. Using white matter skeleton [4] alleviates the requirement of accurate image registration, and is, therefore, effective for cross-subject comparison. Regardless, both the ROI and voxel-wise approaches are for group-wise comparisons but do not directly assess the likelihood of individual mTBI.

Fiber tractography that represents white matter fiber bundles and bundle densities [13] is another potential metric for mTBI prediction. By connecting distant brain ROIs with fiber tracts along diffusion directions, tractography can be used to quantify changes in connectivity across regions in a given subject, or connectivity patterns across different subjects. However, the accuracy of fiber tractography relies on the particular tracking algorithm which depends on image quality such as resolution, noise, distortion and partial volume effects [14]. This poses challenges in mTBI prediction.

Given the current state-of-the-art in DTI analysis, a conclusive mTBI prediction technique remains lacking. In this study, we resort to a novel deep learning approach to predict mTBI based on DTI.

3 Methodology

3.1 Overview

The MICCAI Challenge of Mild Traumatic Brain Injury Outcome Prediction (mTOP Challenge, 2016) provided a DTI dataset from 27 subjects (9 subjects in each of the three distinct categories: healthy, patient I, and patient II). Each DTI dataset was composed of four DTI measures: FA, MD, MO, and AD. A subset of the ground-truth subject labels (i.e., healthy, patient I or II) were leaked (5 per group leaked at three time points, resulting in a total of 15 known subject categories). They were split into "training" and "cross-validation" datasets to train and validate the classifier, as well as to assess the prediction accuracy. The remaining 12 subjects (4 per group) were "unknown".

The mTBI outcome classification pipeline contained two components: classification deep networks and modality-combined permutation tests (Fig. 1). The two components interacted with each other during the training stage as further described below.

Training stage:

1. Training of the multi-modal classification deep networks. For a set of given training dataset, we first extracted the skeletonized representations of the four DTI measures via FSL [15], and used them as the network input. Two multi-modal networks were trained to differentiate the healthy vs. patient groups (i.e., H vs. P), and further between the two patient groups (i.e., P I vs. P II), themselves. The classical layer-wise training procedure in deep network [16] was used. Initial subject labels were obtained upon training convergence.

2. Label update using modality-combined permutation tests. By feeding the trained networks with data from all subjects, the subjects were classified into two groups (H vs. P or P I vs. P II) in each binary classification. TBSS [4] was then conducted for each individual DTI measure between the two groups. The TBSS results were voxelized skeletons whose values represented t-statistic test, $(1\text{-}p)$, denoting the significance of the spatial differences between the two groups. The TBSS skeletons obtained from the four DTI measures were then combined into one by voxel-wise joint multiplication. Large significance values or group differences were expected if the two subject groups were correctly classified. Conversely, low significance values indicated an incorrect classification that required revision. The TBSS analysis enabled an iterative, quantitative feedback of the deep network performance so that to allow further refinement in classification.

Testing stage:

3. mTBI outcome prediction via cascade binary classifications. A two-step classification was conducted. The first, H vs. P classification, also served as a diagnostic prediction in practice. For subjects labeled as P (i.e., patients), a second classification, P I vs. P II, was conducted to further differentiate injury severity.

We chose a two-step classification (i.e., separate binary classifications of H vs. P and P I vs. P II) instead of treating it directly as a three-class (H, P I, P II) prediction problem. This was because the invariance in FA/MD values in the H class [17] made it easier to distinguish with respect to the other two groups that had variant FA/MD values. The subsequent P I vs. P II classification could be improved by removing the interference from data in the H class. In addition, binary classification labels (0-1) were easier to switch in a feedback update than a three-class label (i.e., 0-1-2).

3.2 Multi-modal Deep Learning Network

The multi-modal deep learning network structures and associated parameters are shown in Fig. 2. The network consisted of two components: a dimension reduction layer for each DTI measure, and a fusion layer to combine results from all measures. The initial network input was a vectorized and skeletonized image after cross-subject joint registration.

Preprocessing. The preprocessing included cross-subject joint registration and skeletonization of the input images. First, FA images from all subjects were aligned with the FMRIB58_FA of the MNI152 template via affine and then nonlinear registrations (FLIRT and FNIRT, respectively [18]). The registered FA images were jointly averaged

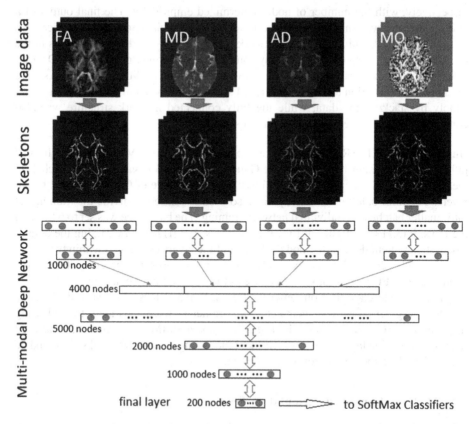

Fig. 2. Overview of the multi-modal deep network structure. Each DTI measure was first individually trained to reduce the dimension. Outcomes from all DTI measures were then linearly stacked to provide input to the lower layers for further layer-wise processing. The final output was a 200-node vector used for classification via SoftMax classifiers.

to construct a spatial skeleton, where local maximum FA values on the surface perpendicular to the tract direction were retained [4]. The resulting skeleton then served as a binary image mask applied to all jointly registered images regardless of the DTI measure. For each image measure, projecting the voxel values onto the skeleton led to a skeletonized representation with much reduced data dimension for subsequent network training and testing. No further registration was necessary as the same skeleton was shared across all subjects and DTI measures.

Network Structure. For the dimension reduction layers, we constructed two fully connected Restricted Boltzman Machine (RBM) layers with 129000 (i.e., the number of skeleton voxels) and 1000 (chosen empirically) nodes, respectively. Combining results from the four input DTI measures led to a vector of 4000 nodes. Four fully connected RBM fusion layers were constructed with 5000, 2000, 1000, and 200 nodes, respectively, with the number of nodes determined empirically. The final output of a 200-node vector was subsequently used for classification via a SoftMax classifier [19].

A RBM-based, fully connected network was used because different regions in the neuroimages (i.e., corpus callosum) may contribute to different ranges of FA/MD variation. In contrast, convolution networks such as CNN and CRBM-based networks were insensitive to the region locations. The RBM structure allowed multi-modal data fusion simply by stacking the data, while the fully connected network structure was also compatible with the skeletonized data representation.

Implementation. The RBM layers were implemented using the Medal package (https://github.com/dustinstansbury/medal). A Gaussian input layer was used for each DTI measure, while all other layers were binary. A learning rate of 0.001 was used for all layers. The mini-batch method [20] was also used to randomly divide the training set into smaller batches for individual network training. The batch size was set to 6 for both the H vs. P (3 H vs. 3 P) and P I vs. P II (3 P I vs. 3 P II) networks. Using the default stochastic gradient descent method [21], most of the layers converged within two hours on a Xeon E5-2630 v3 (8 cores, 16 GB memory) computer. The computation was conducted in CPU instead of GPU because of the large memory consumption required. The two cascade classification networks (H vs. P and P I vs. P II) shared the same structure (Fig. 2). However, their network parameters were separately trained using different data (H and P, P I and P II). The conventional SoftMax classifier [19] was used in the classification layer, which was further tuned using an iterative label switch/update mechanism described in the following section.

3.3   Modality-Combined Permutation Tests

TBSS analysis [4] was applied to enhance and fine-tune the binary classifications. First, an initial group-wise significance map was generated using classified subjects based on a subset of training dataset. Remaining subject labels in the training dataset were then iteratively switched to retrain the deep learning network. Decrease or increase in the voxel sum from the updated TBSS significance map would indicate the correctness in subject classification.

TBSS Processing. The classified subjects were grouped accordingly (e.g., H vs. P) to conduct TBSS analysis independently for each DTI measure. First, voxel-wise permutation tests were performed for each pair of skeletonized image groups. The result was a skeletonized significance map whose voxel values were $(1-p)$, where p was the significance value from the permutation tests. The significance map represented the spatial differences between the image group pair. Combining the significance maps from all of the DTI measures (FA, MD, AD, MO) via voxel-wise multiplication led to a unified map (Fig. 3), which was expected to be a stronger indicator for group-wise differences than each individual map alone.

Classification Label Update. The voxel sum of the modality-combined significance map was used as a feedback to fine-tune the deep network classifiers. First, using the

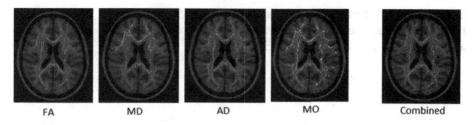

FA   MD   AD   MO   Combined

Fig. 3. Skeleton maps of the significance values of the four DTI modalities and their combined map overlaid on the MNI152 standard atlas.

given leaked subject labels as the training set, all subjects were classified (i.e., H or P) upon the classification network convergence. The TBSS analysis for the classified H vs. P group led to a modality-combined significance map, whose voxel sum indicated their group-wise differences. Then, we individually switched the label of each testing subject (i.e., not used for training) to extract the combined significance map via the TBSS analysis. Each time a subject label was switched (i.e., from H to P and vice versa), the resulting voxel sum of the combined significance map was revised accordingly. An increased voxel sum indicated that the label switching enhanced the group-wise differences. Therefore, the corresponding label-switched subject was added to the training set to re-train the deep network. Otherwise, the label switching reduced the group-wise differences if the voxel sum decreased. The corresponding subject was then switched back. A feedback update was accomplished when all testing subjects were switched and tested. To satisfy the constraints of the given numbers of subjects in each category, the first n switched labels resulting in the largest increase in voxel sum were retained, where n was determined to remain the given total numbers of the H/P groups. To mitigate overfitting concerns, at most 2 updates ($n = 2$) were empirically found to be sufficient for the feedback update.

4   Performance Analysis

Training and Cross-Validation Datasets. Five sets of ground-truth labeled subjects (total of 15 from the 3 groups) were provided to cross-validate the proposed technique. A Monte-Carlo Cross-Validation with 20 repeated random samplings was performed by setting the size of H vs. P training set to be either 3 (1 per mTBI category), 6 (2 per category), or 9 (3 per category), respectively. Conversely, the P I vs. P II training set had a size of 2, 4, or 6, respectively. The remaining subjects with known labels served as cross-validation datasets.

Random Cross-Validation. During cross validation, we randomly selected training samples from the leaked 15 labeled subjects, following the training-updating procedure to construct the classifiers. The cross-validation errors for H vs. P and P I vs. P II classifiers are shown in Figs. 4 and 5. The loss functions of the corresponding deep networks are also shown to progressively minimize the classification errors during the layer-wise deep learning process. The lowest cross-validation errors were obtained when using 9 subjects for training: 0.167 for the H vs. P and 0.222 for the P I vs. P II classification. However, over-fitting also occurred, as the error in the latter increased to 0.416 after 200 layer-wise iterations (arrow in Fig. 5).

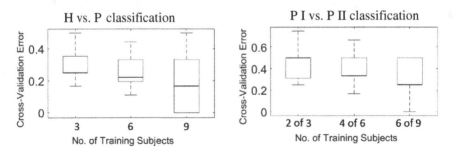

Fig. 4. Cross-validation errors of the deep networks for H vs. P (**left**) and P I vs. P II (**right**).

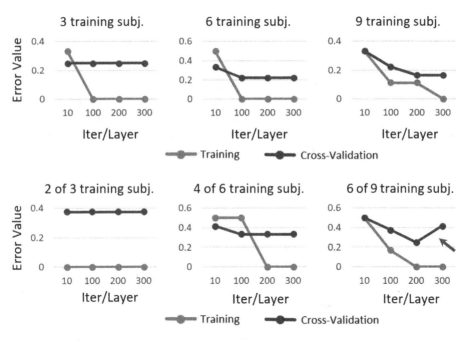

Fig. 5. Model losses (mis-classification error values) of the deep networks for the H vs. P (**top**) and P I vs. P II (**bottom**) classification using the leaked 15 labeled subjects. Using 9 subjects for training led to the lowest cross-validation error but with a higher risk of over-fitting (see arrow).

Over-Fitting Mitigation. When more than one third of the subjects (i.e., 9 of the 27 total) were used for training, risk of over-fitting increased (arrow in Fig. 4). To minimize this problem, we used the mini-batch method [20] to train the network. We randomly selected smaller subsets from the pool of labeled subjects to train the networks while further limiting the number of training iterations. For example, 6 samples (2 subjects per category; as determined to have the best robustness via cross-validation, see Sect. 3) were randomly selected to train the networks. The number of deep learning training iterations were empirically limited to 50 for all layers. Subsequently, another batch of 6 random samples were selected to re-train the networks. The process continued until the deep networks converged. This scheme was applied to both the H vs. P and P I vs. P II binary classifiers. Conceptually, the random selection was analogous to a classical cross-validation method for performance analysis. Label updates via permutation tests were also applied to refine the classification (see Sect. 3.3). The final classification for all of the 27 subjects is reported in Table 1 (Appendix).

5   Discussions

DTI Measures vs. T1-weighted MRI. It is well-known that subtle changes in the brain as a result of mTBI especially diffuse axonal injury cannot be detected using conventional anatomical images alone such as T1-weighted MRI. Therefore, unlike other studies [22, 23], we resorted to the four DTI measures exclusively without employing the T1-weighted MRI. Nevertheless, the additional anatomical images may serve as an auxiliary for brain region segmentation and image volume registration.

White Matter Skeleton vs. Whole Brain. Detecting axonal abnormalities using whole-brain tractography to assess its connectivity was straightforward. However, fiber tracing could be noisy and not reliable [4]. Therefore, here we focused on the white matter skeleton for injury analysis. This was obtained from the mean FA map from the co-registered image dataset [4]. The skeleton preserved the most common voxels in the image dataset where major fiber tracts traversed. Unlike other studies that employed whole brain FA/MD and T1 image volumes [22, 23], the feature space in our study was significantly smaller and much more concentrated. Nevertheless, we achieved similar classification performance. This was not surprising given that most of the injury cases in the mTOP Challenge dataset provided were diffuse axonal injuries, presumably only occurring in the white matter.

Further Mitigate Over-Fitting via Early Stopping. Over-fitting may be further mitigated by monitoring the increase/decrease of the optimization loss function and labeling error rate on the cross-validation dataset in order to identify the best training results. The validation subset can be repeatedly re-subsampled from the training dataset. The final subject labeling can then be obtained by averaging their separate classifications over the unknown testing dataset. We arranged the 15 subjects with known leaked labels into groups of "6 training + 3 validation + 6 testing", similarly to the previous mini-batch approach. The 3 validation samples were used to monitor the training of the 6 training samples, while the 6 testing cases were used to assess the classification accuracy. By repeating 9 training trials, we achieved average error rates of 0.19 (H vs. P) and 0.222 (P I vs. P II). They were similar to the previous direct training approach (i.e., "9 training + 0 validation + 6 testing", with mean error rates of 0.167 and 0.222, respectively), but with a reduced standard deviation (0.131 vs. 0.182).

Summary: To summarize, we developed an mTBI outcome prediction pipeline by combining multi-modal deep learning networks with permutation tests serving as a classification feedback. The deep learning networks provided an initial classification of the input dataset, which was further strengthened and refined using a label update scheme via TBSS-based permutation tests. A number of techniques were devised to address the challenges resulting from the limited number of subjects but relatively diverse categories (three distinct subject groups). The proposed technique may be used to provide an objective diagnosis of mTBI, and further prognosis and evaluation of the severity of mTBI, based on DTI neuro-images alone.

Acknowledgement. Funding is provided by the NIH grants R01 NS092853 and R21 NS088781.

Appendix

Table 1. Summary of subject classifications along with the corresponding confidence (obtained by the Softmax function of the classifier) levels. Shaded entries represent leaked labels.

Subject	Final Label	Confidence (H vs. P)	Confidence (P I vs. P II)
1	P I	0.7862	0.7040
2	H	0.6476	N/A
3	P I	0.6779	0.9670
4	P II	0.9163	0.6100
5	H	0.6787	N/A
6	P II	0.7862	0.9293
7	P II	0.7862	0.9741
8	P II	0.9364	0.9491
9	P I	0.9177	0.9483
10	P I	0.7159	0.9671
11	H	0.5387	N/A
12	P I	0.7862	0.9706
13	P II	0.9414	0.5528
14	P II	0.8202	0.9338
15	P I	0.8480	0.9670
16	P I	0.7862	0.9779
17	H	0.5303	N/A
18	P II	0.7862	0.9284
19	P II	0.6973	0.9170
20	P I	0.9050	0.9484
21	H	0.6910	N/A
22	H	0.6076	N/A
23	H	0.6972	N/A
24	H	0.6721	N/A
25	P II	0.8924	0.9407
26	P I	0.5505	0.9682
27	H	0.6787	N/A

References

1. Mitra, J., Shen, K., Ghose, S., Bourgeat, P., Fripp, J., Salvado, O., Pannek, K., Taylor, D.J., Mathias, J.L., Rose, S.: Statistical machine learning to identify traumatic brain injury (TBI) from structural disconnections of white matter networks. Neuroimage **129**, 247–259 (2016)
2. Levin, H.S., Li, X., McCauley, S.R., Hanten, G., Wilde, E.A., Swank, P.: Neuropsychological outcome of mTBI: a principal component analysis approach. J. Neurotrauma **30**, 625–632 (2013)
3. Alexander, D.C., Barker, G.J., Arridge, S.R.: Detection and modeling of non-Gaussian apparent diffusion coefficient profiles in human brain data. Magn. Reson. Med. **48**, 331–340 (2002)
4. Smith, S.M., Jenkinson, M., Johansen-Berg, H., Rueckert, D., Nichols, T.E., Mackay, C.E., Watkins, K.E., Ciccarelli, O., Cader, M.Z., Matthews, P.M., Behrens, T.E.J.: Tract-based spatial statistics: voxelwise analysis of multi-subject diffusion data. Neuroimage **31**, 1487–1505 (2006)
5. Nichols, T., Holmes, A.: Nonparametric permutation tests for functional neuroimaging. In: Human Brain Function, 2nd edn., pp. 887–910 (2003)
6. Nichols, T.E., Holmes, A.P.: Nonparametric permutation tests for functional neuroimaging: a primer with examples. Hum. Brain Mapp. **15**, 1–25 (2002)
7. Arfanakis, K., Haughton, V.M., Carew, J.D., Rogers, B.P., Dempsey, R.J., Meyerand, M.E.: Diffusion tensor MR imaging in diffuse axonal injury. AJNR Am. J. Neuroradiol. **23**, 794–802 (2002)
8. Rutgers, D.R., Toulgoat, F., Cazejust, J., Fillard, P., Lasjaunias, P., Ducreux, D.: White matter abnormalities in mild traumatic brain injury: a diffusion tensor imaging study. AJNR Am. J. Neuroradiol. **29**, 514–519 (2008)
9. Kraus, M.F., Susmaras, T., Caughlin, B.P., Walker, C.J., Sweeney, J.A., Little, D.M.: White matter integrity and cognition in chronic traumatic brain injury: a diffusion tensor imaging study. Brain **130**, 2508–2519 (2007)
10. Mayer, A.R., Ling, J., Mannell, M.V., Gasparovic, C., Phillips, J.P., Doezema, D., Reichard, R., Yeo, R.A.: A prospective diffusion tensor imaging study in mild traumatic brain injury. Neurology **74**, 643–650 (2010)
11. Ilvesmäki, T., Luoto, T.M., Hakulinen, U., Brander, A., Ryymin, P., Eskola, H., Iverson, G.L., Öhman, J.: Acute mild traumatic brain injury is not associated with white matter change on diffusion tensor imaging. Brain **137**, 1876–1882 (2014)
12. Niogi, S.N., Mukherjee, P., Ghajar, J., Johnson, C.E., Kolster, R., Lee, H., Suh, M., Zimmerman, R.D., Manley, G.T., McCandliss, B.D.: Structural dissociation of attentional control and memory in adults with and without mild traumatic brain injury. Brain **131**, 3209–3221 (2008)
13. Wang, J.Y., Abdi, H., Bakhadirov, K., Diaz-Arrastia, R., Devous, M.D.: A comprehensive reliability assessment of quantitative diffusion tensor tractography. Neuroimage **60**, 1127–1138 (2012)
14. Farquharson, S., Tournier, J.-D., Calamante, F., Fabinyi, G., Schneider-Kolsky, M., Jackson, G.D., Connelly, A.: White matter fiber tractography: why we need to move beyond DTI. J. Neurosurg. **118**, 1367–1377 (2013)
15. Jenkinson, M., Beckmann, C.F., Behrens, T.E.J., Woolrich, M.W., Smith, S.M.: FSL. Neuroimage **62**, 782–790 (2012)
16. Ngiam, J., Khosla, A., Kim, M., Nam, J., Lee, H., Ng, A.Y.: Multimodal deep learning. In: Proceedings of 28th International Conference on Machine Learning, pp. 689–696 (2011)

17. Wilde, E.A., McCauley, S.R., Hunter, J.V., Bigler, E.D., Chu, Z., Wang, Z.J., Hanten, G.R., Troyanskaya, M., Yallampalli, R., Li, X., Chia, J., Levin, H.S.: Diffusion tensor imaging of acute mild traumatic brain injury in adolescents. Neurology **70**, 948–955 (2008)

18. Andersson, J.L.R., Jenkinson, M., Smith, S.: Non-linear registration aka Spatial normalisation FMRIB Technical report TR07JA2. In Pract. 22 (2007)

19. Nowlan, S.J.: Maximum likelihood competitive learning. In: Advances in Neural Information Processing Systems, vol. 2, pp. 574–582 (1990)

20. Cotter, A., Shamir, O., Srebro, N., Sridharan, K.: Better mini-batch algorithms via accelerated gradient methods. In: NIPS, pp. 1–9 (2011)

21. Bengio, Y., Lamblin, P., Popovici, D., Larochelle, H.: Greedy layer-wise training of deep networks. Adv. Neural Inf. Process. Syst. **19**, 153 (2007)

22. Kao, P., Rojas, E., Chen, J., Zhang, A., Manjunath, B.S.: Unsupervised 3-D feature learning for mild traumatic brain injury. In: MICCAI Workshop:mTOP Grand Challenge (2016)

23. Bellotti, R., Lombardi, A., Amoroso, N., Tateo, A., Tangaro, S.: Semi-unsupervised prediction for mild TBI based on both graph and K-nn methods. In: MICCAI Workshop:mTOP Grand Challenge (2016)

Mild Traumatic Brain Injury Outcome Prediction Based on Both Graph and K-nn Methods

R. Bellotti[1,2], A. Lombardi[3], C. Guaragnella[3], N. Amoroso[1,2],
A. Tateo[1,2], and S. Tangaro[2(✉)]

[1] Dipartimento Interateno di Fisica "M. Merlin",
Università degli studi di Bari "A. Moro", Bari, Italy
[2] Sezione di Bari, Istituto Nazionale di Fisica Nucleare, Bari, Italy
sonia.tangaro@ba.infn.it
[3] Dipartimento di Ingegneria Elettrica e dell'Informazione,
Politecnico di Bari, Bari, Italy
angela.lombardi@poliba.it

Abstract. Cognitive impairment has mainly two, non mutually exclusive, etiologies: structural or connectivity lesions. Analogously, we present here a methodology aimed at investigating magnetic resonance imaging (MRI) scans of subject after a traumatic brain injury (TBI) to detect the presence of these heterogeneous lesions and access the information content within. In particular, we use (i) complex network topological features to capture the effect of disease on connectivity and (ii) morphological brain measurements to describe anomalous patterns from a structural perspective. This integrated base of knowledge is then used to emphasize differences arising within a cohort including normal controls and patients labeled as category-I and category-II according to their outcome after TBI. Results suggest that topological measurements provide a suitable measurement to detect category-I subjects, while structural features are effective to distinguish controls from category-II subjects.

Keywords: TBI · MRI · Complex networks · Graph theory · K-nn

1 Introduction

Machine learning algorithms and multivariate data analysis methods have been widely utilized in recent years exploring several validation strategies and classifiers, several feature extraction and selection methods, applied especially to structural MRI measurements [2,4,18]. Besides, the development of more and more accurate algorithms for DWI analysis has encouraged the investigation of connectivity - based studies, especially basing on the mathematical framework of graph theory.

Graph theory can be a suitable tool to reveal the topological brain network properties [5,33]. The investigation of which measurements and properties can

© Springer International Publishing AG 2016
A. Crimi et al. (Eds.): BrainLes 2016, LNCS 10154, pp. 271–281, 2016.
DOI: 10.1007/978-3-319-55524-9_25

better detect and model the alterations depends on the data used and the connectivity definition adopted.

In our previous work, we investigated a complex network framework to describe the topological brain organization and to distinguish Alzheimer's disease from control subjects [3, 22]. Our findings suggested that topological measures could accurately detect patterns of mild impairment, emphasizing differences that structural measurements seem to less efficiently outline.

The purpose of this work is to predict outcomes for two categories of subjects suffering from mild Traumatic Brain Injury (TBI) and a group of normal controls (NC).

A traumatic brain injury occurs when an external force causes a focused and sudden impact upon the head.

The effects following a brain trauma may be structural and morphological damages whose locations depends on the impact and secondary events due to changes in intracranial pressure and cerebrospinal fluid.

Unlike a neurodegenerative disease, it does not have any connection with the genetic makeup of an individual. However, taking into account the different structural implications, it is reasonable to assume that a traumatic injury can affect the integrity of the brain connectivity and, therefore, that the identification of TBI outcomes can be improved by investigating the network organization of the brain.

So, even if in a different context, in this work some connectivity measurements, such as strength or clustering coefficient, are evaluated to identify the category-I patients and then, once this diagnostic class is excluded, category-II patients are diagnosed with respect of normal controls using structural measurements.

2 Materials

This work uses an magnetic resonance imaging (MRI) dataset of 27 subjects including 15 labeled subjects divided into three classes (5 subjects per group). For each subject, raw T1-weighted and DWI scans are available, besides preprocessed data is also provided, it includes T1 scans rigidly normalized to the MNI152 template, the gross segmentations of white matter, gray matter and cerebrospinal fluid, the mean diffusivity (MD) map and the fractional anisotropy (FA) map.

We focused our model on the analysis of T1 scans, MD and FA maps. In fact, the rationale underlying this choice is that the information content provided from these three images is not redundant, since they are three different, complementary descriptions of the brain morphology and its connectivity. T1 captures morphological changes, MD measurements are sensitive to the cerebral spinal fluid (CSF), while the values of FA to white matter pathways [1].

3 Methods

The proposed approach consists of four main steps shown in Fig. 1:

1. Each brain, for each considered imaging modality (T1, FA and MD), is parceled in a collection of patches representing the nodes of a network; edges of each network are the absolute pairwise Pearson's correlation between the supervoxels, thus resulting in an undirected weighted network;
2. from each network a number of statistical graph features are collected;
3. a k-nearest neighbors (*k-nn*) machine learning classification is used to differentiate the category-I patients from remaining subjects;
4. structural feature extraction is performed with FreeSurfer on NC and category-II patients;
5. k-nn machine learning classification is used for NC and category-II patients discrimination.

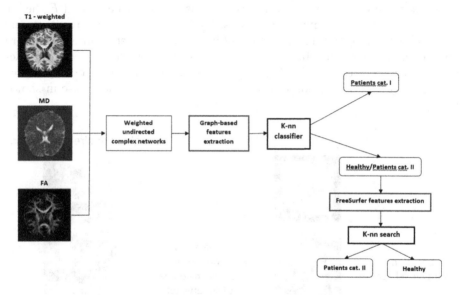

Fig. 1. A schematic overview of the proposed framework is presented.

3.1 Complex Network Construction

Once MRI scans had been co-registered, they were segmented in rectangular boxes, *supervoxels*. Firstly, brain hemispheres were separated, then each hemisphere was covered with an equal number of supervoxels. Using the brain mask of the template we discarded all supervoxels overlapping with the mask for less than 10%. As scans had been spatially normalized it was reasonable to assume that:

1. within each brain the corresponding supervoxels included roughly the same regions;
2. gray level distributions of corresponding supervoxels should remain substantially unchanged unless heavy morphological variations.

Supervoxels were chosen to not represent pre-defined anatomical areas. In contrast to region of interest approaches, therefore, they do not rely on the segmentation accuracy of the anatomical regions. Moreover, as they collect the information related to thousands of voxels they are robust to typical artifacts of voxel based morphometry approaches.

The supervoxel size D was chosen considering that supervoxels too small could be considerably affected by registration noise; on the contrary, extremely large supervoxels could conceal subtle differences making it harder to differentiate the groups. To investigate how the size of the supervoxel affected the accuracy of the analysis, D was varied from a minimum of 2000 to a maximum of 4000 voxels.

The proposed framework naturally introduces a graph description. By definition, a graph $\mathcal{G}$ is a couple (N, E) where N is the set of *nodes* and E the set of *edges*. Nodes are the fundamental constituents of a graph, they represent the elements interacting within the system of interest. The existing interactions are represented by the edges. In this way, no matter the complexity of the interactions involved nor the nature of the constituents, a graph allows a compact but formally rigorous description of a generic system; the presented case in shown in Fig. 2.

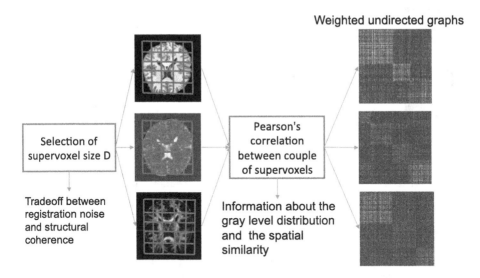

Fig. 2. Complex networks construction.

The supervoxels were considered nodes of a network whose connections represented the grade of similarity between them. Pearson's correlation r was the chosen metric:

$$r = \frac{D\sum_{j=1}^{D} x_j y_j - (\sum_{j=1}^{D} x_j)(\sum_{j=1}^{D} y_j)}{\sqrt{[D\sum_{j=1}^{D} x_j^2 - (\sum_{j=1}^{D} x_j)^2][D\sum_{j=1}^{D} y_j^2 - (\sum_{j=1}^{D} y_j)^2]}} \tag{1}$$

where the sums are extended to all D voxels within a supervoxel; x_j and y_j are the intensity of the j-th voxel. This choice has the fundamental advantage of combining not only the information deriving from the gray level distribution similarity between two supervoxels, but also their spatial similarity.

For each modality (T1, FA, MD) we built a weighted undirected complex network whose connections had been calculated through the absolute value of the Pearson's correlation coefficient between pairs of supervoxels.

3.2   Graph Features

For each node i of a network, the following local topological metrics were computed:

– the sum of weights of links connected to the node i.e. its *strength*:

$$s_i = \sum_j w_{ij} \tag{2}$$

– the *clustering coefficient* which represents the fraction of closed triplets around a node and it quantifies the tendency of a node to create clusters with its neighbors [25]:

$$c_i = \frac{2t_i}{s_i(s_i - 1)} \tag{3}$$

where t_i is the number of triplets attached to the node.

Moreover, *the characteristic path length* was used to characterize the overall efficiency of the network.

The Newman's spectral community detection algorithm [24] was used to partition each network into non-overlapping communities of nodes in order to reflect their modular organization. Therefore some features based on the detected communities were extracted to describe the role of each node in relation to each community and to objectively outline the strength of the connections between and within the modules. In particular we considered:

– *the participation coefficient* of each node [16]:

$$P_i = 1 - \sum_{s=1}^{N_M} \left(\frac{\kappa_{is}}{k_i} \right)^2 \tag{4}$$

where κ_{is} is the number of links from node i to nodes in module s, k_i is the degree of node i and N_M is the number of communities. It is an index of the degree of participation of a node to the network communities since its value is close to 1 if the connections of the node are uniformly distributed among all the modules or 0 if all the connections are confined within a module.

– Defined the inter-community strength of a community l as the sum of the weights of links connecting the community l with all the other communities:

$$S_{INTER,l} = \sum_{\substack{m=1 \\ m\neq l}}^{N_M} W_{lm} \tag{5}$$

we used its average value over all the communities to measure the *inter-community strength* of the network.

– At the same manner, defined the intra-community strength of a community l with N_l nodes as the sum of the weights of links within it:

$$S_{INTRA,l} = \sum_{i=1}^{N_l} \sum_{j=i+1}^{N_l} w_{ij} \tag{6}$$

its average value is used to quantify the global *intra-community strength*.

For each subject and each modality, median, standard deviation, range and interquartile range of the distributions of strength, clustering coefficient and participation coefficient were calculated resulting in a 27×45 feature matrix used for k-nn prediction.

3.3   K - Nearest Neighbors

The working principle of a k-nn algorithm is the following: it identifies an established number (k) of closest training examples to a query point and assigns it the label of the class that has the most instances in the set of nearest neighbors of the point. The metric used to evaluate distances between points is cosine.

This technique offers some advantages over other unsupervised classification methods:

– it is a non-parametric instance-based learning method: it does not build a model so it might be more suitable in some particularly complex classification problems;
– it also works even in the presence of a small number of training examples. In this case, an unsupervised algorithm such as k-means or k-medoids, which makes decisions mainly based on the distance of a query point from a centroid or medoid of a class, could introduce a significant bias in the presence of outliers.

In this work, a k-nn classifier was used with a one-class discrimination logic in order to identify the category-I subjects against all the other subjects in a semi-unsupervised manner. For this purpose, given the matrix of the graph-based features, the k-nn algorithm performs an exhaustive search to calculate the distance between the feature vectors of the subjects with unknown labels and those relating to the subjects of the category-I. This search provides a ranking of the subjects among which the closest ones are selected.

3.4   Structural Feature Extraction

We performed our analysis using volumetric and cortical thickness features computed with FreeSurfer [12]. FreeSurfer[1] is an image analysis software commonly adopted for the analysis and visualization of structural and functional neuroimaging data developed by the Laboratory for Computational Neuroimaging at the Athinoula A. Martinos Center for Biomedical Imaging. In particular, we have employed FreeSurfer tool v5.1 in the cortical reconstruction to estimate the volumetric features in MRI. Specifically, we have extracted only 180 features provided by the recon-all freesurfer command. To name a few: Left-Latera-Ventricle, Right-Latera-Ventricle, Left-Inf-Lat-Vent, Right-Inf-Lat-Vent, Left Hippocampus, Right Hippocampus, and many more. We have run FreeSurfer tool on the ReCaS infrastructure located at the Physics Department at University of Bari. This infrastructure includes 1200 CPU cores, 4.5 TB of RAM, 4.5 PB of disk space, and all computer node have a connection of 10 Gbit/s wire-speed. The FreeSurfer image processing time is of 12 h for each MRI nevertheless the distributed method and the computational power of Data Center employed has allowed us to obtain the output for all considered subjects in a time slightly higher than that for a single subject. A specific software tool was performed to automatically manage jobs in case of casual segmentation failure.

3.5   NC/Category-II Patients Discrimination

In the final step, the features extracted with FreeSurfer Tool were taken into account to distinguish controls from category-II subjects. Among all the features, those with high correlation values ($r > 0.9$) and those with low variance values (less than 0.2) were not considered. Starting from the two known sets, the k-nn algorithm builds two kd-trees to identify the subjects belonging from each group.

4   Discussion and Conclusions

In this paper, a framework to perform semi-unsupervised outcome prediction for two categories of Mild TBI is presented. In particular, a two-steps classification pipeline is adopted to emphasize the differences between the healthy control group and the two patient groups.

In the first step, a complex network approach was applied to construct graphs from available scans and to extract the topological features used to identify category-I patients amongst all subjects. The mathematical model underlying the graph theory was chosen because it provides a direct description of the structural properties of a network. Furthermore, a multimodal analysis was carried out to reflect the heterogeneity of injury patterns that can affect the patient cohorts. More specifically, bearing in mind that an early detection of changes in white matter tracts and in distribution of cerebrospinal fluid could improve

---

[1] freesurfer.nmr.mgh.harvard.edu

significantly diagnoses and prognoses in case of diffuse axonal injury, contusions, edema and hemorrhages [20], MD and FA maps were considered as well as T1-weighted images. From each graph relating to each modality, topological features able to capture different relational aspects of the network elements, were computed. Besides the metrics commonly used to quantify the strength of the topological connections and the total efficiency of the network (i.e., strength and characteristic path length), a special focus was addressed to measures that reflect the modular organization of the interacting elements. So other measures such as the clustering coefficient, the participation coefficient, the intra-community and inter-community strength, were introduced with the aim of assessing the degree of weakening of the structural connections caused by injuries and the resulting configuration changes. Finally, second-level statistical features were extracted from the distributions of such metrics in order to provide a general description of all the sample images. Indeed, in principle, traumatic injuries could affect several brain regions causing extensive damage or they could be focal, compromising a specific functional area.

In the second step, we performed the discrimination between controls and category-II patients by means of a k-nn classifier. At this stage, FreeSurfer volumetric and cortical thickness features proved to be effective in detecting morphological differences between the two groups of subjects. However, given the small number of examples for the two classes (five known labels for each group), dimensionality reduction of the feature set was performed with minimum variance and maximum correlation criteria. As a matter of fact, a binary k-nn classifier relies on building two distance-trees, by calculating the distances between the training examples of each of the two groups and the unlabeled instances and subsequent by ranking these unknown instances. If the adopted distance metric is affected by noise due to the presence of low-significance features, the computation of the actual distance among the examples and the instances could be compromised, causing worse performances [23]. In fact, a dimension of the feature space much greater than the number of samples, would cause a problem of data sparsity, making inconsistent the computation of the distance between couple of points in the metric space.

In the context of the mTOP Challenge 2016, as winner, the performances of the proposed method have proven to be higher than those of other approaches based on Convolutional Network and Deep Learning. Our framework has good generalization properties as is not constrained by the knowledge of the areas involved in the traumatic injury. However, future developments may require a greater number of training examples in order to validate the obtained results and improve the classification accuracy.

Aknowledgement. Cortical reconstruction and volumetric segmentation were performed with the FreeSurfer image analysis suite, which is documented and freely available for download online. The technical details of these procedures are described in prior publications [6,7,9–15,17,19,30]. Briefly, this processing includes motion correction and averaging [26] of multiple volumetric T1 weighted images (when more than one is available), removal of non-brain tissue using a hybrid watershed/surface deformation procedure [30], automated Talairach transformation, segmentation of the subcortical white matter and deep gray matter volumetric structures (including hippocampus, amygdala, caudate, putamen, ventricles) [12,13] intensity normalization [32], tessellation of the gray matter white matter boundary, automated topology correction [11,31], and surface deformation following intensity gradients to optimally place the gray/white and gray/cerebrospinal fluid borders at the location where the greatest shift in intensity defines the transition to the other tissue class [6,7,9]. Once the cortical models are complete, a number of deformable procedures can be performed for in further data processing and analysis including surface inflation [6], registration to a spherical atlas which utilized individual cortical folding patterns to match cortical geometry across subjects [15], parcellation of the cerebral cortex into units based on gyral and sulcal structure [8,10], and creation of a variety of surface-based data including maps of curvature and sulcal depth. This method uses both intensity and continuity information from the entire three-dimensional MR volume in segmentation and deformation procedures to produce representations of cortical thickness, calculated as the closest distance from the gray/white boundary to the gray/CSF boundary at each vertex on the tessellated surface [9]. The maps are created using spatial intensity gradients across tissue classes and are therefore not simply reliant on absolute signal intensity. The maps produced are not restricted to the voxel resolution of the original data thus are capable of detecting submillimeter differences between groups. Procedures for the measurement of cortical thickness have been validated against histological analysis [28] and manual measurements [21,29]. Freesurfer morphometric procedures have been demonstrated to show good test-retest reliability across scanner manufacturers and across field strengths [17,27].

References

1. Alexander, A.L., Hurley, S.A., Samsonov, A.A., Adluru, N., Hosseinbor, A.P., Mossahebi, P., Tromp, D.P., Zakszewski, E., Field, A.S.: Characterization of cerebral white matter properties using quantitative magnetic resonance imaging stains. Brain Connect. **1**(6), 423–446 (2011)
2. Allen, G.I., Amoroso, N., Anghel, C., Balagurusamy, V., Bare, C.J., Beaton, D., Bellotti, R., Bennett, D.A., Boehme, K.L., Boutros, P.C., et al.: Crowdsourced estimation of cognitive decline and resilience in Alzheimer's disease. Alzheimer's Dement. **12**(6), 645–653 (2016)
3. Amoroso, N., Monaco, A., Tangaro, S.: Topological measurements of DWI tractography for the Alzheimers disease detection. In: Computational and Mathematical Methods in Medicine (2016, in press)
4. Bron, E.E., Smits, M., Van Der Flier, W.M., Vrenken, H., Barkhof, F., Scheltens, P., Papma, J.M., Steketee, R.M., Orellana, C.M., Meijboom, R., et al.: Standardized evaluation of algorithms for computer-aided diagnosis of dementia based on structural MRI: the CADDementia challenge. NeuroImage **111**, 562–579 (2015)
5. Daianu, M., Jahanshad, N., Nir, T.M., Toga, A.W., Jack Jr., C.R., Weiner, M.W., Thompson, P.M.: Breakdown of brain connectivity between normal aging and Alzheimer's disease: a structural k-core network analysis. Brain Connect. **3**(4), 407–422 (2013). For the Alzheimer's Disease Neuroimaging Initiative
6. Dale, A.M., Fischl, B., Sereno, M.I.: Cortical surface-based analysis: I. Segmentation and surface reconstruction. Neuroimage **9**(2), 179–194 (1999)

7. Dale, A.M., Sereno, M.I.: Improved localizadon of cortical activity by combining EEG and MEG with MRI cortical surface reconstruction: a linear approach. J. Cogn. Neurosci. **5**(2), 162–176 (1993)
8. Desikan, R.S., Ségonne, F., Fischl, B., Quinn, B.T., Dickerson, B.C., Blacker, D., Buckner, R.L., Dale, A.M., Maguire, R.P., Hyman, B.T., et al.: An automated labeling system for subdividing the human cerebral cortex on MRI scans into gyral based regions of interest. Neuroimage **31**(3), 968–980 (2006)
9. Fischl, B., Dale, A.M.: Measuring the thickness of the human cerebral cortex from magnetic resonance images. Proc. Natl. Acad. Sci. **97**(20), 11050–11055 (2000)
10. Fischl, B., van der Kouwe, A., Destrieux, C., Halgren, E., Ségonne, F., Salat, D.H., Busa, E., Seidman, L.J., Goldstein, J., Kennedy, D., et al.: Automatically parcellating the human cerebral cortex. Cereb. Cortex **14**(1), 11–22 (2004)
11. Fischl, B., Liu, A., Dale, A.M.: Automated manifold surgery: constructing geometrically accurate and topologically correct models of the human cerebral cortex. IEEE Trans. Med. Imaging **20**(1), 70–80 (2001)
12. Fischl, B., Salat, D.H., Busa, E., Albert, M., Dieterich, M., Haselgrove, C., Van Der Kouwe, A., Killiany, R., Kennedy, D., Klaveness, S., et al.: Whole brain segmentation: automated labeling of neuroanatomical structures in the human brain. Neuron **33**(3), 341–355 (2002)
13. Fischl, B., Salat, D.H., van der Kouwe, A.J., Makris, N., Ségonne, F., Quinn, B.T., Dale, A.M.: Sequence-independent segmentation of magnetic resonance images. Neuroimage **23**, S69–S84 (2004)
14. Fischl, B., Sereno, M.I., Dale, A.M.: Cortical surface-based analysis. II: inflation, flattening, and a surface-based coordinate system. Neuroimage **9**(2), 195–207 (1999)
15. Fischl, B., Sereno, M.I., Tootell, R.B., Dale, A.M., et al.: High-resolution intersubject averaging and a coordinate system for the cortical surface. Hum. Brain Mapp. **8**(4), 272–284 (1999)
16. Guimera, R., Amaral, L.A.N.: Functional cartography of complex metabolic networks. Nature **433**(7028), 895–900 (2005)
17. Han, X., Jovicich, J., Salat, D., van der Kouwe, A., Quinn, B., Czanner, S., Busa, E., Pacheco, J., Albert, M., Killiany, R., et al.: Reliability of MRI-derived measurements of human cerebral cortical thickness: the effects of field strength, scanner upgrade and manufacturer. Neuroimage **32**(1), 180–194 (2006)
18. Inglese, P., Amoroso, N., Boccardi, M., Bocchetta, M., Bruno, S., Chincarini, A., Errico, R., Frisoni, G., Maglietta, R., Redolfi, A., Sensi, F., Tangaro, S., Tateo, A., Bellotti, R.: Multiple RF classifier for the hippocampus segmentation: Method and validation on EADC-ADNI harmonized hippocampal protocol. Phys. Medica **31**(8), 1085–1091 (2015)
19. Jovicich, J., Czanner, S., Greve, D., Haley, E., van der Kouwe, A., Gollub, R., Kennedy, D., Schmitt, F., Brown, G., MacFall, J., et al.: Reliability in multi-site structural mri studies: effects of gradient non-linearity correction on phantom and human data. Neuroimage **30**(2), 436–443 (2006)
20. Kumar, R., Husain, M., Gupta, R.K., Hasan, K.M., Haris, M., Agarwal, A.K., Pandey, C., Narayana, P.A.: Serial changes in the white matter diffusion tensor imaging metrics in moderate traumatic brain injury and correlation with neurocognitive function. J. Neurotrauma **26**(4), 481–495 (2009)
21. Kuperberg, G.R., Broome, M.R., McGuire, P.K., David, A.S., Eddy, M., Ozawa, F., Goff, D., West, W.C., Williams, S.C., van der Kouwe, A.J., et al.: Regionally localized thinning of the cerebral cortex in schizophrenia. Arch. Gen. Psychiatry **60**(9), 878–888 (2003)

22. La Rocca, M., et al.: A multiplex network model to characterize brain atrophy in structural MRI. In: Mantica, G., Stoop, R., Stramaglia, S. (eds.) Proceedings of the XXIII International Conference on Nonlinear Dynamics of Electronic Systems Emergent Complexity from Nonlinearity, in Physics, Engineering and the Life Sciences. Springer Proceedings in Physics, vol. 191, Como, Italy, 7-11 September 2015. Springer International Publishing, Cham (2017)

23. Marimont, R., Shapiro, M.: Nearest neighbour searches and the curse of dimensionality. IMA J. Appl. Math. **24**(1), 59–70 (1979)

24. Newman, M.E.: Finding community structure in networks using the eigenvectors of matrices. Phys. Rev. E **74**(3), 036104 (2006)

25. Onnela, J.P., Saramäki, J., Kertész, J., Kaski, K.: Intensity and coherence of motifs in weighted complex networks. Phys. Rev. E **71**(6), 065103 (2005)

26. Reuter, M., Rosas, H.D., Fischl, B.: Highly accurate inverse consistent registration: a robust approach. Neuroimage **53**(4), 1181–1196 (2010)

27. Reuter, M., Schmansky, N.J., Rosas, H.D., Fischl, B.: Within-subject template estimation for unbiased longitudinal image analysis. Neuroimage **61**(4), 1402–1418 (2012)

28. Rosas, H., Liu, A., Hersch, S., Glessner, M., Ferrante, R., Salat, D., van Der Kouwe, A., Jenkins, B., Dale, A., Fischl, B.: Regional and progressive thinning of the cortical ribbon in Huntingtons disease. Neurology **58**(5), 695–701 (2002)

29. Salat, D.H., Buckner, R.L., Snyder, A.Z., Greve, D.N., Desikan, R.S., Busa, E., Morris, J.C., Dale, A.M., Fischl, B.: Thinning of the cerebral cortex in aging. Cereb. Cortex **14**(7), 721–730 (2004)

30. Ségonne, F., Dale, A., Busa, E., Glessner, M., Salat, D., Hahn, H., Fischl, B.: A hybrid approach to the skull stripping problem in MRI. Neuroimage **22**(3), 1060–1075 (2004)

31. Ségonne, F., Pacheco, J., Fischl, B.: Geometrically accurate topology-correction of cortical surfaces using nonseparating loops. IEEE Trans. Med. Imaging **26**(4), 518–529 (2007)

32. Sled, J.G., Zijdenbos, A.P., Evans, A.C.: A nonparametric method for automatic correction of intensity nonuniformity in MRI data. IEEE Trans. Med. Imaging **17**(1), 87–97 (1998)

33. Tijms, B.M., Wink, A.M., de Haan, W., van der Flier, W.M., Stam, C.J., Scheltens, P., Barkhof, F.: Alzheimer's disease: connecting findings from graph theoretical studies of brain networks. Neurobiol. Aging **34**(8), 2023–2036 (2013)

Unsupervised 3-D Feature Learning for Mild Traumatic Brain Injury

Po-Yu Kao[1(✉)], Eduardo Rojas[1], Jefferson W. Chen[2], Angela Zhang[1], and B.S. Manjunath[1]

[1] University of California, Santa Barbara, Santa Barbara, CA 93106, USA
{poyu_kao,manj}@ece.ucsb.edu
[2] University of California, Irvine, Irvine, CA 92697, USA
jeffwc1@uci.edu

Abstract. We present an unsupervised three-dimensional feature clustering algorithm to gather the mTOP2016 challenge data into 3 groups. We use the brain MR-T1, diffusion tensor fractional anisotropy, and diffusion tensor mean diffusivity images provided by the mTOP2016 competition. A distance-based size constraint method for data clustering is used. The proposed approach achieves 0.267 adjusted rand index and 0.3556 homogeneity score within the 15 labeled subjects, corresponding to 10 correctly classified data items. Based on visual exploration of the data, we believe that a localized analysis of the lesion regions, using the computed tractography data, is a promising direction to pursue.

1 Introduction

This paper addresses the challenge of feature detection and classification of subject data based on brain imaging, as described in the mTOP challenge. The imaging data include the MR-T1 and diffusion weighted images (DWI). While there is extensive work on applying unsupervised learning to clustering 2-D image features [1–3,6], the problems posed by the mTBI data set are particularly challenging since the features of interest are likely very localized. Furthermore, the subject categorization is derived not necessarily from the image data but from other observations, making this problem very distinct from the traditional works in natural image processing.

We propose a fully unsupervised methodology to learn the 3-D features from the data, a 3-D convolutional network to extract the feature representation for each subject, and a distance-based size constraint methodology for data clustering.

2 Unsupervised 3-D Feature Learning

Our proposed workflow includes four stages. The first stage performs data preparation and pre-processing on mTOP 2016 data set. The second stage performs learning 3-D features from brain MR-T1, diffusion tensor fractional anisotropy

© Springer International Publishing AG 2016
A. Crimi et al. (Eds.): BrainLes 2016, LNCS 10154, pp. 282–290, 2016.
DOI: 10.1007/978-3-319-55524-9_26

(DT-FA) and diffusion tensor mean diffusivity (DT-MD) images from 27 subjects of mTOP2016 data set. The third stage performs feature representation for each subject, and the last stage performs group clustering based on these feature representations.

2.1 Data Preparation and Pre-processing

The mTOP data consists of MR-T1, DT-FA and DT-MD images, see Fig. 1. This data set contains 27 subjects belonging to 3 different categories (healthy, patient category 1 or patient category 2) each consisting of 9 subjects. mTBI Patients are categorised into one of two groups based on their long term recovery status following the injury. The imaging data includes for MR-T1 image at $182 \times 218 \times 182$ voxels, with $1\,\mathrm{mm} \times 1\,\mathrm{mm} \times 1\,\mathrm{mm}$ voxel resolution, and the dimension for DT-FA and DT-MD image is $91 \times 109 \times 91$ with $2\,\mathrm{mm} \times 2\,\mathrm{mm} \times 2\,\mathrm{mm}$ voxel resolution.

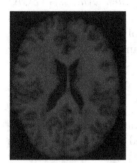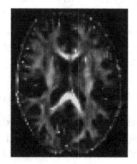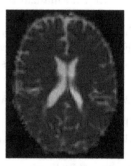

Fig. 1. Left: MR-T1 image, Middle: DT-FA image, Right: DT-MD image

Data preparation for MR-T1 images is shown in Fig. 2. For MR-T1 images, we consider $8 \times 8 \times 8$ voxel volume represented as a 512 dimensional vector of voxel values, $\tilde{x}_{T1}^{(i)} \in \mathbb{R}^{512}$, where i indexes the 3-D patch. The overlap between the volumes in a sliding window is 50%, and those volumes that have more than 75% zero values are discarded. Thus, a large number of data vectors are generated that are the organized as column vectors in a matrix.

Moreover, these vectors are normalized to zero mean and unit standard deviation:

$$x^{(i)} = \frac{\tilde{x}^{(i)} - mean(\tilde{x}^{(i)})}{std(\tilde{x}^{(i)})}$$

where $\tilde{x}^{(i)}$ is a unnormalized column vector and "mean" and "std" are the mean and standard deviation of the element of $\tilde{x}^{(i)}$. Let X_{T1} represent this matrix that includes data from all of the 27 subjects. Similarly, two other matrices X_{FA} and X_{MD} are constructed. However, since the spatial resolution of the data for

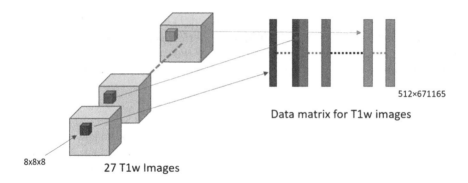

512×671165

Data matrix for T1w images

8x8x8

27 T1w Images

Fig. 2. Data preparation for MR-T1 images

these two cases are different from the MR-T1, we use a $4 \times 4 \times 4$ voxel volume. Therefore, the data vectors all represent a $512\,\mathrm{mm}^3$ spatial volume.

After normalization, we apply the standard *Zero Component Analysis* (ZCA) whitening transform [5] on each of the datasets X_{T1}, X_{FA}, and X_{MD}. This helps minimize the correlation among the components of the column vectors. For contrast-normalized data, we set the whitening parameter ϵ_{zca} to 0.01 for $8 \times 8 \times 8$ voxel patches and 0.1 for $4 \times 4 \times 4$ voxel patches.

2.2 Dictionary Learning via K-means Clustering

The next step is to learn a dictionary for each of the data matrices using the standard K-means clustering. A separate dictionary is learned for each of the three matrices. Let the data matrix be $X \in \mathbb{R}^{N \times M}$ and the corresponding dictionary be $D \in \mathbb{R}^{N \times K}$. Then,

Loop until convergence:

$$c_j^{(i)} = \begin{cases} D^{(j)\top} x^{(i)}, & \text{if } j = \arg\min_l |D^{(l)\top} x^{(i)}| \quad \forall i, j. \\ 0, & \text{otherwise.} \end{cases}$$

$$D := XC^\top + D$$

$$D^{(j)}/||D^{(j)}||_2 \quad \forall j$$

where $c_j^{(i)}$ is the code vector associated with the input $x^{(i)}$ (i^{th} column of X), and $D^{(j)}$ is the jth column of the dictionary D that is a 3-D feature we learned. In the end, we will learn K 3-D features from a dataset ($D \in \mathbb{R}^{N \times K}$). Note that $C \in \mathbb{R}^{K \times M}$. Let the three corresponding dictionaries be D_{T1}, D_{FA}, and D_{MD}.

2.3 Feature Representation

Feature computation workflow schematic is shown in Fig. 3. Input data includes the three types: brain MR-T1, DT-FA and DT-MD, for each of the subjects.

Each of these datasets is first normalized by subtracting the mean voxel value and dividing by the standard deviation within the brain region. The dictionary code words learned from the K-means clustering above are used as the weights for the first convolutional layer. The stride for MR-T1 is 2 voxels, and for DT-FA and DT-MD is 1 voxel. This is followed by a 3-D max-pooling layer of size $3 \times 3 \times 3$. The final merge layer concatenates the features from the three different pooling layers, thus constructing a single feature vector for each of the subjects. The dimensions of the resulting 3-D feature vector is $1536 \times 25 \times 32 \times 23$.

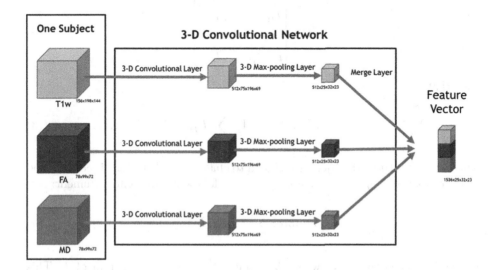

Fig. 3. 3-D Convolutional network for feature extraction

2.4   Group Clustering with Size Constraints

Ideally one would like to train the convolutional network to adjust the weights for discriminating the three different classes. However, given the number of data points, this is currently not feasible. We explored training an SVM with cross-validation but the initial results were not promising. Instead, we now consider this problem as one of unsupervised clustering in the feature space computed by the above hand-tuned convolutional network.

For clustering, we use the standard K-means clustering with distance-based size-constraint, building upon the method described in [8]. However, [8] does not provide a unique solution as it only uses the cluster labels. Instead, we modify the method to account for both labels and distances to the centroid as follows.

Given a dataset of N objects with P centroids (number of clusters), let $Dist$ be the $N \times P$ distance matrix,

$$Dist = \begin{bmatrix} d_{11} & d_{12} & \dots & d_{1P} \\ d_{21} & d_{22} & \dots & d_{2P} \\ \vdots & \vdots & \ddots & \vdots \\ d_{N1} & x_{N2} & \dots & d_{NP} \end{bmatrix} \qquad (1)$$

where d_{ip} is the distance between i object and p-th centroid. The objective is to compute a constrained $P \times N$ binary label matrix L,

$$L = \begin{bmatrix} l_{11} & l_{12} & \dots & l_{1N} \\ l_{21} & l_{22} & \dots & l_{2N} \\ \vdots & \vdots & \ddots & \vdots \\ l_{P1} & l_{P2} & \dots & l_{PN} \end{bmatrix} \qquad (2)$$

such that

$$\sum_{i=1}^{P} l_{ij} = 1, \quad j = 1, \dots, n, \quad \text{and} \quad \sum_{j=1}^{N} l_{ij} = N_i, \quad i = 1, \dots, p \qquad (3)$$

where $l_{ij} = 1$ if the j-th object is assigned to cluster i, and cluster i is constrained to have exactly N_i points. This results in the following problem statement:

$$\text{minimize} \sum_{k=1}^{n} Dist_{(k)} L^{(k)} \qquad (4)$$

where $Dist_{(k)}$ is the kth row of $Dist$, and $L^{(k)}$ is the kth column of L. This binary integer linear programming problem can be easily solved by any existing solver. The mTOP2016 data set has 27 subjects which are belonged to three different classes, and each class has nine subjects. Therefore, for this data set, we set $N = 27, P = 3$, and $N_i = 9$ for each class.

3   Experiments and Discussions

Experiments are carried out with the following parameter settings: (i) whether to use whitening (ii) the size of 3-D patches (iii) the size of 3-D max-pooling kernel (iv) the number of 3-D features. We use adjusted rand index (ARI) [4] and homogeneity score (HS) [7] to measure the performance. The adjusted rand index measures the similarity of two assignments (clustered labels vs. ground truth labels), which is invariant to permutations and normalised to chance. Similarity score is between 1.0 and -1.0. Random labelings have a ARI close to 0.0, and 1.0 stands for perfect match. Homogeneity score measures the purity of ground truth labels within cluster. HS is between 1.0 and 0.0. 1.0 stands for perfectly homogeneous labeling.

3.1 Effect of Whitening

In general, the whitening transformation helps improve the accuracy. Figure 4 shows some example dictionary elements learnt from K-means clustering and contrasts that to the original data. We observe that the ZCA transformation results in a sharper dictionary kernel. Figure 5 shows the clustering performance with and without whitening. The x-axis here shows the size of the dictionary. With the ZCA transform the results improve considerably as evidenced by the corresponding ARI and HS scores. This experiment used a stride size of 4 voxel and $8 \times 8 \times 8$ patch size for MR-T1 images, a stride size of 2 voxel and $4 \times 4 \times 4$ patch size for DT-FA and DT-MA image, and a $25 \times 32 \times 23$ kernel in the max-pooling layers.

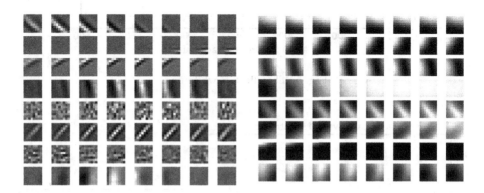

Fig. 4. 3-D features learned by K-means algorithm from MR-T1 images. Each row stands for a 3-D feature and different columns stand for different axial planes. Left: Learned from whitened image patches. Right: Learned from un-whitened image patches

3.2 Effect of 3-D Patch Size

We also computed features at different 3-D patch (volume) size settings and the results are plotted in Fig. 6. Similar to the previous figure, the x-axis shows the size of the dictionary. The 3-D feature size in the inset corresponds to the MR-T1 images. This experiment used ZCA transformed (whitened) data and $3 \times 3 \times 3$ kernels in max-pooling layers, 2 voxel stride size for MR-T1 image and 1 voxel stride size for DT-FA and DT-MD images. Overall, the $8 \times 8 \times 8$ features for MR-T1 image and the $4 \times 4 \times 4$ features for DT-FA and DT-MD image worked best. Therefore, increasing the max-pooling kernel decreased the classification accuracy.

3.3 Effect of the Size of 3-D Max-pooling Kernel

In Fig. 7, we compared the results between $3 \times 3 \times 3$, and $25 \times 32 \times 23$ maximum pooling kernel size. The x-axis also shows the size of the dictionary. In our

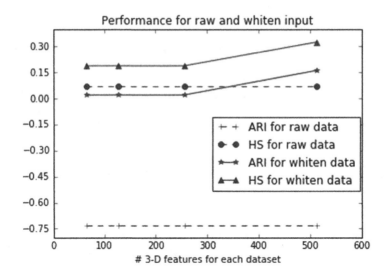

Fig. 5. The effect of whitening

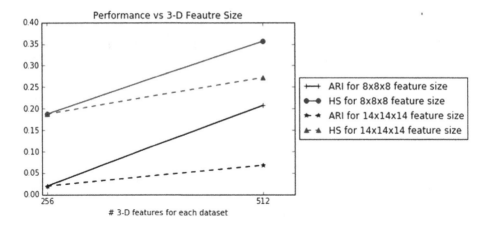

Fig. 6. The effect of 3-D features size

experiments we observe that $3 \times 3 \times 3$ maximum pooling kernels have the best performance. This experiment used whitened data sets, $8 \times 8 \times 8$ feature kernels, and a stride size of 2 voxel for MR-T1 image, and $4 \times 4 \times 4$ feature kernels and 1 voxel for DT-FA and DT-MD images.

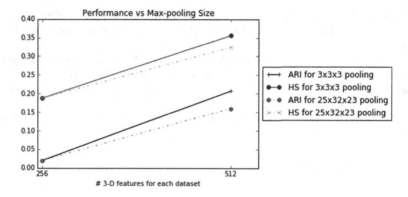

Fig. 7. The effect of max-pooling size

3.4   Effect of Dictionary Size

We considered feature representations with 64, 128, 256, and, 512 3-D dictionary items. Figures 5, 6 and 7 clearly show that a dictionary size of 512 gives the best results. Going beyond 512 did not result in much improvement.

4   Conclusion

We explored unsupervised classification of the mTBI challenge data set. Given the small number of samples, it is not feasible to train a deep learning network for feature extraction and classification. Instead we focused on computing volume features and using it for classification. In the end, the best classification results correctly classified 10 out of 15 samples for which the labels are known, and the corresponding unsupervised clustering scores are $ARI = 0.267$ and $HS = 0.3556$. We are currently working on extending this to use the tractography data computed from the DWI. Here we notice that there are significant discontinuities in the computed tracks at several potential lesion locations. Future work includes developing automated methods to detect such discontinuities and score them.

Acknowledgments. This research was partially supported by HD059217 from the National Institutes of Health.

References

1. Coates, A., Lee, H., Ng, A.Y.: An analysis of single-layer networks in unsupervised feature learning. Ann. Arbor **1001**(48109), 2 (2010)
2. Coates, A., Ng, A.Y.: Learning feature representations with K-means. In: Montavon, G., Orr, G.B., Müller, K.-R. (eds.) Neural Networks: Tricks of the Trade. LNCS, vol. 7700, pp. 561–580. Springer, Heidelberg (2012). doi:10.1007/978-3-642-35289-8_30
3. Hinton, G.E., Osindero, S., Teh, Y.-W.: A fast learning algorithm for deep belief nets. Neural Comput. **18**(7), 1527–1554 (2006)

4. Hubert, L., Arabie, P.: Comparing partitions. J. Classif. **2**(1), 193–218 (1985)
5. Krizhevsky, A., Hinton, G.: Learning multiple layers of features from tiny images (2009)
6. Olshausen, B.A.: Emergence of simple-cell receptive field properties by learning a sparse code for natural images. Nature **381**(6583), 607–609 (1996)
7. Rosenberg, A., Hirschberg, J.: V-Measure: a conditional entropy-based external cluster evaluation measure. In: EMNLP-CoNLL, vol. 7 (2007)
8. Zhu, S., Wang, D., Li, T.: Data clustering with size constraints. Knowl. Based Syst. **23**(8), 883–889 (2010)

Author Index

Printed in the United States
by Bookmasters

Printed in the United States
By Bookmasters